Health Informatics

Kathryn J. Hannah Marion J. Ball
Series Edit

D1039510

DATE DUE

Health Informatics Series
(formerly Computers in Health Care)

Series Editors
Kathryn J. Hannah   Marion J. Ball

(continued after Index)

Eliot L. Siegel   Robert M. Kolodner
Editors

Filmless Radiology

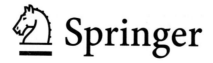 Springer

Eliot L. Siegel, M.D.
Department of Radiology
Baltimore Veterans Administration
  Hospital
Baltimore, MD 21201, USA

Robert M. Kolodner, M.D.
Department of Veterans Affairs
810 Vermont Avenue NW
Washington, DC 20420, USA

Series Editors:

Kathryn J. Hannah, Ph.D., RN
Vice President, Health Informatics
Sierra Systems Consultants, Inc.
and
Professor, Department of Community
  Health Science
Faculty of Medicine
University of Calgary
Calgary, Alberta, Canada

Marion J. Ball, Ed.D.
Professor, Department of Epidemiology
University of Maryland School of
  Medicine
and
Vice President
First Consulting Group
Baltimore, MD, USA

Cover photograph courtesy of Medical Media Production Service,
VA Maryland Health Care System, Jordon M. Denner, RBP.

Library of Congress Cataloging-in Publication Data
Filmless radiology / [edited by] Eliot L. Siegel, Robert M. Kolodner.
    p.   cm.—(Computers and health care)
  Includes bibliographical references and index.
  ISBN 0-387-98515-8   (hardcover : alk. paper)
    1. Radiography, Medical—Digital techniques.   2. Telecommunication
in medicine.   I. Siegel, Eliot L.   II. Kolodner, Robert M.
III. Series: Computers in health care (New York, N.Y.)
    [DNLM: 1. Radiology Information Systems.   2. Technology.
Radiologic.   WN 26.5 F487 1998]
RC78.7.D35F55 1998
616.07′572′0285—dc21

                                                                    98-3823

ISBN 0-387-95390-6

Printed on acid-free paper.

Printed in the United States of America.

9 8 7 6 5 4 3 2

springer.com

Series Preface

This series is directed to healthcare professionals who are leading the transformation of health care by using information and knowledge. Launched in 1988 as Computers in Health Care, the series offers a broad range of titles: some addressed to specific professions such as nursing, medicine, and health administration; others to special areas of practice such as trauma and radiology. Still other books in the series focus on interdisciplinary issues, such as the computer-based patient record, electronic health records, and networked healthcare systems.

Renamed Health Informatics in 1998 to reflect the rapid evolution in the discipline now known as health informatics, the series will continue to add titles that contribute to the evolution of the field. In the series, eminent experts, as editors or authors, offer their accounts of innovations in health informatics. Increasingly, these accounts go beyond hardware and software to address the role of information in influencing the transformation of health care delivery systems around the world. The series also will increasingly focus on "peopleware" and the organizational, behavioral, and societal changes that accompany the diffusion of information technology in health services environments.

These changes will shape health services in the next millennium. By making full and creative use of the technology to tame data and to transform information, health informatics will foster the development of the knowledge age in health care. As coeditors, we pledge to support our professional colleagues and the series readers as they share advances in the emerging and exciting field of Health Informatics.

Kathryn J. Hannah
Marion J. Ball

Preface

The replacement of the old Baltimore Department of Veterans Affairs (VA) Medical Center by a new ultramodern, high-tech facility on the campus of the University of Maryland School of Medicine provided a once-in-a-lifetime opportunity. We were given the chance to propose, design, and implement a totally digital imaging department, hospital, and healthcare network.

During the past six years, since we have moved into the new hospital, we have had the privilege of sharing our experiences with a large number of visitors. These visitors have included such diverse groups as radiologists, technologists, clinicians, administrators, information technology specialists, nurses, architects, business leaders, medical and technology vendors, politicians, patient advocacy groups, lawyers, and the media.

In addition to a tour of the department, we are often asked questions about our experiences with the purchase and implementation of our Picture Archival and Communication System (PACS), and the impact of filmless radiology on the cost and quality of patient care. Although we often provide reprints of our previous articles and scientific papers concerning filmless radiology, we have not, until the publication of this book, been able to provide a more comprehensive reference on the subject.

The subject for this book has thus been inspired by the questions and concerns of visitors who have been seeking practical advice and answers to questions about filmless radiology. The first section of the book addresses the current state of the art and expected trends in PACS, offers a history of PACS, and provides a detailed guide and template for formal specifications for such a system. In the second section, we stress very practical issues including medical–legal considerations, productivity, economic impact, and challenges associated with filmless radiography. The third section addresses issues related to the acquisition of high-quality digital images in general radiography and mammography. The fourth section emphasizes the use of the PACS and specifically, the computer workstation itself, by nonradiologists, while the fifth section focuses on more technical considerations, including advanced workstation design, image compression, and the current standard for communication of medical images, DICOM. The seventh section provides a more detailed description of medical imaging and telemedicine in the VA System, as well as case studies of filmless radiology implementations at the Hammersmith Hospital in London, at UCLA, and other academic medical centers. Finally, we have been given permission to reproduce the extraordinarily well-received glossary of terms related to filmless imaging initially presented at the annual meeting of the Radiological Society of North America.

Rob Kolodner and I are grateful to our distinguished colleagues for sharing their tremendous expertise and experience with us and for their contributions to this book. The success of the PACS at the Baltimore VA Medical Center can be largely attributed to our collaboration with many of these wonderful people.

Acknowledgments

Rob Kolodner and I are indebted to Marion Ball, who provided the inspiration for this series and the encouragement to pursue this project. We would also like to express our deep gratitude to Judy Douglas, whose organizational skills, enthusiasm, encouragement, and initial editing provided the framework for the entire book. We also want to acknowledge the superb editing provided by Barbara Chernow and the extraordinary patience and guidance provided by Kelley Suttenfield, assistant editor, Springer-Verlag. We also want to offer special thanks to our contributing authors who managed to find time to contribute and refine their chapters despite incredibly hectic work and travel schedules.

Our success at the Baltimore VA Medical Center would not have been possible without the unbelievable indulgence and enthusiasm of our radiologists (particularly Drs. Briscoe and Diaconis) and our administrator, Robert Cox, chief technologist, Wayne Mazan, and our superb staff of radiology and nuclear medicine technologists. These staff members in our department have been the true pioneers in our early exploration with filmless radiology.

Above all, I would like to express my love and sincere thanks to my wife, Susan, and my son, Stephen, who have provided invaluable support and have even maintained their sense of humor despite my crazy clinical, administrative, and travel schedule.

Eliot L. Siegel

Contents

Section 1

Section 2

Section 3

Section 4

Section 5

Section 6

Contributors

Dorothy Steller Artz
ISIS Center, Georgetown University Medical Center, Washington, DC 20007, USA

Roger A. Bauman, M.D.
Journal of Digital Imaging, Winchester, MA 01809, USA

Scott B. Berger, M.D.
Department of Diagnostic Imaging, Yale University School of Medicine, New Haven, CT 06504, USA

Barry B. Cepelewicz, M.D., J.D.
Meiselman, Farber, Packman & Eberz, P.C., 118 North Bedford Road, Mount Kisco, NY 10549, USA

Ruth E. Dayhoff, M.D.
Director, Advanced Technology, Veterans Health Administration, Silver Spring, MD 20910, USA

Charles D. Flagle, Ph.D.
Health Services Research and Development Center, Johns Hopkins University, Baltimore, MD 21201, USA

Matthew T. Freedman, M.D.
ISIS Center, Georgetown University Medical Center, Washington, DC 20007, USA

Steven L. Fritz, Ph.D.
Director, Imaging Physics Lab, University of Maryland Medical School, Baltimore, MD 20201, USA

Günther Gell, Prof. Dr.
Department of Medical Informatics, University of Graz, A-8036 Graz, Austria

Fred Goeringer, Col.
710 Bridgeport Avenue, Shelton, CT 05484-0918, USA

Mitchell Goldburgh
Loral Medical Imaging Systems, Hoffman Estates, IL 60195, USA

Jaquelyn Hogge
ISIS Center, Georgetown University Medical Center, Washington, DC 20007,
USA

Steven C. Horii, M.D.
Department of Radiology, University of Pennsylvania Medical Center, Philadelphia, PA 19104, USA

H.K. Huang, Ph.D.
Laboratory for Radiological Informatics, Department of Radiology, University of California, San Francisco, CA 94143-0628, USA

Rebecca L. Kelley
Technology Services, Veterans Health Administration, Silver Spring, MD
20910, USA

Robert M. Kolodner, M.D.
Department of Veterans Affairs, 810 Vermont Avenue NW, Washington, DC
20420, USA

Peter M. Kuzmak
Computer Specialist, Veterans Health Administration, Silver Spring, MD
20910, USA

Seong Ki Mun, Ph.D.
ISIS Center, Georgetown University Medical Center, Washington, DC 20007,
USA

John Perry
48 W880 Chandelle Drive, Hampshire, IL 60140, USA

Stephen M. Pomerantz, M.D.
Department of Radiology, University Hospital, Baltimore, MD 21201, USA

Fred Prior, Ph.D.
Integrated Clinical Solution, Philips Medical Systems North America,
Shelton, CT 06484-0917, USA

Zenon Protopapas, M.D.
Department of Radiology, Hospital of St. Raphael, New Haven, CT 06511, USA.

Bruce I. Reiner, M.D.
Department of Radiology, Saint Mary's Hospital, Leonardtown, MD 20650, USA

Eliot L. Siegel, M.D.
Department of Radiology, Baltimore Veterans Administration Hospital, Baltimore, MD 21201, USA

Nicola H. Strickland, M.D.
Department of Radiology, Hammersmith Hospital, The Royal Postgraduate Medical School, London W12 0HS, UK

John C. Weiser, Ph.D.
Department of Radiology, Byrd HSL Center, West Virginia University, Morgantown, WV 26506-8150, USA

Charles E. Willis, Ph.D.
Department of Radiology, University of Texas Houston Medical School, Houston, TX 77030, USA

Michael Wilson
Veterans Administration Hospital, Baltimore, MD 21201, USA

Rebecca A. Zuurbier, M.D.
ISIS Center, Georgetown University Medical Center, Washington, DC 20007, USA

Section 1

1
Current State of the Art and Future Trends

ELIOT L. SIEGEL

Although I am convinced that the first chapter of a book about filmless radiology should include a discussion about the current state of the art and predictions about the future, this has been an interesting challenge. In some ways it feels like pulling out a diary in the middle of a rollercoaster ride and trying to write down what is happening at any particular moment and trying to look ahead at all of the hidden loops and curves and predict where the ride is going. With the state of the art changing so rapidly, this chapter can only serve as a snapshot of a technology that is in tremendous flux.

The explosion in computer and information technology and the ongoing overhaul of our health care delivery system have created both the opportunity and the mandate to reinvent the way in which diagnostic imaging has been practiced. However, despite the many advances in the art and science of radiology since the discovery of the x-ray by Wilhelm Corad Röntgen on November 8, 1895, the acquisition of conventional radiographs and the management and display of images has changed very little.

The acronym PACS stands for Picture Archival and Communication System. In common usage, the term PACS refers to a computer system that is used to capture, store, distribute, and then display medical images. For diagnostic imaging applications, PACS technology can be utilized to achieve near filmless operation.

During the past 100 years, film has played a heroic role as a one man *tour de force* in which it has been versatile enough to capture, store, move, and display radiographic images. It has taken a full century for a worthy successor to emerge in the form of late twentieth-century computer technology, which has provided attractive alternatives to film. This has been accomplished using innovative approaches for image capture, high-speed networks, powerful computer "servers" and workstations, and ultrahigh resolution monitors.

The transition to filmless radiology provides the opportunity to break free from the century-old constraints of film with regard to the acquisition, communication, storage, and display of images. Unfortunately, the phrase has been overutilized to the point where it has almost become a cliché, with its meaning applied to a bewildering spectrum of different technologies and applications. In this chapter, filmless radiology refers to a hospital or network-wide environment in which film has either completely or at least largely been replaced by an electronic system that acquires, archieves, and communicates and displays images.

Filmless radiology has the potential to provide two major benefits. The first is the improved accessibility, integration, and efficiency made possible by the incorporation of images into the patient's electronic medical record. The second is the creation of new techniques to take advantage of the recent developments in image acquisition, display and image processing. These technologies can be used to redefine the radiologist's basic toolkit, analogous to the internist's stetchoscope or the surgeon's scalpel. The reinvention of conventional radiology represents more than just an improvement in technology; it provides medical facilities and hospital networks with the opportunity to redesign the way in which they practice.

The majority of medical facilities will likely make the transition to filmless radiology during the next ten to twenty years. Figure 1.1 represents my guess of the rate at which the transition to near (at least 90%) filmless operation will occur in the United States. Although this estimate is a bit more conservative than those made by others with regard to the speed of the transition, previous predictions during the past 20 years have consistently proven to be optimistic. Despite expectations of a wide-scale conversion to filmless operation during the 1990s, there are still arguably just a half a dozen nearly filmless facilities in the United States.

Why has the transition to filmless operation been so relatively slow? This is likely the result of a number of factors, but in my opinion, the most im-

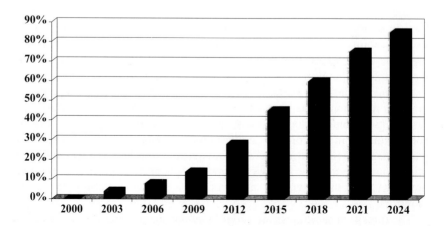

FIGURE 1.1. Rate of transition to filmless (>90%) radiology in the United States.

portant has been that the purchase of a PACS requires a complete reengineering of the operations of the radiology department. The entire workflow of the radiologists, technologists, and other clerical and technical personnel needs to be redesigned to achieve a successful PACS. Additionally, a high-level of integration of PACS into the health care enterprise is required to ensure its optimal function. This typically requires a tremendous amount of planning and implementation with computer personnel, engineers, and the administration as well, of course, as other clinical departments. This is far more complex to achieve than any other acquisition process for the radiology department and the hospital. It is comparable but more difficult than, the transition to a new radiology or hospital information system or billing system. Finally, there continues to be relatively little data that has been published on the impact of PACS, especially in the area of cost benefit analysis.

Image Acquisition Technology

Introduction

Although the newer modalities, such as Magnetic Resonance Imaging (MRI), Computed Tomography (CT), Ultrasound, digital angiography, digital fluoroscopy, and nuclear medicine, directly obtain images in a digital format, approximately 70% of a radiology department's workload continues to be in the area of conventional radiography (plain films). General radiography, with its high volume and detailed images, represents a special challenge for PACS. This challenge has been met by the introduction of new modalities, such as computed radiography, direct radiography, and film digitization.

Current Technology

Most imaging equipment for the digital modalities, such as CT, MRI, ultrasound, nuclear medicine, CR, direct radiography (DR), angiography, and digital fluoroscopy, is currently purchased with a standard interface that uses a communication protocol and image format known as DICOM. This protocol preserves the original full fidelity (spatial and contrast resolution) generated by the modality during the transfer to the PACS. However, it has been recently estimated (I believe somewhat pessimistically) that only 4% of diagnostic radiology equipment currently in worldwide use is fully DICOM compliant. In the absence of a DICOM interface, images can be captured for transmission into a PACS using video capture boards that can intercept the video output to a monitor or camera.

This frame-grabbing technique is still used for digital modalities such as ultrasound, nuclear medicine, and angiography, as well as fluoroscopy when a digital interface is not available, and is usually required for nonradiological modalities such as pathology, endoscopy, and bronchoscopy. Unfortunately, there is a good deal of variability in the quality of video capture units and even the best ones may introduce artifacts that degrade image quality. These units are limited to capture of only 8-bits (256 shades of gray) which is insufficient for 12-bit (4,096 shades of gray) modalities such as CT and MRI. Thus, for example, a CT of the thorax acquired by such a frame-grabbing device would need to be captured and archived as multiple images using 8-bit lung, mediastinal, bone, and abdominal settings rather than as a single, digital, 12-bit image.

General Radiography: Computed Radiography, Direct Radiography, and Film Digitization

Approximately 70% of the examinations in a typical radiology department fall into the category of general radiography, often referred to as plain films. These studies are particularly challenging in a filmless environment not only because of the large volume of studies performed but also because of the fact that they require a very high level of spatial and contrast resolution resulting in large (6–16 megabyte) image files. In a filmless environment there are only three currently available methods for the acquisition of general radiographic studies: CR, DR, and film digitization.

Computed radiography, also known as storage phosphor radiography (SP), is currently the only widely available commercial solution for the digital acquisition of conventional radiographs. With this technology, a reusable phosphor plate is placed in an imaging cassette in lieu of film. The image on the phosphor plate is extracted using a CR plate reader (analogous to a film processor), which is used to convert the pattern of radiation on the phosphor plate into a mathematical matrix corresponding to the amount of radiation that fell on each picture element (pixel). The major advantage of CR is its wide dynamic range and its use of computer image processing, which result in the potential to decrease image retake rates and improve the diagnostic quality of radiographs, particularly in challenging areas such as the emergency room and the intensive care unit. There are, however, a number of limitations of the technology. The throughput of the CR plate readers (currently up to about 70 plates per hour) is substantially slower than dark room or daylight film processors. The lower spatial resolution of 2.5 line pairs per millimeter for large field of view studies, such as chest and abdominal radiography, is less than one third of that theoretically achievable using film. It should be noted that this decreased spatial resolution seems less important in actual practice than contrast resolution, which is greater with computed radiography than conventional film. The technology is expensive, with costs ranging from $150,000 to $450,000 for a CR system and a $700 to $800 cost for replacement of each phosphor plate and similar cost for the cassettes. Finally, these phosphor plates have a limited life expectancy of only 2,000 to 6,000 exposures before they need to be replaced; this adds to the cost of ownership of CR.

There is a strong consensus that storage phosphor radiography, at least for high volume general radiography applications and fluoroscopy, will be replaced over the next ten to twenty years with what is currently referred to as DR. With DR, a large, flat-panel x-ray detector or array of detectors is utilized to directly capture the radiographic image. This eliminates the need to process or read the detector (film in a conventional system; the phosphor plate in a CR system) in another location, thereby eliminating this step. With a DR system that is fully integrated with the hospital information system, a technologist can obtain a series of images and then immediately review and send the images to a PACS. This filmless and plateless system has the potential to increase productivity. As of this date, no studies have been performed to determine the extent to which this translates into improved efficiency in a real-world environment, but improvements on the order of ten to twenty five percent seem feasible. The DR technology also has the potential to increase spatial resolution in comparison with currently implemented CR systems and to decrease artifacts associated with the physical damage that can occur over time with storage phosphor plates. The major disadvantages of the technology are the high costs (over $350,000 per room), the relatively high vulnerability to damage of the detector systems, and the lack of portability. These disadvantages will limit the use of DR to relatively high volume, single radiographic room replacements during the next few years.

In the absence of a digital acquisition device or a digital or frame-grabber interface, film can be digitized using a high-end device which, in some ways, is analogous to a facsimile machine. A film digitizer is a device that scans a film and then sends the resulting electronic image to a storage device or PACS. Conventional films can theoretically be digitized to a relatively high level of both spatial and contrast resolution using a high quality film digitizer. In practice, however, the digitization process introduces a number of artifacts that can degrade image quality. In addition to these artifacts, the image quality is limited by the quality of the original film. The film digitization process is often found to be unexpectedly time consuming because of the need to identify each patient, the study performed, and the date and time of the examination, and to enter that information into the PACS database. We performed an analysis of the time required to digitize our last five years of films at the Baltimore VA Medical Center and concluded that the process would take approximately seven years using four full-time employees! The perception of radiologists at our facility is that image quality is significantly limited for digitized films resulting in decreased diagnostic confidence. These limitations have resulted in the adoption of computed radiography rather than film digitization in facilities with PAC systems.

Mammography

Mammography represents the biggest challenge of all in a filmless radiology department. The current generally accepted requirements for mammography exceed five line pairs per millimeter and thus probably cannot be met by the resolution currently available using CR. Consequently, full-breast dedicated mammography units have recently been developed and are just becoming commercially available. These units acquire images at a matrix size of approximately 4,000 by 4,000 pixels, resulting in a 32-megabyte data set (four × the current size of a CR image). The challenges presented by these units are related to the large data set. Current monitors are limited in their resolution to 2,500 by 2,000 pixels and consequently images would have to be magnified or "zoomed" to reveal the full resolution. This can be time consuming and unwieldy using current PACS workstations. Additionally, the current generation of video display cards is insufficient to store and display a large number of these very large images for image navigation and display. The strategy utilized by most large-scale PACS installations has been to perform conventional film screen mammography, have the radiologists interpret the films, and then digitize the films into the PAC system for subsequent review by surgeons and other clinicians. Recent developments in mammography soft copy review workstations seem promising, but have not yet been commercially implemented.

Image Acquisition: Clinical Requirements

When planning for a filmless imaging department, it is critical to specify, in detail, that all modalities will have digital interfaces to the PACS. These interfaces should utilize the DICOM standard for communication with the PACS. Additionally, image acquisition devices should be purchased with the ability to communicate directly with the hospital or radiology information system (HIS/RIS) to facilitate electronic entry of patient and study information. All new radiology equipment purchases should specify the ability to obtain a worklist from the hospital information system based upon either a patient name, identification, or a list of recently ordered studies. Additionally, all new HIS/RIS purchases should specify the ability to communicate with a PACS or medical imaging device. This will eliminate the relatively inaccurate and inefficient manual entry of this data that is currently required. Image acquisition devices must be able to send images to the PACS rapidly to minimize radiologist and clinician waiting times. This requires, for example, that a CR image be transmitted in less than thirty seconds and a sixty image CT study in less than two minutes.

Video capture or frame-grabbing technologies should be avoided because of the potential for significant degradation of image quality. Film digitization should be avoided when possible because of digitization artifacts and the relatively slow speed of this process.

Image Acquisition: Current State of the Art

The current state of the art in image acquisition is for modalities to be fully DICOM compliant with the ability to communicate bidirectionally (i.e., both send images to and receive images from) with the PACS. The various imaging modality vendors are just beginning to implement modality worklists. Mammography units from a number of vendors will acquire 4,000 by 4,000 pixel images and store and display them locally and send them to a PACS. Computed radiography systems are becoming highly reliable, with improved plate reader capacities of 70 to 100 plates per hour. CR image processing, is beginning to be optimized for soft-copy interpretation rather than for printing to film. Direct radiography is just coming into use and has shown promising results with regard to image quality and potential productivity gains.

Image Acquisition: Future Trends

All imaging modalities will become primarily digital during the next few years. Full-breast digital mammography units with replace conventional film screen units because of their improved contrast resolution for use with dense breasts and their clinically acceptable spatial resolution. CR will become the dominant modality for general radiography in digital departments for the next ten years and will gradually be replaced by direct digital radiographic units. These DR systems will also provide high frame rate (up to 30 frames per second), high-resolution (at least 2K by 2K) alternatives for general fluoroscopy rooms.

For lower volume applications, CR prices will drop substantially (below $60,000) which will result in the gradual elimination of film digitizers for this application. This will result in the eventual replacement of conventional film, even in the relatively lower volume clinic setting.

PACS Interfaces

One of the most important lessons of early PACS implementations has been the critical importance of smoothly functioning and reliable interfaces. These interfaces can be thought of as communication highways that permit the modalities, the PACS, and the hospital and radiology information systems (HIS/RIS) to communicate with each other.

Three types of interfaces or gateways are required for the successful operation of a large-scale PACS. The first of these is the modality to PACS interface, which permits transfer of medical images and patient and study information from the acquisition devices (such as a CT scanner), to the PACS and potentially image transfer from the PACS to the modality. The second is the HIS/RIS to PACS interface, which permits transfer of patient information such as name, identification, and study type to and from the PACS. The third type of interface is the HIS/RIS to modality interface, which permits direct communication between a medical imaging device and the hospital or radiology information system.

PACS/Modality/HIS/RIS Interfaces: Clinical Requirements

The most important requirement of a clinical gateway is reliability. These gateways should be fully operational more than 99.5% of the time. When feasible, the hospital information system and/or radiology information system should serve as the master database. All patient and study transactions should initially occur on the HIS/RIS. This information on the HIS/RIS should be automatically communicated across an interface to both the PACS and the modalities (either simultaneously or in series) or should be made available on the HIS/RIS for use by the PACS and/or modalities. This information should include patient identifying information, patient location, scheduled examinations, and previous examinations and reports, and ideally allergy information, recent laboratory values such as creatinine value, as well as a patient problem list and recent progress notes or discharge summaries when available. Both the PACS and the modalities should keep the HIS/RIS updated as to exam status (e.g., let the HIS/RIS know when an examination has been completed and sent or if an examination has not yet taken place).

The modalities must have the ability to rapidly transfer patient images and accurate patient and study data to the PACS. Transfer rates of modality interfaces should be at least 2 megabits per second. This will result in transfer of a CT image in about 2 seconds and a computed radiography, 8-megabyte study in approximately 30 seconds. The modality interface and image output must comply with the DICOM standard and include some type of conformance statement that describes the specifics of the way that the vendor has implemented DICOM. This conformance statement is important because vendors vary considerably in their support for all of the many facets of the complex DICOM standard. Unfortunately, the DICOM standard is limited in its ability to handle communication errors. This topic should be discussed at length with potential PACS and modality vendors. The vendors should be given functional specifications, such as percentage of images sent over successfully and time required to send the study, and should be strongly motivated contractually to meet these specifications.

PACS/Modality/HIS/RIS Interfaces: Current Technology

Virtually all CT, MR, and nuclear medicine vendors directly support the DICOM standard with an increasing number of the major manufacturers of ultrasound, angiography, and digital fluoroscopy equipment supporting the standard as well. The major computed radiography vendors either support DICOM directly or provide third party DICOM interfaces.

Support for modality worklists, which would permit a modality such as CT to query the HIS/RIS for patient and study information, is currently minimal, but is expected to become commonplace in the next few years. The limiting step currently seems to be reluctance on the part of the major HIS/

RIS vendors to agree on a standard means of communication between their information systems and the individual modalities and the PACS. Thus, it seems likely that large-scale PACS sites will continue to endure the problems associated with manual entry of patient data. This manual entry has been reported to be associated with a 15 to 20% error rate and is a relatively time-consuming process. The currently utilized interfaces are surprisingly slow, given the theoretical bandwidth of even conventional Ethernet connections. Actual throughput rates are often 50 to 100 K bytes per second. The concept of plug and play has not yet been realized in current commercial systems, which often require third-party vendors to translate from one version of DICOM to another.

Future Trends in PACS Modality Interfaces

Modality interfaces of the future will become bidirectional, permitting a modality to query the HIS/RIS or PACS, upload patient and examination information and then display a list of patients to be imaged. In the next few years, there will be full support for DICOM features, such as subfolders for individual MRI sequences, and for ultrasound, nuclear medicine, and MRI cine loops. Plug and play capability will become more common, eliminating the need for third-party vendors to translate from one interpretation of DICOM to another. The next few years will bring about changes in HIS/RIS interfaces as well. HIS/RIS vendors will provide greater support for HL-7 and/or DICOM and eventually for a distributed object-oriented architecture such as Corba (Common Object Request Broker Architecture). These HIS/RIS to modality interfaces will allow the modalities to directly query the HIS/RIS for a broad range of information including patient and study identification. Finally, it will become routine to transfer a much greater scope of information including recent laboratory studies, the patient's problem list, and other information from a patient's electronic medical record.

PACS Archival Technology

Introduction

Once images are acquired, they must be stored (archived) for subsequent image review by radiologists and clinicians. Image storage has traditionally been divided into short and long term (and in some cases, medium term), although the distinctions between these are becoming blurred as larger short-term and faster long-term image storage become available. There is a tremendous difference in speed of retrieval between long- and short-term storage, with the difference on the order of 20:1 to 100:1 or more in the time required to retrieve an image or set of images. The typical PACS archive has, at any one time, at least 95% of its images in the much slower long-term archive. This makes it very important to utilize intelligent algorithms to maximize the likelihood that the required current and comparison studies are available in short-term storage.

PACS Archival Clinical Requirements

The short-term archive should permit retention of images for a period of at least two to three weeks and optimally should have the capacity to store at least one to three months of images. Retrieval times should be two seconds or less for CR images and ten seconds or less for a twenty-image CT study when retrieving a study from a central image repository (central PACS architecture) or from a local workstation (distributed PACS architecture). These speeds are necessary to maintain acceptable levels of radiologist and clinician productivity. Image retrieval reliability should be 100% at all times of the day and week with no down or slow times associated with preventative maintenance operations. The long-term archive should have the capacity to store at least five to six years of medical imaging studies. This period corresponds to the requirements that many institutions have for retention of conventional films. Because of the relatively high costs and possible delays and errors associated with a human operator for off-line platters, off-line storage of optical platters should be avoided if possible. The retrieval times for a CR image from long-term storage should be less than one minute. A thirty image CT study should be available within two minutes. To maximize the likelihood that comparison images are located in short-term storage, a method should be in place to transfer these old examinations from long- to short-term storage when they are likely to be required. This process, known as prefetching, should occur after a request for a new examination is made in the HIS/RIS and should result in retrieval of relevant previous studies. Other events that trigger transfer of old studies into faster short-term memory include hospital admission, a scheduled appointment with a health care provider, and patient transfer or discharge. Using a well-designed prefetch strategy, it should be very unusual for a radiologist or clinician to have to stop or slow down to wait for old studies to be retrieved from long-term storage.

PACS Short-Term Storage: Current Archival Technology

Short-term images are typically stored on magnetic disks with a redundant data storage scheme such as RAID (redundant array of inexpensive disks). Most current systems have short-term storage capacity in the range of 20 to 256 gigabytes. Nondestructive compression used by some systems can increase this capacity by a factor of two to threefold. Retrieval times for images vary widely with a number of different commercial PAC systems, ranging from 1 to 15 seconds or more for a single portable chest radiograph. Many systems currently require that images be prefetched to an individual work-station for retrieval from the local hard drive. This requires the system to anticipate the workstation or workstations that might be used to view a particular study, which may be difficult.

PACS Long-Term Storage: Current Archival Technology

The majority of large-scale PAC systems currently use an optical jukebox for long-term storage of images. Storage capacities typically range from 20 gigabytes to slightly more than 2 terabytes with retrieval times ranging from 20 seconds to about 5 minutes for a single computed radiography image (8 megabytes). The optical jukebox, perhaps because of the multitude of mechanical parts, has often been one of the less reliable components of a large-scale PACS. A few PAC systems use helical or other tape storage devices with capacities ranging from one to a hundred or more terabytes. Retrieval times for these tape units have been quoted as comparable to, or in new units, somewhat faster than the current generation of optical jokebox systems. The degree of image compression currently utilized in these long-term storage devices ranges from 2 to 3:1 using lossless compression, and up to 10:1 using so-called lossy, or destructive, compression algorithms.

PACS Image Storage: Future Trends

In the next few months, there will be a further blurring of the distinction between long- and short-term storage. This will occur as short-term storage capacity increases to between 250 gigabytes and 1 terabyte, permitting storage of many weeks or months of images with retrieval of images requiring only a few seconds. This will result in a situation in which long-term storage is primarily used for archival purposes with retrievals occurring infrequently. In addition, long-term storage devices of from 1 to 100 or more terabytes will become much faster, permitting rapid archiving and retrieval times in the range of 10 to 30 seconds or less for a CR image. With long-term storage capacities this large, image compression might be unnecessary in the archive, but would continue to be used dynamically (on the fly) to save time and money for such applications as teleradiology. Although shelf lives of optical disks are quoted as 100 years, it is likely that technical obsolescence of the previous standards will make replay of these old disks difficult. Digital Linear Tape (DLT) can provide transfer rates of as much as three times that of optical disk once the image has been located and may be a viable option, particularly for transfer of large imaging studies. Digital versatile disks (DVD) will provide an inexpensive, higher capacity alternative to the current generation of optical disks as standards for their use in the archival of medical images are set.

PACS Image Display

The image display system, or workstation, is the component of the PACS that has traditionally received the most attention. Indeed, for most users, it is the only component of the PACS with which they will directly interact. The PACS workstation functions as a window into the images and the patient and study databases.

PACS Image Display: Clinical Requirements

The imaging workstation must be able to retrieve images rapidly and easily and to permit rapid and intuitive navigation of the database to facilitate retrieval and comparison of relevant historical or related exams. The display monitors should have resolution of at least 2,000 by 1,500 pixels for use in the diagnosis of general radiography (preferably 2.5K by 2K pixels) and should have a display surface that is comparable in size to a conventional 14" by 17" film. The American College of Radiology standard for teleradiology suggests that conventional radiographs be reviewed using a resolution of at least 2K pixels.

Our research suggests that radiologists are significantly more productive using a two-monitor configuration in comparison to a single monitor and are slightly more efficient using a four-monitor configuration comparison to a two-monitor system. In the interpretation of CT and MR studies, a four-monitor 2,000 pixel configuration is recommended for those radiologists that read studies in a manner analogous to film in frame mode (images are displayed on each monitor, typically 9, 12, or 15 images per monitor). However, primary interpretation of CT and MR is increasingly being made in stack mode, in which images from a given MRI or CT series are electronically stacked together and reviewed in a sequential or cine fashion. Images from multiple dates or in related series (such as axial pre- and post-contrast MR images) can be matched and advanced and reviewed together in a logical manner. A number of studies have suggested that interpretation of cross sectional exams. Additionally, review of images in stack mode can be perfomed efficiently with only two monitors.

The software for image display and image manipulation, such as window/level and magnify, and for distance and angle measurements should be intuitive and thus easy to use and learn. Computer based training (CBT) and, ideally, on-line, context sensitive CBT should be included with the purchase of a PACS given the difficulty in scheduling formal training for radiologists and clinicians.

PACS Image Display: Current Technology

Workstation technologies for image display, image enhancement, and special processing, such as 3D rendering, have become very sophisticated, with hundreds of products available using a wide variety of processors and displays. Most current modality specific (e.g., CT) workstations use a single 1,000 by 1,000 pixel display and software designed to facilitate review of a single imaging study. Most of these non-PACS, modality displays are designed for image review or processing by the technologists rather than for primary diagnosis by radiologists and perform poorly when used to compare a current study to previous or related examinations.

The workstations designed for PACS typically utilize 1 to 4 monitors with from 1,000 by 1,000 pixel to 2,000 by 2,500 pixel resolution. Standard image manipulation software includes window/level, zoom and magnify, distance and angular measurement, and pixel value display. Less standard, but common, are cine or movie capability, area and perimeter measurement, edge enhancement, and histogram equalization.

Image navigation, or the ability to retrieve and display images for comparison purposes from, current as well as related examinations has been relatively disappointing on most PAC systems, although this has improved considerably during the past year or two. Currently, many steps are still required to retrieve prior studies for comparison with current exams. Additionally, many systems do not support the ability to easily compare subfolders, such as MRI individual sequences with images from other examinations.

High-resolution monitors (i.e., 2K) are currently very expensive and have difficulty maintaining acceptable levels of image brightness without adversely affecting image sharpness. These monitors also have a tendency to drift, or change brightness or clarity over time. Thus, a careful quality control program is absolutely essential for any large-scale PACS.

PACS Image Display Future Trends

The intensive research and development that will occur before the introduction of high-definition television into the consumer marketplace should have a very positive effect on monitor technologies and costs. It is very likely that they will become increasingly reliable and stable with improvements in the life span of the display systems. There will also be a continuing trend toward increased graphics speed and overall performance in the workstation platforms used for image display, thereby permitting more rapid image manipulation. Also, support for intuitive navigational features such as drag and drop for imaging studies and portions of studies, will become standard. Tools for image enhancement based on indication for the study or patient diagnosis will provide special processing for detection of central lines or endotracheal tubes in an ICU patient, or for detection of a pneumothorax, for example. More sophisticated image enhancement techniques, such as segmentation and texture analysis, will also be available at the standard workstation. This will be supplemented by computer aided diagnostic tools, such as an algorithm to assist in the detection of microcalcifications of certain sizes and shapes that would be characteristic for neoplasm. Many of these tools for computer assisted diagnosis will require very high performance systems that will not be practical to include in every workstation. This high-performance processing could take place on a system that would be shared by workstations on a network. Thus, users may perform 3D reconstruction or computer-aided diagnosis on images at any workstation on the network by sharing time on a black box located on the network, capable of performing these functions.

It is likely that in the future there will be a greater separation between radiology and clinical workstations. PACS of the future will probably be incorporated into hospital and radiology information systems, which will take responsibility for dissemination of images throughout the medical center or network. Radiology workstations will become increasingly specialized as high-end workstations are optimized for rapid image display, manipulation, and analysis. PACS workstations of the future will also become much more secure with better password checking and new verification procedures to ensure patient confidentiality and image security such as fingerprint or retinal scanning.

The trend in workstation design has been toward the use of personal computers running software such as Windows NT. These computers and operating systems have matured to the point where they offer comparable speed to a more traditional high-end workstation, especially when equipped with a high performance video card. A major advantage of the use of a PC workstation is the ability to add commercial off-the-shelf (COTS) software, such as voice recognition, electronic mail, televideoconferencing, and structured reporting packages.

PACS Networks

The PACS network can be though of as a "highway" that has been constructed to carry images to the PACS from acquisition modalities and from the PACS to workstations, the HIS/RIS gateway, and the image archive. Current network designs utilize either a central or a distributed architecture. In a PACS with a "central architecture" images are available using a shared short-term storage device (typically a RAID or redundant array of inexpensive disks). The advantage of this architecture is that all images in short-term storage are available at all workstations typically with a very rapid retrieval rate. The disadvantage is the vulnerability of this configuration to a system wide failure associated with a failure of the central storage system. The alternative design is a distributed architecture in which images are stored in multiple servers distributed throughout the medical center or health care enterprise. The major disadvantage of this configuration is the requirement that images need to be automatically or manually sent to individual servers or workstations in order to achieve acceptable performance. With this architecture, one must know, in advance, which images to have available to which workstations, which can be a major challenge. No studies have been performed to date which have documented a significant difference in system down time between the two architectural approaches. The unscheduled system "downtime" at the Baltimore VA Medical Center, which uses a central architecture, has been approximately 1%, with a scheduled down time for system upgrades and maintenance of approximately 1% as well.

PACS Network: Clinical Requirements

The PACS network must be able to support dozens or more simultaneous users without a significant degradation of throughput. Fortunately, according to the data collected at the Baltimore VA, workstation utilization is typically only 20 to 25% even during peak periods of activity. It must also be reliable with sufficient redundancy to maintain network traffic despite a malfunction. Finally, the network must provide a high level of security to ensure that only authorized users have access to patient information and must also provide protection from those who might tamper with the PACS database.

PACS Networks: Current Technology

A large variety of network topologies have been utilized successfully in small- and large-scale PACS. Fiberoptic networks are used almost exclusively for current large-scale PACS. Current off-the-shelf networks can deliver network performance in the range of 100 to 155 megabits per second, and proprietary and nonstandard networks can deliver 2 to 10 times that throughput. The recent trend has been to utilize a network protocol known as ATM (Asynchronous Transfer Mode). One of the limitations with regard to network performance is that of limited hospital infrastructures, which have been traditionally designed for text and billing requirements and not for imaging. A number of facilities have found that PC network or intranet-based systems that have relied on existing hospital network infrastructure have been plagued with unacceptably slow performance.

PACS Networks: Future Trends

In the next two to five years, the general use of higher performance networks will permit images to be distributed on multiple servers to maximize performance and reliability, but will offer the capability of retrieval of any imaging study at any workstation in less than two seconds. These high performance networks will also be able to support such functions as real-time transmission of cine images, such as ultrasound, and will be able to support high-resolution video conferencing at the PACS workstations. As standards evolve for high-speed networks, proprietary architectures will disappear. Gigabit network performance will be affordable and commonplace in the near future, resulting in the elimination of waiting time for static imaging studies. The combination of these very fast networks with real time compression will result in the ability to display cine cardiac, angiography, and ultrasound studies.

Teleradiology

Teleradiology in a PACS environment refers to the transmission of radiology and nuclear medicine images to and from another "site" for evaluation. This technology permits other hospitals or clinics (spokes) to send images to a central hub for evaluation, for the central PACS site (hub) to distribute workload to multiple sites, or for multiple hubs or spokes to share workload and staff.

Teleradiology: Clinical Requirements

Requirements vary depending on the teleradiology application. Teleradiology workstations for radiologists and clinicians should have similar requirements as those for an "in-hospital" PACS. For most teleradiology applications, communication speeds are limited, especially when sending images to a radiologist's or practitioner's office or home. This lack of high-speed communication lines necessitates the use of prefetching strategies that send images to the workstation well in advance of their being reviewed and/or high rates of image compression to reduce transmission times. When using teleradiology for primary interpretation of radiographic studies, historical images and patient demographic information should be available just as they are in the hospital. The reliability of image transmission must be very high. The phrase lossy image compression refers to a computer algorithm that is used to reduce the size of image files by a factor of between 3:1 to 100:1 or more while accepting minimal loss of the original image data. The goal with lossy image compression is to reduce the size of the image file to speed up transmission while not sacrificing any clinically significant features of the image. Lossy image compression can be performed using standard published algorithms at ratios of 10:1 and possibly up to 80:1 for general radiography and at ratios of 5:1 to 30:1 for CT and MR studies. Compression ratios of up to 300:1 or more can be achieved for cine studies, such as ultrasound or angiography.

Teleradiology: Current Technology

Most current teleradiology systems transmit the new examination, but often do not send the previous examination database or the prior imaging studies. Images are often transferred into the computer's hard drive before the radiologist or clinician reviews them. Because of a combination of proprietary network configurations and limitations in network speeds, most systems do not permit remote uses to log onto the PACS as though they were within the hospital using a workstation on the main network. Thus teleradiology systems in current use are relatively slow and diagnosis cannot usually be made as rapidly as from a workstation within the hospital directly connected to the network.

The cost of high-speed telecommunications is currently very high, with T1 or frame relay speeds of 1.5 megabits expensive ($740 per month in Baltimore) for a very small clinic or a radiologist's or clinician's home. ISDN telephone lines can be relatively inexpensive ($35 per month in the Baltimore Metropolitan area) and can deliver baud rates of 128,000 bits per second. This is much faster than the 28,800 to 56K baud rates that are currently achieved in most teleradiology systems. Satellite communications have been plagued with problems with reliability and are often even more expensive than other alternatives.

The American College of Radiology standard recommends a 2,000-pixel monitor for interpretation of digitized film or computed radiography images. However, the majority of teleradiology systems use monitors that display images using a matrix size of 1,000 by 1,000 pixels or less. These monitors are, however, adequate for interpretation of most digital modalities such as CT, MRI, nuclear medicine, and ultrasound. Many systems use lossless compression (an algorithm that reduces the size of an image file without any loss of data) achieving reductions in image file sizes of 2:1 or 3:1. Many systems do not take advantage of so called "lossy" compression with ratios of 10 to 30:1 despite a large amount of literature suggesting that there are no clinically significant differences in the diagnostic quality of these compressed images.

Teleradiology: Future Trends

During the next few years, demand for high-speed internet access will result in substantial increases in telecommunication speeds. Teleradiology systems in the future will use faster telecommunications technologies, such as ADSL (Asymmetric Digital Subscriber Line), cable modems, and home satellite systems. These fatter pipes will soon permit image download rates of 400 kilobits to 6 megabits per second for the home and physician's office (about 10 to 100 times faster than with a 56 K modem) resulting, when combined with appropriate compression technologies, in acceptable on-demand image retrieval rates. The availability of these high-speed communications will permit primary interpretation of radiographic images at home or in any other location. This is likely to result in substantial changes in the way that radiology is practiced.

Conclusion

Current large-scale PACS are only beginning to take advantage of the tremendous advances that have taken place in computer and network technology. During the next few years, nonproprietary, standards-based systems with performance within acceptable clinical parameters will proliferate as mainstream academic and private radiology practices make the transition to filmless imaging. These systems will become much better integrated with hospital information systems and will also be able to readily exchange information with other PAC systems.

Filmless radiology provides the potential to completely reinvent the way in which diagnostic radiology is practiced. This will result in a complete redesign of the radiologists reading rooms and the location of radiologist reading areas within a hospital and throughout the health care enterprise. The transition to filmless radiology should not be thought of as an endpoint but rather as an essential admission pass to the next phase in the history of diagnostic imaging. In the future, all PACS will become smoothly integrated into the entire health care enterprise, resulting in the availability of a patient's electronic medical record as well as vast image and text libraries. There will be almost instant access to any image within the health care system at any time, with improved image security, consistently higher quality and more diagnostic images, and a new generation of tools for the radiologist. These tools will enable the future radiologist to enhance the quality of existing images and combine multiple images from one (e.g., dual energy image subtraction) or more (e.g., nuclear medicine with CT and MRI) modalities into a single image or study to improve diagnostic accuracy. Finally, a new set of decision support features will be available in the future. These will use clinical information from the electronic medical record in conjunction with images from the radiology database and combine them with clinical and image information associated with a new study to help find and even suggest a diagnosis.

2
Large-Scale PAC Systems

GÜNTHER GELL AND ROGER A. BAUMAN

Traditionally the term PACS has been used to denote systems in radiology departments that deal with radiological images, although some PACS have expanded beyond those limits to contain images from other sources, such as pathology and endoscopy (Dayhoff and Kuzmak, 1994; Dayhoff, Maloney, and Kuzmak et al., 1991). Interest in PACS was triggered by the introduction of digital imaging methods such as computed tomography (CT) and magnetic resonance (MR), in which the "original" image is derived by a computational process from detector measurements, and the production of a hard copy on film is only a secondary process. This is in contrast to traditional radiology, where the film and image cannot be separated, and film itself is the detector.

If images are directly produced by a digital process without film, it seems logical to replace film as the medium for image transport, archiving, and display and to use electronic networks, digital storage media, and electronic displays. A complete PACS therefore aims at filmless radiology.

Greinacher (cited in Bauman, 1994) proposed the following definition of a PACS: "A PACS consists, at least, of one or multiple imaging modalities (acquisition devices), a communication network, an intermediate and/or long-term storage device, and an image review and/or post processing workstation." This definition covers the full range of PACS; a PACS with one modality, archive, and one workstation would today be called a mini-PACS, if not a micro-PACS.

A picture archiving and communications system (PACS) should fulfill the following functions by using digital technology:

- Image acquisition.
- Image communication (transfer).
- Image storage (archiving).
- Image display.
- Image processing.

The implementation of such an ambitious project presents many difficulties. For early PACS developers, the first step was to overcome the problems connected with the huge amount of data generated in radiology. A recent paper (Honeyman, Hude, Frost et al., 1996) estimated the yearly data volume of a

TABLE 2.1. University of Graz-Storage capacity needed for one year (1995) for text of reports and for images.

Type	No (in 1995)	Total storage		
MR reports	8500	10MB	1.2KB/report	
MR images	740,000	180GB	0.25 MB/image	87 images/report
CT reports	13,000	14 MB	1.1 MB/report	
CT images	600,000	300 GB	0.5 MB/image	46 images/report

It should be noted that the number of reports is not equal to the number of examinations. Every examination is reported, but one report may be on more than one examination (e.g., with and without contrast medium). Images (uncompressed) are for four CT and two MR. The ratio between text and images in terms of storage capacity is approximately 1:20,000 uncompressed

radiology department that performs 160,000 imaging examinations per year as 3,943 gigabytes (i.e., circa 4 terabytes) with a peak acquisition rate (if all images are digital) of about 1.8 gigabytes per hour. Well in line with other estimates, these reflect a gigantic increase when compared to the data volumes handled by a conventional radiology information system (RIS) without images. Table 2.1 compares the data volumes for the text reports and for images for CT and MR in 1995 for the Department of Radiology of the University of Graz. The ratio is on the order of 1:20,000!

The computer technology of the 1980s could not easily cope with such large data volumes. Therefore, early PACS pilot projects included only parts of a full system. For example, a pilot system would archive and transmit images of all patients for a certain type of modality or it would process images from different modalities for a selected subset of patients or a specific function like an emergency room.

Two Surveys

This chapter is largely based on two surveys of PACS, one in 1993 and one in 1995 (Bauman, 1994; Bauman, Gell, and Dwyer, 1996a, 1996b). In the earlier survey, Bauman discussed the following parameters for defining a large PACS:

- Daily clinical use.
- Whether the system includes three or more modalities.
- Availability of images in and outside of radiology.
- Number and percentage of included studies.
- Number and percentage of interfaced primary acquisition devices.
- Archive size.
- Whether the PACS is limited to a single "campus".
- Whether the interfaces are exclusively digital.
- Filmless operation.
- Level of complexity.
- Departmental volumes.

The first survey found 13 institutions with a PACS operational on November 1, 1993, which met the first three criteria: in daily clinical use, three or more modalities, and images available inside and outside radiology. These systems had from 5 to 17 image acquisition devices and up to 6 types of imaging modalities such as CT and MR. However, daily clinical use meant daily acquisition of selected examinations, but did not necessarily include long-term archiving or filmless reporting. Only four systems archived more than 80 percent of the examinations in the PACS; six archived fewer than 25 percent of their examinations.

The second survey is much more detailed. The definition of a large PACS was not changed except that an additional criterion was added, namely that a large PACS must handle a minimum of 20,000 exams annually. Using this definition, 23 large PACS were identified as of February 1, 1995; 12 of them had already been in the first survey. They are listed in Table 2.2.

As shown in Table 2.3, every large PACS includes at least one CT, and approximately 85 percent have at least one CR and one MR. These percentages did not change between 1993 and 1995. The presence of other modalities increased, particularly digital angiography, which went from 38 to 77 percent. In 1995, almost every PACS (22 out of 23) had an operational interface between the PACS and either a HIS or a RIS or both.

TABLE 2.2. Large PACS in clinical use as of February 1, 1995.

First clinical use	In 1993 survery	Hospital name
1988	Yes	University Hospital Graz
1989	Yes	Hokkaido University Hospital
1989		The Credit Valley Hospital
1992	Yes	Danube Hospital-SMZO
1992	Yes	Free University of Brussels, PRIMIS
1992	Yes	Madigan Army Medical Center
1992	Yes	UCLA Health Sciences Center
1992	Yes	University Hospital of Geneva
1992	Yes	University of Florida
1992	Yes	Wright Patterson AFB Medical Center
1993	Yes	Baltimore VA Medical Center
1993	Yes	Brooke Army Medical Center
1993	Yes	University of Pittsburgh
1993		Viborg Country Hosptial
1994		Brigham & Women's Hospital
1994		Conquest Hospital
1994		Houston VA Medical Center Hospital
1994		Osaka University Hospital
1994		Samsung Medical Center
1994		Toshiba Hospital
1994		University of California San Francisco
1994		University of Virginia
1995		Hospital of the University of Pennsylvania

Source: Bauman, Gell, and Dwyer (1996a).
The first column lists the year of first clinical use. A yes in the second column indicates, that the system was already listed in the first (1993) survey as a large PACS

TABLE 2.3. Interfaces to PACS by modality.

	CR	CT	DA	DF	MR	NM	US
1993 N = 13	11	13	5	6	11	5	6
% of total	85%	100%	38%	46%	85%	38%	46%
1995 N = 22	19	22	17	10	18	10	13
% of total	86%	100%	77%	45%	82%	45%	59%

Source: Derived from Bauman (1994) and Bauman, Gell, and Dwyer (1996a).
Abbreviations include: CR = computed radiography; CT = computed tomography; DA = digital angiography; DF = digital fluoroscopy; MR = magnetic resonance; NM = nuclear medicine; US = ultrasound.

An important feature concerns primary interpretation on PACS, that is, filmless reporting from diagnostic workstations. Three institutions (Danube Hospital—SMZO, Vienna, Austria; Baltimore Veterans Affairs Medical Center, Baltimore, Maryland; Viborg County Hospital, Denmark) reported that all primary interpretation, except for mammography, was on PACS. Four more hospitals reported much of the interpretation was done on PACS. The remainder did only some interpretation on PACS. In six of the large PACS installations, development was done inhouse; eight different vendors installed the rest of the systems.

The 1995 survey also gathered technical information regarding networks, archives, workstations, and so on. Some interesting trends or facts that emerge from the technical details include:

- External Access: One-third (seven) of the large PACS have more than 20 workstations for review outside of radiology, giving increased access to images. This is important if faster communication and filmless operation are to be realized.
- C Network: FDDI is the leading network supported by the main vendors as a backbone in connection with Ethernet and TCP/IP.
- Archive: Jukeboxes with optical disks (OD) and, to a lesser extent, magneto-optical disks (MOD) are the standard means for long-term archiving. The capacities of OD-jukeboxes range from 76 to 2400 gigabytes with an average of 786 gigabytes. The capacities of single ODs vary between 0.6 and 10 gigabytes with 10 different values given. This diversity seems to indicate that the technology is reliable, but not yet stable. New technologies (e.g., jukebox-like tape archives) and enhanced recording densities and formats may make current archive equipment obsolete. Although the media themselves remain readable, recopying of archives will be necessary because the reading equipment must be replaced to benefit from enhanced technology.
- Compression: With one exception, all large PACS installations avoid the use of lossy compression before interpretation. One-third (seven) of the installations use 1:10 lossy compression for the long-term archive.

Early Development Patterns

Early large PACS prototypes were for the most part developed at academic hospitals, often in cooperation with industry. Usually a stepwise approach was chosen, whereby PACS was introduced into an existing department with existing modalities and well-established organizational patterns. In these instances, PACS prototypes encompassed only part of a department's images and a subset of PACS functions, for example, images for selected patients or from selected modalities. The lack of standards in the past and the need to adapt to existing equipment and habits often made ad hoc solutions and compromises necessary. Some developments led to dead ends and had to be abandoned. For example, one major manufacturer of radiology equipment correctly concluded from an analysis of the future transfer rates generated by image communication in a completely digital radiology department that unsegmented Ethernet, the standard network then available, would be insufficient. Since FDDI was only emerging and not really stable, the manufacturer developed and installed special network technology for PACS at several hospitals. Retrospectively, this was an error. On the one hand, commercial standard network technology evolved rapidly enough to carry the workload of existing PACS in combination with prefetching techniques. On the other hand, the substitution of conventional film by computed radiography and consequently the increase of the digital workload developed slower than anticipated.

A second approach was based on experiences of the pilot projects and undertook the implementation of a complete PACS in one step, often in connection with the building of a new department of radiology or at least a deep reorganization of an existing department. An example of each approach follows. Other systems will be described in detail in later chapters and elsewhere in the literature (DeValk, 1992; Huang, 1996; Osteaux, 1992).

Graz PACS: The Stepwise Approach

In 1985 the Department of Radiology of the University of Graz and Graz General Hospital, a 2,500 bed university hospital, entered into collaboration with Siemens. Their purpose was to develop a PACS based on existing modalities (CT, MR) from different manufacturers to use with the comprehensive RIS that had been developed in-house. Together they developed, implemented, and tested many important concepts, including grouping images into folders, routing and prefetching policies, linking to the RIS, and essential functionalities of diagnostic workstations (Gell, Schneider, and Wiltgen, 1989; Wiltgen, Gell, and Graif et al., 1993).

In 1987/1988 the PACS went into routine operation with an emphasis on image acquisition, communication, and archiving; soft copy interpretation was limited to selected cases. Since then the system has grown continuously. Today it is a heterogeneous PACS with components from different vendors and complex functionalities.

The responsibility for planning, integrating, and operating the overall system lies with the University Department of Medical Informatics, which began as the informatics section of the Department of Radiology. The department maintains a friendly customer-vendor relationship with Siemens, which supplies most of the workstations and archives. The network was planned and installed locally as part of the hospital wide network. Some modalities and modality oriented subsystems with workstations and archives (e.g., for CR or nuclear medicine) come from other vendors and are integrated via DICOM interfaces or via ACR/NEMA. The RIS controls rearchiving and image distribution (to neurology, neurosurgery, radiotherapy planning, for maxillafacial surgery three-dimensional models, and so on). To keep prices down, the Department of Medical Informatics has developed software for image viewing on normal PCs and for paper hard copies. Inexpensive, the hard copies are of reasonable quality for review purposes as an illustration to the report, not for primary interpretation. The percentage of soft copy interpretation has increased rapidly during the last few years and film consumption has decreased correspondingly.

The main reasons for better acceptance of primary interpretation from workstations are:

- More high quality workstations are available for interpretation. Continued economic and space constraints and increasing demands for numerical post processing, e.g., to produce three-dimensional models may limit this availability.
- More radiologists are trained primarily in soft copy reporting.
- The high number of images produced by modern spiral CTs calls for dynamic viewing (scrolling) methods provided only by displays.
- Paper hard copy replaces the film in the conventional patient image jacket and serves as a quick reference when electronic displays are not at hand or occupied.

SMZO-Donauspital, Vienna: The Integral Approach

In the 1980s the City of Vienna decided to build a completely new hospital with 933 beds to better serve the northeastern parts of the city. The heads of the future departments were appointed at an early stage and were able to influence the planning process. Dr. W. Hruby, the appointed chief radiologist, convinced the authorities of the potential of digital radiology. Siemens was awarded the contract to build a filmless digital radiology department. Based on the experience with PACS in Graz and other pilot sites, the company developed an integrated system including various modalities, except MR. The PACS and an RIS became operational in 1991/1992, thereby creating one of the first filmless departments. The PACS became a product, Sienet, which is now sold worldwide. Another example of the integral approach is the PACS in Hokkaido, Japan. The Medical Diagnostic Imaging System (MDIS) system developed by Loral and Siemens for the U.S. Army shows a mixed approach, involving integral planning and stepwise integration.

Large PACS: Present State

Communications at several recent conferences (Kilcoyne, Lear, and Rowberg, 1996; Lemke, Vannier, Inamura, and Farman, 1996) suggest that the trend toward large and comprehensive PACS is continuing, if not accelerating. Several factors have contributed to this development.

Standards

DICOM is now firmly established as the relevant standard for the communication of radiological images. Almost all the manufacturers of radiological equipment, radiological workstations, and PACS (or parts of PACS) have committed themselves to DICOM and have followed up by demonstrating interoperability at major conferences (RSNA, CAR, and so on) and by documenting their DICOM interfaces in DICOM conformance statements (Clunie, 1996; Clunie, http://www.rahul.net/dclunie/dicom-conformance/survey.html). The ComitJ EuropJen de Normalisation (CEN) has adopted DICOM as an official European standard. More and more hospitals require DICOM as part of their procurement policy. Still, DICOM is not yet a "plug-and-play" standard. Integrating a system from different vendors requires technical knowledge and commitment on the part of the buyer and vendor or the involvement of an experienced external system integrator.

Maturity

PACS systems have moved from the status of prototypes and pilot projects to the status of products. There are now many vendors selling mature components, such as workstations, and a few companies with enough experience to sell a "turnkey" PACS.

Technology

The technology for many PACS components has developed rapidly over the last few years. High-speed networks like FDDI and ATM have become a robust standard, and jukeboxes and RAID storage with high capacities are now off-the-shelf products. Powerful workstations and personal computers with high-resolution displays and user-friendly graphical interfaces are common and affordable. A PACS can be built with standard commercial hardware

components with the possible exception of specialized diagnostic workstations with multiple screens, very high resolution, and high luminance and
contrast. But this rapid development impacts stability.

Stability

Because the underlying technology for most PACS components is developing rather rapidly, components become obsolete in a few years. There are,
however, differences. For example, present investments in networks such as
Ethernet or FDDI will not be lost if ATM becomes the leading technology;
they will instead be integrated via gateways. Workstations may become outdated but will remain usable if they have a DICOM conformant interface.
The most crucial problem will arise in archiving, where, as already mentioned, the technology is not yet stable, and there is competition among
different methods (OD, MOD, tape), data formats, and recording densities.
In a few years the installations may face the unpleasant alternative of either
copying their archived data on new media (expensive and time consuming)
or maintaining outdated and inefficient equipment at high cost. The situation is somewhat alleviated by the fact that the medical indication to retrieve old images decreases rapidly with time; it may, therefore, be sufficient
to maintain one reading station in case a special need arises.

Large PACS: Trends

The definition of a large PACS will always be somewhat arbitrary, but in the
future the distinction between stand alone and integrated systems may be
more meaningful. PACS in general and in particular large PACS have a tendency toward integration—to merge with other information systems. From a
logical point of view, a PACS is a subsystem of a hospital information system (HIS) or a larger healthcare network information system (HNIS) (Greenes
and Bauman, 1996). The purpose of such an IS is to provide all staff members with the information they need to perform their duties effectively and
efficiently. This, of course, includes images, when and where they are needed.
The large PACS of the future will be a system that is seamlessly integrated
into the HIS or the HNIS. For practical reasons, however, a distinction between PACS and IS may remain; problems of image acquisition, softcopy
interpretation, and medical image processing will require specific solutions.

A Scenario to Illustrate an Integrated PACS of the Future

Description

Using an HNIS or HIS-station, the clinician requests a radiological examination. Depending on local policies and the type of examination, the infor-

mation system books an appointment either immediately or after confirmation by an authorized person in the imaging department. Alternately, rather than request a specific examination, the clinician may ask the imaging department for a diagnosis and leave the selection of the appropriate examinations to the radiologist. In this latter case, the radiologist may request additional information from the information system such as laboratory results, clinical data, histology reports, or previous images, before deciding which procedures should be performed. Again the system books the examination, checks with the referring department, and asks for clinical confirmation if required (e.g., for angiography). The system also produces worklists for the department (for preparing the patient), for the patient transport system, and for the examination room (for preparing contrast media, catheters, and so on).

The technologist at the MR scanner or other modality has one workstation, with one or more large graphical user interface monitors, which provides seamless access to the information systems, the PACS, and the scanner controls. The technologist selects a patient from the worklist on the display and starts the procedure. Images and image parameters are transferred to the information system, linked to the patient, and routed to the archive, to diagnostic workstations, and elsewhere as needed, for example, to the referring clinician. The focal point in the imaging department is the radiology workstation, an assembly of large screens with high resolution, luminance, and contrast. This workstation displays images from the actual exam alongside selected images from relevant prior exams. The images are prearranged according to stored rules that take into account the type of examination, the organ, the clinical problem, the predilections of the radiologist, and so on.

The radiologist may request clinical data, laboratory results, endoscopic images, or any other part of the electronic patient record. The radiologist has access to tools and programs for image processing and quantitative evaluations, large databases containing interactive reference books, and image databases with collections of reference images that may be selected according to symptoms or diagnoses and to the current literature. During interpretation, the radiologist selects illustrative images to become part of the new "integrated radiology report." Those images may be annotated with graphics and speech. The report is dictated to the system, which displays the transcribed text for verification. The radiologist authorizes the results, which immediately become available to the referring clinician.

The clinician viewing this report sees (and hears, if so desired) the report and the selected images. Graphical symbols appear and highlight part of the images as they are being explained, giving the clinician a kind of animated consultation which maybe stopped, interrupted or repeated at any time. Despite access to all the images, as well as any other part of the patient record, the referring physician seldom chooses to view all images. The integrated radiology report provides the key information in a short time. The selection of images by the radiologist is a valuable service that spares the clinician the time-consuming task of viewing hundreds of images on a relatively slower PC workstation, using a smaller monitor.

The radiologist may also use the system to request advice or confirmation by sending annotated images to another radiologist's workstation. Advice may be given asynchronously, sent back by text or voice. Alternately, workstations may be used to set up teleconferences, enabling radiologists to discuss images displayed simultaneously on all workstations along with a moving cursor, annotations, and so on. Such a consultation may also be held between the radiologist and a clinician. All these features may be operated over any distance using generally available networks (Bauman, 1996; Gell 1994; Greenes and Bauman, 1996).

Obstacles

The scenario is somewhat futuristic and optimistic. Almost every single feature—and more could be added—has already been implemented somewhere in a pilot project. Integration is certainly feasible, albeit a very large task. Nonetheless, particularly in Europe, PACS causes apprehension among radiologists who perceive it as a threat to their specialty. According to one German radiologist, "It would be a horrible vision for the year 2000 to see the radiologist as the administrator of an electronic image archive, where everybody has free access. We needed almost 100 years to develop from a very technical discipline to clinical radiology, we do not want to lose this positive development by a new technology" (Peters, 1991; translated from German).

The underlying fear is that, instead of waiting for the radiological report (which tends to lag after the examination because of working habits and the delay between dictation and transcription), clinicians will use the images from the PACS immediately for diagnosis and therapeutic decisions. The situation in Europe differs somewhat from that in the United States. Clinicians in the United States who base a therapeutic decision on their own interpretation of radiological images and not on an expert opinion have a higher risk of facing and losing a malpractice suit. This kind of litigation is very rare in Europe.

Summary

Clearly a PACS integrated with an HNIS or HIS has the potential to change the way radiologists and clinicians interact. An integrated PACS also offers radiologists the opportunity to provide better patient care by providing clinicians with timely and instructive information and by improving the quality of radiological diagnosis itself.

Large integrated PACS can serve effective and efficient patient care. Among the capabilities that PACS provides are the following:

- Improved diagnostic quality by full utilization of the total information content of images: windowing, zooming, scrolling, quantitative measurements, modeling.
- Improved diagnostic quality by access to computer guided diagnosis, reference image data, interactive textbooks, online literature searches (Gell, 1993).
- Better service to remote areas by teleradiology and teleconsulting.
- Decreased delays because of fast and reliable digital archives, fast access to images and the full patient record, electronic transmission of results.
- Better service to clinicians by the use of multimedia reports and teleconsultation.
- Economic savings by decreasing film consumption, reduced archival space, less handling and overhead.

If not used astutely, these capabilities carry some risk. For instance, electronic communication could supersede clinical conferences with important personal contacts. Indiscriminate image distribution and unqualified interpretation could diminish diagnostic quality.

Radiology can look to the ACR Standard for Teleradiology (http://www.acr.org/standards.new/teleradiology-standard.html) for its proactive attitude towards a new technology. This standard explores new possibilities, defines the goals that can be reached, and states the conditions that must be fulfilled in order to use the technology safely without risk of damage. The attitude in this standard can serve radiology well, as it studies possible integrated PACS scenarios and maps how to implement and use these new technologies safely and securely.

References

American College of Radiology. ACR Standard for Teleradiology (Res. 21–1994), http://www.acr.org/standards.new/teleradiology- standard.html.

Bauman RA. World-wide experience with large PACS systems. Proc SCAR 1994, 17–21.

Bauman RA, Gell G, Dwyer SJ. Large picture archiving and communication systems of the world—part 1. J Digital Imaging 1996a, 9, 99–103.

Bauman RA, Gell G, Dwyer SJ. Large picture archiving and communication systems of the world—part 2. J Digital Imaging 1996b, 9, 174–177.

Bauman RA. Reporting and communications. Radiol Clin North Am 1996, 34, 597–606.

Clunie DA. DICOM Conformance Statement Survey, http: //www.rahul.net/dclunie/dicom-conformance/survey.html.

Clunie DA. Survey of DICOM Conformance Statements. In: Kilcoyne RF, Lear JR, Rowberg AH, eds. SCAR96, Computer Applications to Assist Radiology. Carlsbad CA: Symposia Foundation, 1996, pp. 217–223.

Dayhoff RF, Kuzmak PM. A network of fully integrated multispecially hospital imaging systems. Proc SPIE 1994, 556–562.

Dayhoff RF, Maloney DI, Kuzmak PM, et al. Integrating medical images into hospital information systems. J Digit Imaging 1991, 4, 87–93.

De Valk JPJ. Integrated Diagnostic Imaging. Amsterdam: Elsevier, 1992.

Gell G. Expert systems as a support to radiological diagnosis. Eur J Radiology 1993, 17, 8–13.

Gell G. PACS-2000. Radiologe 1994, 34, 286–290.

Gell G, Schneider GH, Wiltgen M. PACS–RIS Interfacing: Experiences and Problems. In: Lemke HU, Rhodes ML, Jaffe CC, Felix R, eds. Computer Assisted Radiology. Berlin: Springer, 1989, pp. 623–627.

Greenes RA, Bauman RA. The era of health care reform and the information superhighway. Radiol Clin N Am 1996, 34, 463–468.

Honeyman JC, Hude W, Frost MM, et al. Picture archiving and communication system bandwith and storage requirements. J Digital Imaging 1996, 9, 60–66.

Huang HK. PACS Picture Archiving and Communication Systems in Biomedical Imaging. New York: VCH Publishers, 1996.

Kilcoyne RF, Lear JR, Rowberg AH, eds. SCAR96, Computer Applications to Assist Radiology. Carlsbad CA: Symposia Foundation, 1996.

Lemke HU, Vannier MW, Inamura K, Farman AG, eds. Computer Assisted Radiology. Proc SCAR, Excerpta Medica Congress Series. Amsterdam: Elsevier 1996, p. 1124.

Osteaux M, ed. A Second Generation PACS Concept. Berlin: Springer, 1992.

Peters PE. Radiologie 2000. Radiologe 1991, 31, 153–157.

Wiltgen M, Gell G, Graif E, et al. An integrated picture archiving and communication system—radiology information system in a radiological department. J Digital Imaging 1993, 6, 16–24.

3

Purchasing a PACS: An RFP Toolkit

JOHN PERRY AND FRED PRIOR

Request for Proposal: An RFP Template

A Picture Archival and Communication System (PACS) represents a long-term commitment on the part of both the system integrator and the customer. The best vehicle for formal communication of requirements from a customer to a PACS supplier is a clear specification. The best time to start that communication is at the time of the request for proposal (RFP). Unambiguous technical communication between the customer and the supplier before both sides are committed to the project is critical to its success. Whenever an RFP leaves the customer's requirements incomplete or undefined, there is a trap for both the customer and the supplier. Incomplete or undefined requirements signal inadequate preparation and analysis. This chapter consists primarily of a template RFP for a PACS procurement, with commentary identifying issues, applications, and technologies that should be considered during the analysis leading up to the procurement.

In purchasing a PACS, there are several basic steps. The buyer should analyze the specific problem, shop around to see what is available, write an RFP, and work with the suppliers who respond to get to the best solution. One way to shop around is to do some of the specification work and then write a request for information (RFI); responses to the RFI can then help shape the final specification.

To coordinate a PACS project, administration, radiology, and the information systems (IS) departments must work together from the time of the RFP. The RFP is crucial to the customer and the supplier. The supplier needs to know unambiguously what the customer wants; the customer needs to be confident that the project will meet its goals. This requires detail. The process of development of a detailed specification serves to focus and discipline the internal analysis. It requires the involvement of all potential users at an early stage in the project; this involvement yields significant political benefits during implementation.

Writing Specifications

The Institute of Electrical and Electronic Engineers (IEEE) has defined a methodology for writing requirements specifications (1984). In the highly simplified version offered here, the term "normative statement" is used to describe a requirement that must be met by the system. Some rules are:

1. Paragraphs shall be separately identified. This may be accomplished by individually numbering the paragraphs.
2. A paragraph shall contain one normative statement.
3. A normative statement shall define one requirement.
4. A normative statement shall contain the word "shall."
5. A paragraph shall contain as much clarifying language as desired.
6. Clarifying language shall not be considered normative.

Defining requirements in normative statements helps tremendously in the analysis of a specification. "Shall language" separates normative statements from clarifying language, which is not binding but which may be helpful in interpreting the normative statement. For example, in rule 1 above, the second sentence is clarifying language. Note that statements using "must," "will," and "should" are not normative. Thus, "The cabinet should be green" is not normative; "The cabinet shall be green" is. The objective of this somewhat stilted and confining language is to communicate the requirements unambiguously, so the customer and supplier have to agree on a clear set of conventions.

When writing a proposal in response to an RFP, the supplier should create a requirements traceability matrix in which every requirement from the RFP is identified and correlated with a statement or statements in the proposal. The separation of requirements into individually identified normative statements simplifies creation of the matrix. The matrix is necessary to confirm that the supplier has responded to every requirement. Having each normative statement contain only one requirement assists in determining whether the requirement has been addressed completely.

When writing any specification, it is important to distinguish between requirements and design. In the case of an RFP, the customer's objective should be not to engineer the details of the solution, but rather to ensure that the PACS will solve the problem. Many specifications define in great detail items of the user interface, file structure, or internal system communication protocols that could be handled in other ways without negatively affecting the customer. Unless a particular problem mandates a specific technical solution (e.g., the goal of the project is to utilize an existing ATM network), it is advisable to focus on the operational requirements from the user's perspective, not implementation details.

Finally, anything left unsaid in the specification is freedom which the supplier may need to adapt the product to the problem at hand. Avoiding unnecessary requirements, whether for extra elegance, extra functionality, or specific design parameters, may provide just the freedom the supplier needs to respond at all.

Overview: RFP Section 1

The remainder of the chapter is organized as a generic RFP template that can be adapted to fit the needs of most PACS procurements. It is not necessary to adhere exactly to the format outlined below. In smaller scale projects, some of the requirements discussed may not be needed.

The RFP starts with a title page that identifies the project (a project name can provide a useful shorthand in future references) and the institution. This is followed by a table of contents. A table listing the document's revision history may appear next or be included later.

Summary: Section 1.1

The first part of an RFP should summarize the project so that a supplier can quickly grasp the scale of the investment and the opportunity. A good beginning is to describe the hospital, including:

- Size of the campus.
- Names and locations of the buildings.
- Number of floors in each building.
- Locations of the key departments.
- Size of the radiology department (number of rooms, key equipment, and so on).
- Total number of beds.
- Number of procedures per year.
- Plans for expansion of the facilities or procedure volume.

The introduction must also include a procedure volume analysis like that in Table 3.1, which details the data volumes involved. Next, there should be a high-level summary identifying the problem to be solved and the objectives of the project. The description should indicate the rough scale of the system. Is it a full-hospital PACS or focused on productivity in a specific department? Is it intended for intrahospital image distribution, or does it have a substantial teleradiology component? The description should also make clear the operational gains to be realized from the project. Finally, the description should indicate the time scale for the project. Is it an immediate procurement or a future project? If it will be implemented in phases over time, what are the planned sequence and the objectives for each step?

Clinical Operations: Section 1.2

In preparing a proposal for any project, questions arise that are not addressed by the normative requirements. A description of the customer's vision of how the system would work in clinical operation can function as a framework for resolving such questions. This description may include design assumptions,

TABLE 3.1. Procedure volume analysis.

Modality	Procedure	Annual volume	Images /study	KB Image	MB /study	MB/year with no compression
Radiography	Chest 1 view	37,500	1	7,500	7.5	281,250
	Chest 2 view	32,000	2	7,500	15.0	480,000
	Portable Chest	6,250	1	7,500	7.5	46,875
	Other Portables	4,100	2	7,500	15.0	61,500
	Upper Extremity	6,900	3	7,500	22.5	155,250
	Lower Extremity -Pelvis	11,000	2.5	7,500	18.8	206,250
	Spine-Cervical	4,000	8	7,500	60.0	240,000
	Spine -Toracolumbar	4,000	2	7,500	15.0	60,000
	Head	1,250	5	7,500	37.5	46,875
	Mammography	6,500	5	7,500	37.5	243,750
	Tomography	50	13	7,500	97.5	4,875
	Miscellaneous	2,300	6	7,500	45.0	103,500
Fluoro	Upper GI /Small Bowel	1,000	25	2,000	50.0	50,000
	Barium Enema /Colon	5,000	25	2,000	50.0	250,000
	Abdomen/KUB	3,900	1	7,500	7.5	29,250
	3-way Abdomen	3,400	3	7,500	22.5	76,500
	IVP	630	15	2,000	30.0	18,900
	Other GU	600	8	2,000	16.0	9,600
	Oral Cholecystogram	20	10	2,000	20.0	400
	Gall Bladder, All other	30	10	2,000	20.0	600
	Myelography	100	20	2,000	40.0	4,000
	Arthrograms	120	15	2,000	30.0	3,600
DSA	Specials/Neuro	325	1200	500	600.0	195,000
	Arteriography, Vascular	3,250	800	500	400.0	1,300,000
	Cardiac	3,300	800	500	400.0	1,320,000
CT	Head + Body	19,000	75	500	37.5	712,500
MR	Head	4,900	128	140	17.9	87,808
	Body	2,100	150	140	21.0	44,100
Nuclear Medicine	Body	7,850	90	3	0.3	2,120
	Heart	7,650	90	3	0.3	2,066
Ultrasound	Cardiac	9,200	36	60	2.2	19,872
	Body	14,000	36	60	2.2	30,240
Total		202,225				6,086,680
Total without DSA						3,271,680

as long as it is clear that the statement is nonnormative and the assumptions are only for the purpose of clarity. In writing this description, customers should be aware that vendors are sensitive to the appearance of what is called a "lock-out spec," which implies that the procurement is not fair. Assembling a full-hospital PACS proposal is costly, and a vendor who thinks the customer is already committed to another company's will be reluctant to make a serious effort. Thus, the RFP should focus on clinical operations and avoid wherever possible technical details that could be interpreted to indicate a preference for one manufacturer's product.

Clinical scenarios require system analysis by the customer to visualize how the hospital operation would handle specific tasks in a PACS environment, making best use of its capabilities. To gain maximum advantage, the hospital may need to change some of its procedures. The development of clinical scenarios is an excellent opportunity to involve all stakeholders in a focused activity that requires each of them to think about how the system will impact their daily work.

Some topics for which individual clinical scenarios may be helpful, along with some illustrative ideas for contents are listed below:

- Portable Exams: Describe the process by which the exams would be ordered; the way the technologists would acquire the exams (film, computed radiography, both, and so on), identify the patients, keep the cassettes straight; and the way the images would be inserted into the system.
- Conventional Exams: Same as for Portable Exams.
- Computed Tomography (CT) and Magnetic Resonance (MR) Exams: Same as for Portable and Conventional Exams.
- Special Procedures: Describe the process by which exams would be ordered, the way the technologists would identify the patients, the way the images would be transmitted into the system, and any diagnostic interpretation to be done on the modality. Requirement 2.6.1 (below) includes some ideas specific to computed radiography (CR).
- Stat Exams: Describe the process by which stat exams would be ordered, the way the technologists would be notified to acquire the exams, and the way the system would identify the exams for attention by diagnostic personnel.
- Quality Control (QC): Describe the quality control process. If QC technologists review films before they are posted, describe how that process will work in a softcopy environment. If exams for some modalities will be automatically accepted for display, describe that process.
- Film File Room Operations: Describe how exams acquired on film would be inserted into the system, including how file room staff would be notified to digitize an archived film folder.
- Intensive Care Unit (ICU): Describe how the ICU would use the system, including how exams would be ordered (possibly automatically in some cases), how exams would be identified (possibly by bed number, in addition to other methods), and how and when exams would be viewed.

- Film Printing: If the system will print films, describe how an exam would be selected for printing, how films would be identified and distributed, and what controls, if any, would be imposed to limit the production of film and charge client departments for its use.
- Diagnostic Reporting: Describe how exams would be reported, including the division of work within the department, the key image presentation functions to be used, and how the report transcription and approval functions would work.
- Clinical Exam Review: Describe how and where exams and reports would be used for review and the key image functions needed.
- External Exam Processing: Describe how the external components like radiotherapy planning systems would find and obtain exams for processing.
- Archived Exam Retrieval: Describe the situations in which exams would be retrieved from the archive, including how the user would identify the exam and the constraints, if any, imposed on certain classes of users.
- Interaction with the Hospital Information System (HIS)/Radiology Information System (RIS): Describe what systems are in place and how the PACS and HIS/RIS would interact, including order entry requisitions, patient identification, report transfer, report approval, and exam billing.
- Teleradiology Operations: Describe how exams would be acquired and transmitted, how reports would be handled, and how exams would be viewed via a telecommunication link.

Note that many of the processes above will be described in normative text later in the RFP. The idea here is not to rewrite the normative text but rather to provide detailed examples of the system working in the clinical environment. Normative text, being focused on operational requirements only, usually does not describe the overall vision very well. The description provides the glue that gives life to the normative text.

Revision History: Section 1.3

Every document needs a history of when revisions were made, by whom, and why.

System Components: RFP Section 2

PACS Architectures

Architecture has been an important distinguishing characteristic of PACS products. Today, however, it is less important. As technology currently in the lab reaches the field, the distinctions between architectural approaches will fade even more.

PACS architectures have generally been classified into two configurations based on how and when they route images (Cho, Huang, and Tillisch, 1989). In a shared file system PACS, all the images are stored centrally, and each workstation looks at the central store when viewing images. This scheme gives every user access to every image, but requires high-speed transmission of image data because transmission occurs after the user selects the image for viewing.

In a distributed file system PACS, the images are distributed across one or more storage systems, and each workstation has its own cache of local image storage from which images are viewed. Autorouting algorithms are used to transmit images from storage to the workstations at which they will be needed in advance of the viewing request. With this system, lower speed networks are satisfactory, although users must wait for transmission when the autorouting algorithm fails to provide the images in advance.

Open Systems

An open system is based on widely accepted standards for which software is readily available from multiple sources. In a sense, an open system is a set of services with standard interfaces distributed on a network and sharing common communication facilities (Wilson, Prior, and Glicksman, 1995). The problem with industry standards is that there are so many from which to choose. Further, there are no standards for the implementation of PACS, so there are no standard PACS applications. Many commercial products marketed as open systems are in fact completely closed applications running on standardized platforms.

For PACS, the objective of open systems is to support interconnection of components from multiple vendors. There are two categories of components. The first includes those internal to the operation of the PACS, such as workstations, storage systems, and so on. The second includes external components with which the PACS must communicate, for example, other imaging modalities, external hospital information systems (HIS) and radiology information systems (RIS), RTP systems, external image processing (3D) systems, and so on. Standards like Digital Imaging and Communications in Medicine (DICOM) have proven extremely valuable for connecting external components to a PACS, and some vendors are beginning to employ DICOM for internal interfaces as well. It remains to be seen whether the standard is sufficiently rich and complete to solve the complex problems that arise in a large scale PACS.

Compression

There are two fundamental kinds of compression: (1) reversible or bit-preserving or loss-less compression, which is guaranteed to return exactly what was put in, and (2) nonreversible (also known as "lossy") compression, which is not. The apparent price paid in the latter case buys higher compression ratios. Customers do not have to care what kind of reversible algorithm the supplier uses, as long as it really is reversible. (The most common reversible algorithm is DPCM with Huffman coding.) There are numerous nonreversible compression algorithms, but their names alone are not enough to describe everything about a specific implementation. (The popular DCT algorithm, for instance, achieves compression by throwing away some of the high frequencies in an image. As more frequencies are thrown away, more compression is achieved.) Other algorithms used for high-rate compression are known as wavelet and fractal. Currently the DICOM standard requires a compression algorithm (named JPEG) which has both reversible and nonreversible versions. Because other algorithms may prove to be superior, it is advisable not to constrain the vendor to a pure DICOM implementation, but rather to require the vendor to justify the algorithm used (if not JPEG). Nonreversible compression, particularly at high compression ratios, could theoretically have a visible effect on an image. In some RFPs, this results in the requirement that nonreversible compression not be performed on an image before primary diagnosis has been completed. As noted below, however, this is probably not the best way to state the requirement.

Data Security

Key considerations in this area include authentication, access control, and encryption. Authentication refers to the validation of the user's identity. The simplest approach to authentication is the use of user accounts with passwords that are required when the user logs in to the system. Other approaches include network-based authorization servers and electronic identification cards, which must be inserted into a workstation before the user may operate it.

Access control refers to methods to restrict the data that a user may access. In some systems, each user has a profile stored in the database that defines the types of data which he or she is authorized to see.

Encryption is a way to protect data from interception while it is being transferred across the network by encoding it so that only the sender and the receiver can understand it.

Data security, at whatever level it is practiced, is meaningful only if it is applied across the entire system. Thus, the best systems allow the definition of user passwords and access control privileges once for the system rather than once for each component of the system.

Character Sets

To achieve interoperability between PACS, imaging modalities, and the radiology information system (RIS), and to permit user interface text to be presented in the native language of the user, requirements must be added to the RFP to specify the character set to be used. For European languages, the International Standard Organization (ISO) 8859 standard is sufficient. DICOM and the character generators of most workstations support this standard. An appropriate requirement might be as follows:

2.0.1. All system components shall support the standard US-ASCII character set as well as the extended ISO 8859 character set appropriate for (the native language of the users).

Network: RFP Section 2.1

Every PACS needs an industry-standard network for communication. Even in a shared file system with a separate high-speed image distribution capability, the network must serve as the channel for database queries and other command and control functions. The network also supports acquisition from some modalities and communication with external systems. Most implementations employ Ethernet and/or FDDI for this purpose. ATM and 100 Mbps Ethernet are growing in popularity.

Although it is usually unnecessary to write any requirements for the network itself, some projects require a particular network protocol or wiring topology. For example, all components within an enterprise-wide network may need to support the Simple Network Management Protocol (SNMP) to permit remote management. Such requirements must be included in the RFP. In general, however, it is best to specify the performance of clinically relevant operations (e.g., image retrieval) and leave the technology to the vendor.

Many institutions already have a routed fiber backbone. Connecting a PACS to the campus net is not advisable, because PACS data volumes will swamp the network. However, the PACS vendor may be able to take advantage of unused fiber pairs (i.e., dark fiber) between buildings or linking outlying areas. If a cable plant that could be used by the PACS vendor already exists in the facility, details of the installation should be included in the RFP. If it can be used to save cost or time, the vendor will do so, but may have another, cheaper solution.

Generally, a hospital information system (HIS) or radiology information system (RIS) connects to a PACS through a local area network (LAN). Any connections between the PACS LAN and any other hospital LAN should isolate the internal traffic on each system's network from the other network. This is generally done with a bridge, but the implementation will depend on the specific situation.

Database: RFP Section 2.2

A full-hospital PACS database is a sophisticated component and expensive to develop. In a sense, any PACS database models the imaging operation of that part of the hospital that it serves. If care is taken in writing requirements not to presume a specific design, describing an implementation can suggest the scope of a PACS database. In one model, the basic object that the system manages is the exam. Exams contain images and may contain diagnostic reports. The exams also include statuses and a host of other parameters grouping them into meaningful categories or describing how they are to be displayed.

Perhaps more than any other element, status models the imaging operation of the hospital. To be precise, an exam often has separate statuses for the images, the report, and possibly other things as well. For example, a newly acquired exam might have the image status ACQUIRED. If an exam must be verified for quality control (QC) purposes before it is made available for general viewing, a qualified person might view the exam on a workstation and take an action that changes the image status to VERIFIED. When a radiologist reads the case and dictates the report, the system might change the report status to DICTATED. After transcription, when the radiologist or two radiologists in a two-phase approval system approve the report, the report status might change to APPROVED. At any point in the flow, a particular query might see, or not see, the exam depending on the status values. The specific set of statuses and the events that cause status change will vary from hospital to hospital, but the underlying mechanisms are general. A PACS should support the states which are used by the hospital's HIS or RIS. Another good starting point is the set of status values defined in the DICOM standard (created, scheduled, arrived, started, completed, verified, read).

Queries can be used to find lists of exams for which the user must take some action. These are sometimes called worklists. A few examples of worklists are:

- All magnetic resonance (MR) exams with the status NOT ACQUIRED: the "MR acquisition worklist."
- All computed radiology (CR) exams with the status ACQUIRED: the "Quality Control (QC) worklist."
- All computed tomorgraphy (CT) exams with the status VERIFIED: the "CT unread worklist."
- All exams with the status DICTATED: the "transcription worklist."
- All exams acquired in the last 24 hours with the status STAT: the "stat worklist."

Most systems also group exams into folders that are defined in many different ways, with an exam possibly appearing in multiple folders. Examples of folders are:

- All exams for a specific patient: the patient's "master jacket."
- All CT exams for a specific patient: the patient's "CT folder."
- Selected exams for a specific patient: the patient's "clinical folder," in which exams may be inserted manually or automatically according to selection rules.
- Manually selected exams for a specific clinical conference.

As may be evident, folders can be implemented as queries of the database. Some systems allow the user to gain additional flexibility by imposing ad hoc constraints on standard queries. This can be a useful way to find exams. Worklists and queries are visible to the user through the workstation's navigation interface. The kinds of worklists and queries that are required should be listed elsewhere in the RFP.

The database typically stores lists of users and their privileges. Systems for primary diagnosis need to identify the user working at a specific workstation so that reports are dictated or approved only by radiologists and exams are verified only by authorized QC technologists. Although specific privileges depend on how a given hospital operates, the concepts involved are general. The categories of users and privileges required should be detailed in this section; definitions should be system wide, not workstation specific.

The performance of the database in query operations is very important in giving a sense of interactivity to the user. Query performance is covered in the specifications for workstations because it is at the workstation that performance will operationally be seen and measured.

Because the database stores data on every exam, it can be used to produce statistical reports required by the hospital administration. Some systems give the user the ability to generate certain kinds of usage reports automatically. If statistical reports from the PACS database are necessary, copies of the desired reports should be included in an appendix and referenced in requirements written in this section. Common requirements include a report that tracks film printing from PACS workstations.

Most hospitals require a PACS to be integrated into the existing enterprise information environment. Often this means a PACS interface to the RIS and sometimes to the HIS. The PACS database is a logical target for information system interfacing. Clearly the PACS and RIS/HIS need to agree on patient and study identification information. However, it is debatable whether the report should be stored in the RIS, in the PACS, or both. Existing commercial PACS implementations differ on this question. The important point to make in the RFP is that reports must be accessible, with specified performance criteria, in conjunction with image access. Depending on the criteria, this often means storing approved reports in the PACS database.

In a full-hospital PACS where reports are stored in the database, the database will grow about 1 gigabyte per year for the life of the system. In addition to the obvious impact on storage, this has the potential to affect database performance. Some years ago, Prior and Nabijee (1989) presented a solution to this "infinite database problem." At that time, the only solution was a form of database archiving. Today, with the tremendous growth of disk capacity and central processing speed, it is reasonable simply to continue to add disk drives to the database engine. This problem should be discussed with any potential PACS vendor to confirm that the supplier has a cost-effective solution and that the initial performance of the system will be maintained over the years.

Although the internal mechanisms used by the PACS components to query the database are perhaps best left to the supplier, it is desirable to require that the database system include a DICOM Query/Retrieve Service Class Provider (SCP) to support access by third-party components (e.g., imaging modalities and specialty workstations). This is probably the most effective way to plan for adding new external components. The requirements might read:

> 2.2.1. The database system shall include a DICOM Query/Retrieve SCP. Support for the Study Root queries at the Study Level is recommended.
> 2.2.2. The supplier shall provide with the proposal a Conformance Statement for the DICOM Query/Retrieve SCP of 2.2.1.

These are generic requirements to handle connections to devices that will be obtained in the future. Note that specific systems that will be connected at the time of the purchase should be handled in their own sections as indicated below.

The Conformance Statement, which describes a product's implementation, is very important. DICOM by itself does not guarantee interconnectability; both ends of the link must have a common implementation of the standard. A comparison of conformance statements can determine that two DICOM compliant systems are not capable of communicating. Unfortunately, it cannot prove that they can communicate. Testing is definitely required.

Storage Systems: RFP Section 2.3

Most PACS have two levels of storage systems: an online storage system that provides relatively rapid access and a large archive that is generally slower. This section covers the former.

Storage Capacity

In specifying how many images can be accessed online and quickly, the RFP should address the time-depth parameter. One approach requires that images remain online for the average length of an inpatient stay. Because requiring such a guarantee can present complications, an alternative approach is to require that the storage system be large enough to hold the volume of images which would cover the time desired. This meets the customer's needs while providing the designer the flexibility to handle load transients gracefully. The requirement might read:

2.3.1. The system shall include sufficient online storage to provide access to 10 days' image production as defined in Table 3.1 plus two dearchived exams for each newly acquired exam.

The time-depth parameter is critical. Some experienced PACS users have found that they want six months' online storage.

Performance

The performance of a PACS is a function of the image request load placed on the storage system and the network. While dependent on the architecture, the request rate is roughly the image production rate multiplied by the number of times each image is accessed in its lifetime.

Dwyer and collaborators have published measured request rates for images as a function of time since original acquisition. These data, combined with internal usage dictated by the system architecture, can be used to determine the total load on the storage system and the network. If data on the image request rates exist, then the information in Table 3.2 should be updated. If not, Dwyer's data, which are for seriously ill patients, offer a reasonable start and, in principle, provide a cushion of conservatism. However, no published data show how image access rates are affected by the easy availability of images afforded by PACS. It is reasonable to expect that access rates in a PACS environment will increase significantly.

To account for the variation in activity which occurs over a 24-hour period, Wilson defined the concept of the "n busy-hour day," in which the full day's activity is compressed into "n" hours' steady-state activity (Meredith, Anderson, Wirsz, et al., 1992). As a response to these factors, the requirement might read:

2.3.2. The system shall meet all performance requirements in this specification with the database storing two years' examinations, the storage system filled to its normal steady-state maximum, under an image request load defined by the daily image production as defined in Table 3.1, multiplied by the number of accesses per image defined in Table 3.2, delivered over a five-hour period.

TABLE 3.2. Image request statistics.

Requests per image	
Diagnostic requests for seriously ill patients[*]	
First 3 days of hospital stay	= 10
Next 6 days of hospital say	= 4
Rest of first year	= 3 (= a)
Outpatient studies	= 2 (= b)
PACS operational load	
Initial acquistion	= 1
QC/exam verification	= 1
Initial archival	= 1
Dearchivals	= 5 (= a + b)
Total Requests Per Image	= 27

The PACS operational load will depend on the system architecture and on some of the hospital's procedures, like the QC (Quality Control) process. Do not try to specify this portion of the table, but do require the vendor to include the correct values for his system in the proposal.
[*]Stewart et al. 1993 (March). IEEE Eng Med Biol.

Storage Management

Most storage systems have an automatic cleanup process to keep a little empty space in the system for new images. Serious problems in system operation occur if that process ever stalls (i.e., tries to make space and fails). In that case, once the storage system fills, new images cannot be acquired until somebody does something manually to allow the process to succeed. A better approach is to require that new images be stored in the storage system reversibly compressed and that they be given priority over dearchived images when space is being made. Here are some template requirements:

2.3.3. The system shall not store any image in the online storage system with nonreversible compression.

2.3.4. The system shall not automatically delete from the online storage system any exam until space for new exams is required. "Is required" can be interpreted to mean "is expected to be required in the near future."

2.3.5. The system shall select exams for automatic deletion from the online storage system in order of priority as follows:

1. Dearchived exams not associated with other exams.
2. Dearchived exams associated with exams for which the primary diagnosis is complete.
3. Archived exams for which the primary diagnosis is complete.
4. Dearchived exams associated with exams for which the primary diagnosis is not complete.
5. Archived exams for which the primary diagnosis is not complete.
6. Exams that have not been archived.

This scheme keeps images online for primary diagnosis until they absolutely must be removed. Although Requirement 2.3.3 may be extreme, in refusing to allow dearchived images to be stored with nonreversible compression in the online storage system, it is just one scheme. The customer should discuss other options with vendors and explore other approaches that achieve the objective.

External Interfaces

The key external interface of the PACS is the one to the imaging modalities. The first priority of this interface is to store images onto a PACS storage device. DICOM is now fairly well accepted as the protocol of choice for new imaging equipment. The PACS storage system, in conjunction with the system database, needs to support key DICOM service classes. Any interface, however, has two sides. Thus, the imaging modalities must also be required to support the complementary DICOM interface. (See Requirement 2.6 on how to handle existing, non-DICOM modalities.)

The storage system should include a DICOM Storage Service Class Provider (SCP) capable of accepting all relevant DICOM image types. More correctly, the Storage SCP must support the SOP classes corresponding to the image types of interest: CT, MR, CR, and so on. Unfortunately, storing images is necessary but not sufficient for PACS operation. The modality and PACS database (as well as the RIS) must agree on the identity of the patient and the study being performed. If this agreement does not occur, experience has shown that the PACS database and storage system can accumulate large volumes of mismatched exams. This is particularly true if the PACS is correlating exam information between the modalities and an RIS. To address this problem and minimize retyping of information on the modality console, DICOM has introduced the concept of a Modality Worklist. A modality worklist is simply the list of exams scheduled to be performed on a given modality system. Each list item identifies the patient and the exam in a manner consistent (hopefully) with the PACS and RIS databases.

Even when a modality can successfully store images and those images contain correct identification information, annoying problems persist. First, the modality would like to know that the images are safely (and to some degree permanently) stored on the PACS so they can be deleted from local storage. The DICOM Storage Commitment service class solves this problem by transferring ownership of sets of images to the Storage Commitment SCP. In addition, the PACS needs to know that it has stored and taken ownership of the complete set of images that comprise the modality's view of a study. A modality and an RIS, it should be noted, may disagree on what constitutes a study. The DICOM Study Component Management SOP class can be used to solve this problem by allowing the modality to identify sets of images as constituents of a study.

To completely support a DICOM interface to imaging modalities, a PACS must provide the following DICOM SCPs: Storage, Modality Worklist Management, Study Component Management, and Storage Commitment. Hence, the requirements might read as follows:

2.3.6. The system shall include a DICOM Storage SCP that supports all of the DICOM Storage SCUs implemented on the image acquisition systems listed in Table 3.3.

2.3.7. The supplier shall provide with the proposal a Conformance Statement for the DICOM Storage SCP of 2.3.6.

2.3.8. The system shall include a DICOM Modality Worklist Management SCP (DICOM/MEDICOM Supplement 10).

2.3.9. The supplier shall provide with the proposal a Conformance Statement for the DICOM Modality Worklist Management SCP of 2.3.8.

2.3.10. The system shall include a DICOM Storage Commitment Push Model SCP.

2.3.11. The supplier shall provide with the proposal a Conformance Statement for the DICOM Storage Commitment Push Model SCP of 2.3.10.

2.3.12. The system shall include a DICOM Study Component Management SCP.

2.3.13. The supplier shall provide with the proposal a Conformance Statement for the DICOM Study Component Management SCP of 2.3.12.

If access to specific external systems is required, the customer should obtain the Conformance Statements for the Storage Service Class User Application Entities from the external system vendors and include those statements as appendices to the RFP.

A word of caution. If a supplier does not have a Conformance Statement for his DICOM interface, the interface product is probably not mature. Customers will find it worthwhile discussing any proposal language received on DICOM with a member of the ACR-NEMA Committee.

Technology

For the PACS customer, the technology used in the storage system is not important, as long as the operational requirements are met. The performance issue is covered in Requirement 2.3.2. Additional requirements for data integrity, reliability, and serviceability could be:

2.3.14. The storage system shall tolerate the failure of a single disk drive without loss of data.

2.3.15. The storage system shall remain operational in the event of the failure of a single disk drive.

2.3.16. The storage system shall remain operational during the service required to correct a failed disk drive.

Although these requirements do not guarantee that the storage system will never cause a system outage, they do protect the system from the most frequent failure. Really good systems also provide protection against failed disk system power supplies and fans, two other particularly obnoxious components. Notice that there can be no blanket requirement like:

x.y.z. The PACS shall remain operational without loss of data in the event of any failure in the storage system.

This is a difficult requirement to verify, and it is very expensive to meet. Infrequent failures which take down the storage system are more cost-effectively handled by the planned failover strategies covered in the discussion associated with Requirement 3.3.

Archive System: RFP Section 2.4

The idea of an archive is to store images for as long as they might be needed. Generally, this is much longer than can be cost effectively supported by the technologies used in the online storage system.

Storage Capacity

If the PACS will provide digital archives, a key parameter is how many images will be accessible. Because any archive system will in principle overflow in time, most systems provide for online and off-line archives. In terms of an optical disk jukebox, online platters are those located in the jukebox; off-line platters are those located on a shelf in a storeroom, ready to be manually inserted in the jukebox on request.

Again, the online archive storage capacity is best thought of in terms of time depth. Studies have shown that fewer than 10 percent of images are accessed ever again after the first year. The requirements might read:

2.4.1. The system shall include sufficient online archive storage to provide access to at least two years' image production, as defined in Table 3.1, without manual intervention by a human operator.

2.4.2. Images older than the limit in 2.4.1 shall be accessible. Accessibility can be satisfied by requiring a human operator to insert storage media into the system.

2.4.3. If a human operator is required to intervene, as in 2.4.2, the archive system shall automatically provide instructions, identifying the location of the media involved and the action to be performed.

Performance

PACS archives handle three kinds of requests. Ad hoc dearchive requests can be made by any user with the necessary privileges. Archive requests are made by the process that queues new images for archiving, providing a backup copy of the image even while it is still in the storage system. Dearchive requests can also be made by a prefetch process that responds to the ordering of new exams by fetching, according to a predefined algorithm, old studies from the archive, placing them in the storage system for rapid access as comparison studies for the new study. The key requirements for handling these requests are:

2.4.4. The archive system shall automatically archive images when they are received into the storage system. This requirement can be interpreted to mean that images are entered into a queue for archiving as soon as all the images for the examination have been received and, if required by the implementation, the exam has been verified, provided that in normal operation, the queue is always actively being served.

2.4.5. In response to the ordering of a new exam, the archive system shall automatically dearchive related exams according to a prefetching algorithm.

2.4.6. The vendor shall include in the proposal a detailed description of the prefetching algorithm.

2.4.7. The archive system shall dearchive exams in response to ad hoc requests from users at workstations.

2.4.8. The archive system shall service ad hoc dearchive requests ahead of any other requests.

The customer may want to expand on the concept of 2.4.8 to define classes of users, some of whom have high priority in ad hoc dearchive requests while others do not.

2.4.9. The archive system shall dearchive a standard exam within 60 seconds. Dearchival time is measured from the time the archive system begins servicing a dearchive request for an exam which is located in the online archive until the exam is completely stored in the storage system, including any mechanical seek time required by the implementation. A standard exam is any one of the following:

- Two images of 2K × 2.5K × 2 bytes
- Twenty images of 512 × 512 × 2 bytes
- Eighty images of 256 × 256 × 2 bytes.

The images are to have been stored with whatever compression is proposed for the system.

2.4.10. The archive system shall be able to service an archive/dearchive request load defined by the daily image production as defined in Table 3.1, multiplied by the number of dearchivals plus one, as defined in Table 3.2, within a 16-hour period.

Early experience with full-hospital PACS showed prefetching to be very important if efficient primary diagnosis is to be rendered. The perfect prefetching algorithm, if there is one, has not yet been discovered. Some suggest fetching all previous studies for the patient. This has significant negative consequences for both the storage and archive systems. Another approach is to fetch only the most recent exam of the same modality plus the first plain film for the current illness. The best approach may be to support a different algorithm for each modality.

Compression

One approach to archival compression is to allow the customer to configure the system to select which algorithm to apply to an image depending on the modality. A reasonable configuration might be to use non-reversible compression on CR images and digitized films and reversible compression on the rest. The requirements might read:

2.4.11. The system shall provide a reversible compression algorithm for use during archiving.
2.4.12. The system shall provide a nonreversible compression algorithm for use during archiving.
2.4.13. The nonreversible compression algorithm shall have one or more configurable parameters that affect the degree of compression.
2.4.14. The system shall allow the user to designate, for each modality, the compression algorithm and any configurable parameters to be used in archiving exams for that modality.

Note that Requirement 2.4.14 does not state that the user be allowed to select the algorithm on an exam-by-exam basis. The intent is for the customer to make a single set of choices that are applied on a system-wide basis. This was found to work in a production clinical environment. The customer should be prepared to test the supplier's nonreversible compression algorithm with a large number of clinical images before making a purchase commitment.

Technology

The most common archive system is based on optical disk drives, usually packaged in a robotic server, also known as a jukebox. Other technologies that have been proposed and, in some cases, implemented are optical tape and various kinds of magnetic tape. A specification should not necessarily force the design choice. For example, the random access feature of a laser disk system is not important to the user, as long as the performance requirements in 2.4.9 and 2.4.10 are met. The only additional requirements are:

2.4.15. The archive system shall store images for seven years without loss of data. This requirement is not intended to imply "with reversible compression," only that the images, in whatever form they are archived, remain accessible for seven years.

2.4.16. The supplier shall include with the proposal the results of studies demonstrating the stability of the storage media and descriptions of any procedures required to assure that 2.4.15 is met.

Some PACS specifications have required time horizons of 10 or 21 years or even forever. The archived images, to be useful, must be retrievable throughout the required time horizon. The customer should discuss with potential vendors how this requirement can be met through guaranteed service and spare parts for key system components or upgrades of components that become unserviceable.

External Information System Interfaces: RFP Section 2.5

The external information systems to which a PACS is usually interfaced are the radiology information system (RIS) and sometimes a hospital information system (HIS). From the perspective of the PACS supplier, the preference is to interface only to the system which handles order entry requisitions and reports and to have that system handle communication with the other one. Perhaps the best possible interface would be one in which the two systems directed queries of each other's databases. Today, the interface is generally implemented as a series of messages passed between processes in the PACS and the external system. The precise definition of the interface requires interaction between the PACS and RIS/HIS suppliers. There are two communication standards that may be of use. DICOM defines a set of services (patient, study, results management) for communication between a PACS and a RIS (with limited HIS interface capabilities), but few if any RIS/HIS vendors support it directly. The Health Level 7 (HL-7) standard tends to be preferred by RIS/HIS vendors. Several people have implemented HL-7-DICOM translators (Kuzmak, Norton, and Dayhoff, 1992). The messages passed between the two systems depend on the functionality which is required in the PACS database. Here are a few examples:

- To implement automatic prefetching in the archive, the PACS must know when an exam has been ordered so that the prefetch process can have time to get the old exams from the archive before the radiologist starts to work on the new one. Generally, this is accomplished by passing an "order entry requisition" message from the HIS to the PACS.
- Some external information systems can also supply pull lists of exams for dearchiving. These are supported through an "exam pull" message or by interpreting admission/discharge/transfer (ADT) information passed from an HIS.
- To support modality worklists, allowing modality operators to acquire exams without entering patient demographic data, the PACS must know that an exam has been ordered. The "order entry requisition" message satisfies this requirement.
- To keep information on patients and exams in sync between the two systems, there can be a collection of messages for changing the patient's demographic data or ADT status, merging two patients, or changing the examination (exam code, scheduled time, and so on). If either side can initiate the update, then some of the messages will have to go both ways.
- To access reports from a PACS workstation, when the PACS keeps a copy of the report in its database, a "report transfer" message is necessary. For the PACS user to be able to update the report and/or approve it from the PACS workstation, this message, or another one like it, has to go both ways.
- To have the PACS notify the RIS that an exam has been finished, a handy way to automate what is often a manual process, an "exam complete" message is needed.

These sample messages suggest the kinds of interactions possible with PACS. The customer should not define the exact form of the interface, but rather only the functionality desired. Customers need to talk to their information system vendor and to prospective PACS vendors to determine what requirements to write in the RFP.

Image Acquisition Systems: RFP Section 2.6

The customer must be sure that all the necessary modalities will work with the new PACS. Frequently the PACS supplier has difficulty estimating the cost of connecting third-party modalities to a PACS because the customer is unsure about what he has. In Table 3.3, each individual modality to be connected to the system should be listed, whether the PACS vendor will supply it. For each modality not to be supplied by the PACS vendor, the appendix should include at a minimum the following:

- Manufacturer.
- Model.
- Software version(s) installed.
- Network interface, if present.
- Communication protocols supported, if any.
- DICOM interface, if present.
- Laser camera interface, if present.
- Other options.

The work done gathering the information for each modality will help the supplier make a more accurate proposal and reduce the probability of later surprises.

DICOM is the preferred interface. It is very important to understand the extent to which a modality vendor who claims DICOM conformance has actually supported the standard. It is still, unfortunately, not uncommon to find that the claim of DICOM conformance is not supported by the product. Often, a modality vendor only supports DICOM storage as a service class user (SCU). This is important and certainly better than no DICOM support at all, but as Section 2.3 indicates, it is not sufficient. It is extremely important in a PACS to close the loop between the PACS database (and/or the RIS database) and the imaging modality in terms of patient and study identification and patient demographics. The modality worklist concept solves this problem.

In order for the DICOM interface recommended in Section 2.3 to work, it is essential that the modality systems to be connected to PACS support the complementary interface. When purchasing a new modality, the customer's standard DICOM modality interface specification should be included in the modality RFP. The customer's standard DICOM modality interface specification should also be included in an appendix of the PACS RFP as additional information for the vendor. In summary, this specification should require each modality system to:

- Act as an SCU of the Modality Worklist Management SOP Class (DICOM/MEDICOM Supplement 10), enabling the modality to retrieve worklist information from RIS/PACS via a query.
- Act as an SCU of the appropriate Storage SOP Class.
- Act as an SCU of the Storage Commitment Push (or Pull if you prefer) Model SOP Class to transfer ownership of the images transferred to the image server in the C-STORE operation above.

- Act as an SCU of the Study Component Management SOP Class to create (at the image server) a Study Component that references the images transferred and the study UID (Unique Identifier) obtained from the modality worklist.

For modalities that do not support DICOM, a common solution is the use of third-party interface boxes from companies such as DeJarnette Research and Merge Technologies. In some cases, even if the modality does not support a network interface, the PACS supplier can interface to it through a laser camera port or a magnetic tape controller. In the worst case, the PACS supplier can provide a video digitizer, but this is decidedly inferior to pure digital approaches. The most important requirement for connection of any modality to the PACS is that the connection not decrease the patient throughput of the modality.

One advantage of coupling a modality to PACS is the possibility of having the modality acquire patient demographic data directly from the database, decreasing the technologist's workload, and increasing throughput. There are several approaches to accomplishing this goal:

- The modality can query the database directly for a list of exams to perform and allow the technologist to choose an exam from the list. This can be implemented using DICOM or SQL or a proprietary mechanism for modalities closely coupled to the PACS (i.e., supplied by the PACS vendor).
- The PACS can print barcode labels which the modality or the modality interface device can read and then either query the database directly for the patient and exam information or pass the barcode ID number to the PACS for updating by the storage system.
- The technologist can enter enough information at the modality for the PACS to make the connection with a preordered exam automatically. This is not foolproof, and it requires a method for handling the exceptions, but it can work with almost any modality. This technique is often referred to as profiling.

All modality interfaces should abide by requirements like the following:

2.6.x.1. The system shall connect to the modalities listed in Table 3.3.

To ensure that the PACS does not limit the image quality on acquisition from digital modalities, add a requirement like:

2.6.x.2. The system shall accept the full, original image dataset transmitted from each modality.

If possible, the requirement should be more specific about the image sizes and bit depths. In any case, to ensure that the modality's productivity is not impacted by the PACS, add a requirement like:

2.6.x.3. The system shall receive images at the full speed available from the modality.

The following subsections contain comments and suggestions for interfacing three special classes of modalities, namely, computed radiography, film digitizer, and modality clusters. These may require special subsections in the RFP.

Computed Radiography (CR): Section 2.6.1

CR is the modality most closely associated with PACS. It provides a way to acquire the bulk of image production in digital format, and it offers significant image quality and convenience benefits in portable exams. In a PACS intended to support primary diagnosis, CR acquisition worklists or their equivalent are especially important to productivity because the CR procedure volume is usually very high. This should be discussed with each prospective PACS vendor, and appropriate requirements should be included.

Film Digitizer (FD): Section 2.6.2

Almost every PACS needs a film digitizer to capture reference films from the film file and to input new studies from other institutions. In some instances, a severe PACS system failure will result in the temporary production of film (e.g., using laser printers). These films need to be captured by the PACS when it is restored to full functionality. For simplicity, the customer should buy one from the PACS vendor as part of the PACS. Here are a few suggested requirements on the film digitizer:

2.6.2.1. The FD shall accept the following radiographic film sizes: 14 x 17, 14 x 14, 10 x 12, 8 x 10 (or their metric equivalents).
2.6.2.2. The FD shall have a sensitive area (spot size) no larger than 175 microns for each pixel.

If the digitizer will handle mammography images or if it is desirable just to get more resolution on smaller films, an optional high-resolution mode should be specified. Here is a possible requirement:

2.6.2.3. The FD shall offer a selectable high-resolution mode with a sensitive area (spot size) no larger than 100 microns for use on 8 x 10 films.

The best digitizers provide 12 bits of data per pixel. With 12 bits, the window width and level functions of the workstation can be used to get information that is simply not visible in an 8-bit image.

2.6.2.4. The FD shall digitize to 12 bits per pixel, with all bits being used, across a range from 0 to 3.5 OD.
2.6.2.5. The FD shall be linear within 0.02 OD across its full dynamic range.
2.6.2.6. The FD shall produce less than 0.01 OD noise at 2.5 OD.

Some digitizers have a problem in that they produce strange patterns in the digitized image at one end of the density range or the other. A defensive requirement might be:

2.6.2.7. The FD shall produce no visible noise pattern in the digitized image of a homogeneous region of a film anywhere in the density range required in 2.6.2.4.

Speed is important, even if the system will be infrequently used.

2.6.2.8. The FD shall process one exam consisting of one film of each size required in 2.6.3.1 in fewer than five minutes. The time will be measured from the beginning of any required operator interaction with the digitizer (entering exam or patient information, adjusting the digitizer, inserting the films, and so on) until the last film has been digitized.

If any substantial number of films will be digitized on a routine basis, an automatic film feeder is needed, as stipulated in the following requirement:

2.6.2.9. The FD shall have a film feeder capable of holding 25 films of a mixture of the sizes required in 2.6.2.1.

As was the case in the CR section, acquisition worklists or their equivalent are very important to productivity.

2.6.2.10. The FD shall allow the operator to acquire the exam and patient identification information necessary for digitizing one exam with a simple action. Such an action may be a keystroke, mouse click, barcode acquisition, or the equivalent.
2.6.2.11. The FD shall automatically associate the exam and patient identification information with all the acquired images for the exam.
2.6.2.12. The FD shall also provide an option for the operator to enter exam and patient identification information manually for unscheduled exams.

A film digitizer can be treated as any other imaging modality and the standard DICOM modality interface specification applied. A film digitizer should support the DICOM Secondary Capture Storage SOP class.

Modality Clusters: Section 2.6.3

Several companies offer products that cluster groups of modalities into a small PACS, often referred to as a mini-PACS. Some of these products are optimized for ultrasound or nuclear medicine modalities. Most have, or will have, DICOM interfaces. A key decision is how closely the system and the PACS should be coupled. A simple approach is to treat the cluster like a single modality and have it transfer images to the PACS for archival. Obviously if the PACS is being used for archival functions, the cluster will want to retrieve images at a later date from the archive. A DICOM Query/ Retrieve SCU in the cluster can be used to retrieve images from a DICOM Query/Retrieve SCP that is part of the PACS storage system.

If the cluster is to be treated as an imaging modality, the standard DICOM modality interface specification could be applied. It is also possible that the cluster will support a direct RIS interface (either DICOM or HL7) instead of the Modality Worklist service interface to PACS.

Image Display Workstations: RFP Section 2.7

There are two basic applications for image display workstations: primary diagnosis and clinical review. The physical requirements (for example, the number and size of the monitors) are different for the two applications. Some people feel that the user interfaces and the functionality of the viewing applications must also differ; others do not.

The rest of this section consists of notes on key issues with respect to workstations. This is another place where the user can go too far in specifying requirements, only to discover that he has ruled out vendors who have products which cleverly solve the underlying problems but which do not meet the letter of the RFP.

Configuration

In modern workstations, the user interface spreads over the surface area of all the monitors. Because it is difficult to read an image that is displayed across the boundary between two monitors, most workstation applications recognize the monitor boundaries and avoid such conditions. To fit images of various sizes on monitors that may be smaller or larger than the images, most workstations provide various mapping schemes. One clever way this is done is to use the metaphor of the multiformat film camera, allowing the user to define a monitor to have one of several formats (called by some companies the "up count") defining a number of areas on the monitor into which an image may be mapped.

In reality, there are basically 1K and 2K monitors. There are benefits and drawbacks to each, but most people have settled on using 1K monitors for review workstations and 2K monitors for primary diagnostic workstations. To allow users to see all the detail in an image too large to fit on a given monitor, workstations usually provide a zoom function that always returns to the original image when repainting the screen, thus providing increased resolution as the zoom increases (up to the limit of the original data).

For primary diagnosis, most people want four monitors in order to hold the current exam and a previous one for comparison. Some diagnostic workstations have only two monitors, because of infrequent use or cost constraints.

For clinical review, most workstations have either one or two monitors. This is not because people want to see fewer images at once, but rather because of the need to conserve space and/or cost.

Performance

The most important workstation issue is this: Does every workstation require rapid access to every image? And naturally, "rapid" must be defined. The answers to these questions may determine what kind of architecture the supplier proposes. The requirement must be clear:

2.7.1. The workstation shall display the first image of any exam in the online storage system within two seconds 90 percent of the time. Display time is measured from the time the user completes selection of the exam to be displayed until the last pixel of the first image is visible on the monitor.

or

2.7.1. The workstation shall display the first image of any exam in the local workstation storage within two seconds 90 percent of the time. The display time will be measured from the time the user completes selection of the exam to be displayed until the last pixel of the first image is visible on the monitor.

The 90 percent loophole is necessary because the instantaneous load on a PACS is subject to statistical variations. The 90 percent is not magic; it could just as well be 95 percent, but that would probably not mean anything to the user's perception of the system. Specification of the display speed might be done like this:

2.7.2. The workstation shall display one 2K × 2.5K × 2 byte image filling one monitor in two seconds.
2.7.3. The workstation shall display all the 512 × 512 × 2 byte images at original resolution to fill a monitor in two seconds.
2.7.4. The workstation shall meet 2.7.2 and 2.7.3 for each monitor in an exam filling several monitors.

Display speed is very important in making the workstation feel interactive. For many people, five seconds per monitor is too slow and two seconds is good. A related issue is the speed with which the database can be accessed to see what exams are available. This is important because the database is queried either manually or automatically before viewing any exam. The query usually results in a list of exams from which one or more may be selected for viewing. These may be presented in various ways, for example, as a list or as a set of tokens. Here are template requirements:

2.7.5. The workstation shall display the first 20 results of any query of the system database within two seconds. The display time will be measured from the time the user completes selection of the query until the 20th result is visible on the monitor.

2.7.6. If the workstation separately stores images in its local storage, it shall display the first 20 results of any query of its local database or directory within two seconds. The display time will be measured from the time the user completes selection of the query until the 20th result is visible on the monitor.

In some systems, 2.7.6 will not be relevant, but 2.7.5 is relevant in all systems. Remember that the fundamental issue is diagnostic throughput by the radiologist. For this reason, it is important to describe in Section 1 the typical diagnostic session, with the approximate number of exams handled and the way the radiologist decides which exam is next. Some systems have special features to automate that process, speeding up the cycle time per exam.

Other important performance issues relate to the monitor's refresh rate, brightness, and spot size.

• Refresh Rate: This is relatively easy. The object is to avoid flicker, which is distracting and fatiguing. Flicker is perceived in the periphery at a lower frequency than in the center of the field of vision. This makes refresh rate more important in a multimonitor workstation, where there will be lots of images in the periphery, than it is in a commercial television set. Every individual has a different flicker frequency. Commercial television paints 60 fields per second on the screen. (Two interlaced fields make up a frame, that is, one complete image, but for flicker perception, the field rate is what matters.) Workstations paint whole images rather than interlaced fields, and they refresh at anywhere from 60 frames per second on up. Generally, the higher the monitor resolution, the slower the refresh rate, because of the larger number of pixels that make up one frame. A reasonable approach is to specify at least 66 Hz for diagnostic workstations and at least 72 Hz for clinical workstations. A more aggressive approach is to require that the monitor refresh rate be high enough so the monitor is flicker-free for 95 percent of observers both at standard viewing intensities and with a SMPTE, or standard image phantom, pattern displayed when adjusted to 90 percent of maximum intensity and observed under maximum ambient illumination of not greater than 10 percent of the monitor intensity, with minima of 66 and 72 Hz as above. It is, however, much harder to test for these more stringent requirements.

• Brightness: This is more subtle. Conventional view boxes put out 300 foot-Lamberts. A very few, very expensive monitors come close to that range. The best of the rest are between 50 and 80. The only way to know what is acceptable is to look at multiple monitors under clinical lighting conditions. The subtle part of the problem is that monitors fade over time. This occurs continuously during the life of the monitor and reaches a significant level well before the average monitor fails for other reasons. Usually, monitors are designed to meet a brightness requirement with some brightness adjustment still available. When the monitor ages, the adjustment is all used up, and the monitor starts dimming. Experience suggests the fair way to deal with this is as a warranty and maintenance issue.

• Spot Size: This refers to the size of a single pixel as painted on the screen. This varies across the face of a monitor, generally getting fuzzier in the corners. Good monitors adjust the focus of the electron beam dynamically to compensate. Spot size is hard to measure well. One way to specify it is:

2.7.7.   The spot size shall vary less than 20 percent from the center to any corer of a rectangle 1/2" inside the perimeter of the monitor.

2.7.8.   The vendor shall supply a test image for use in measuring the spot size as in 2.7.7.

In a workstation with multiple monitors, matching the brightness and contrast of the monitors to each other is very important. One way to address this requirement is:

2.7.9.   The brightness and contrast adjustment range of the monitors shall support matching the monitor grayscale displays within five percent.

2.7.10.   The change of monitor brightness and contrast shall be less than five percent over a three-month period.

2.7.11.   The vendor shall supply a QC procedure and any required images and calibration equipment to assure that 2.7.9 and 2.7.10 are met.

Functionality

The list of functions offered by most workstations is long—longer than is really required for clinical operations. Here are comments on the most common ones.

• User Interface Devices: Almost every workstation has a keyboard and a pointing device (mouse, trackball, light pen, graphics tablet), but not all do. For diagnostic workstations, enough functions are required to necessitate a fairly general interface. For review workstations, a restricted function set makes the operation of the workstation easier. This is especially true for workstations used in an intensive care unit (ICU). One key requirement is that it be easy to select images for subsequent operations. Most RFPs say something about having the cursor move smoothly over all the monitors, although there is an implied design in such a requirement.

• Navigation: Part of the user interface is the presentation of the contents of the database so the user can find what he needs. At the top level, many systems employ a folder metaphor. An exam is generally contained in one kind of folder that may not be altered in contents after it is acquired. (Other folders were mentioned in the discussion of Requirement 2.2.) The folder metaphor is very powerful, and some RFPs specifically require it. The user may access exams by patient name, exam date, modality, exam status, or relation to another exam (e.g., as an exam for comparison to a new exam), or by a combination of the preceding. The workstation must provide a rapid and easy way to select the presentation. The importance of connecting new exams to older ones for comparison should not be overlooked. Because comparison is done during most primary diagnostic work, anything that slows down finding the comparison exam decreases throughput.

- Reports: Access to the report for a comparison exam is at least as important as access to its images. The specification must state whether the PACS is to present the report as part of the user interface. As noted in conjunction with requirements 2.2 and 2.5, this has an effect on the system database and the external information system interface. An alternative is to provide report access via an HIS or RIS workstation in the same area as the PACS workstation, but this is decidedly second best. If reports will be presented on the PACS workstation, the specification should make clear whether reports should be seen by all classes of users before they are approved.

- Reporting: If the PACS will handle reports, the specification should define whether the workstation will support report entry. In that case, there must be an easy way to select predefined text reports for normal cases. If there will be an interface to an external information system, report entry at the workstation implies that the interface support uploading reports from the PACS as in Section 2.5. Reporting can also include report approval, which places requirements on the interface to the external information system. Report approval must conform to the mechanisms used in the hospital; therefore, if two approvals are required (for example, resident plus staff), the specification should require that the PACS support a two-phase approval cycle.

- Interactive Grayscale Operations (Window Width and Level): The tool used most often on an image is the window width and level operation. There are many approaches to implementing such tools, including knobs, buttons, switches, trackballs, and mice. Because this operation is frequently used, the key requirement is that it be easy to use. Another requirement is that it be possible to use the tool only on selected images.

- Preset Windows: Another grayscale operation is the preset window function. This is frequently used on selected images to jump between, for example, bone windows and soft tissue windows in CT. At the very least, there should be five or ten user-defined windows that are quickly selectable. Function keys are good for this purpose because the user can toggle back and forth easily, but other implementations might do as well.

- Automatic Window Selection: If an image is received from a modality along with a window width and level for viewing, the window width and level parameters should be used for the initial display on the PACS workstation. If an image is displayed for which no window width and level is available, the workstation should pick a set of values that make the image visible as a starting point for subsequent manual changes. If the exam has been saved (see below), the workstation should use the parameters from the save operation when displaying the exam.
- Grayscale Inversion: Grayscale inversion, also called inverse video, is another grayscale operation frequently used to make certain structures more conspicuous. The key requirement is that it be easily applied to individually selectable images.
- Display Protocols: For productivity during primary diagnosis, the most important function may be a set of display protocols that automatically arrange images on the screens in the patterns appropriate for the types of exams displayed. The display protocol is determined by local practice and depends on the modality of the current exam and of any exams to be displayed concurrently for comparison. Although not all vendors offer automatic display protocols, there is little doubt that such protocols significantly improve productivity.
- Image Rearrangement: Manual rearrangement of the images on the display is sometimes necessary for comparison, even if the display protocol has arranged the images well. The main requirement is that it be easy to do.
- Image Comparison: This describes a fertile field for development of softcopy methods for comparing images by, for example, overlaying two images and providing a simple user interface for transitioning between them. Few commercial systems include such features, but it is worth surveying vendors as the field evolves.
- Image Orientation: This function is not used frequently, but it is a necessary tool, not only for flipping and rotating images that may have been acquired in the wrong orientation but also for reorienting images as necessary for comparisons.
- Next Exam: To minimize the time necessary to transition from one exam to the next during primary diagnosis, a next exam function is desirable. The alternative is to require the user to redisplay the worklist and select the next exam. Productivity functions like this only save a few seconds per exam but are significant, given the large number of exams.
- Zoom: To allow inspection of all parts of an image in detail, the workstation should have a zoom function. Zooming by redisplaying from the original image provides the best resolution, and should be required. Continuous zoom should be required rather than accepting only powers of two. Two different methods have been used to display the zoomed image: pixel replication and interpolation. Despite the common belief that interpolation is better, it may not make much difference for small

zoom factors on high-resolution monitors on which individual pixels are nearly invisible. If the user does not have an opinion already, vendors should be asked for demonstrations. When displaying images that have more pixels than the displays, the workstation should also have a minification function that subsamples the image so that the entire image appears to fit on the display.

- Roam: Roam, sometimes called pan, goes hand-in-hand with zoom. It should be easy to switch quickly between them.
- Magnifying Glass: Most workstations offer a magnifying glass function in addition to zoom. This can be a powerful tool, especially when it includes the options of variable magnification, resizability, internal window width and level, and grayscale inversion.
- Cine and Stack Display: One useful way to manipulate groups of related images is to order them in some way (e.g., by time or position) and display them sequentially. Cine displays with variable frame rate are common. Another useful display approach is to couple the selection of the image from the group to the movement of the mouse. This allows the user to move forward and backward through the stack of images, stopping to focus on anything of interest.
- Distance and Angle Measurement: Distance and angle measurements are important, especially for orthopedists. Almost all workstations have this function.
- Region of Interest (ROI): The ability to obtain statistics on the pixels within an area outlined on an image can be useful both in diagnosis and in calibrating radiographic equipment. The key statistics are area, mean, standard deviation, and number of pixels. To avoid confusion, the statistics function should convert the pixel values to the native units of the modality (for example, Hounsfield units for CT). A similar useful function is the ability to print the pixel values within the ROI.
- Annotation: Textual and graphical annotation is useful in combination with film printing or the ability to save the annotations for future viewers. Nevertheless, it is not used a lot.
- Image Identification: The workstation must display enough information with each image on the screen for the user to identify it quickly. Examples are, depending on the modality, patient name and identification, kVp, mAs, pulse sequence, slice position, and so on. A function to remove the identification from the screen is useful for controlling clutter. Most modalities pass far more information in their image headers than workstations display on the screen with each image. Another useful function is one that displays the entire header of a selected image on command, usually as a series of DICOM elements in a text window.
- Image Printing: If there is a requirement to print images on film, the workstation should provide the option to print a selected exam in any of the formats allowed by the camera. Because of the cost of film, the hospital may want to require that the print function be specially privileged.

A networked laser camera indicates who printed the film so that copies are properly routed; for example, the camera can print the user's name on the edge of the film. Some workstations provide a WYSIWYG user interface to allow the user to place each image on the screen where it will appear on the film before committing to print the full sheet of film. When CR or FD images are printed on laser film, they are usually slightly minified because most laser film printers leave a small border around the edge of the film. Some systems provide a "life-size" format, which prints such images slightly enlarged to compensate for the minification. Other requirements are possible: that the workstation display the status of the selected film printer (what job is printing, out-of-film indication, and so on); that the printer print not only the images but also any overlays (ROIs, annotations, measurements, and so on); that the workstation allow multiple copies up to a fixed limit; and that printing not interfere with the use of the workstation for viewing and diagnostic work. In addition to laser film printers, some systems support 35 mm slide cameras. Some systems make the 35 mm camera a network resource while others attach it to a single workstation. The key is to have the right presentation software on the workstation (for example, Photoshop and PowerPoint). The requirements for professional-looking slides are beyond what any PACS company would be able to invest, so this function should be met with third-party applications running either on PACS workstations or on a specialty workstation connected to the PACS.

- Image Enhancement Functions: Users often request, sometimes in great detail, all sorts of image processing functions, including histogram equalization (global and adaptive) and other nonlinear presentation operations as well as various filtering tools for edge enhancement and smoothing. These toys are rarely used. After the initial excitement wears off, the user's interest returns to productivity, and image processing falls by the wayside because it takes a lot of time. More importantly, people learn quickly that the interactive grayscale operations are incredibly powerful; if the answer is in the image, the user can find it with window width and level.

- Undo: Many workstations support an Undo command. This makes the workstation less intimidating, especially for the novice user, who quickly learns that there is not much danger in experimenting.

- Cancel: Whenever an operation takes a long time, the workstation should indicate that the system is working and provide a way to cancel. This includes especially tedious queries, computationally intense image processing functions, and loading very large exams, although as much as possible, the last two should be hidden from the user by doing them in the background.

- Save: This function provides the ability to save the display state of an exam, including the image arrangement and each individual image's window width and level values, orientation, zoom value and roam position, and any annotations. This data is usually saved in the database so it is available to any user who redisplays the exam after it has been saved.

- Screen Saver: A screen saver is mandatory. The monitors are very expensive, limited lifetime components and should be protected wherever possible.
- Specialty Functions: People have talked of requiring 3D surface rendering, radiotherapy planning, and stereotaxis functions in PACS workstations, but such operations are better done by companies which specialize in them. If such functionality is desired, the PACS vendor should be required to provide connectivity to external systems for these functions.

Film Printers: Section 2.8

For applications that require a film printer, most PACS suppliers offer laser film printers connected to the network through interfaces sometimes called camera servers or spoolers. There are several high-quality laser camera vendors whose products vary in functionality, convenience, and size. Among the things to consider in writing requirements are:

- Decide what multiformat options are necessary. The n:1 terminology specifies the number of images which can be printed on one sheet of film. Everyone needs 1:1. Most systems support 2:1, 4:1, 6:1, 9:1, and 12:1. There are sometimes other options as well, such as 15:1 and 25:1. Some people have talked about using 25:1 (or similar format) to create slides. However, a real 35 mm camera produces slides with increased resolution and better color and is definitely worth the money.
- Decide what film sizes are necessary. Obviously, 14 × 17 is required. It may be desirable to add 8 × 10, 10 × 12, 11 × 14, or 14 × 14 as well, but the specification should require only what is necessary.
- Require a daylight bulk load system with loading magazines for each film size.
- Stipulate that the film printer should be connected to a processor.
- Decide what throughput rate is necessary. Most systems can print more than 30 films per hour; some can print 75.
- It is probably not necessary to specify the bit depth of the interface. Some RFPs have specified 12-bits; others allow eight or more. The most common laser cameras only have 8-bit interfaces, and there is no evidence that there is a clinical difference.
- Be aware that all the major manufacturers' cameras provide about 4K × 5K resolution on a 14 × 17 film.
- Look into interpolation with the various PACS vendors. Because laser cameras are such high-resolution devices, they have to zoom small images to fit them to the multiformat space they are assigned. Interpolative zoom, preferably cubic spline, is desirable.
- Ask for a test image that can be kept in the storage system and printed to test the printer.

- The discussion of image display workstations (above) includes comments on 35 mm slide printers. The key hardware requirement is that the PACS vendor supply a commercial slide printer.

Telecommunications: Section 2.9

There are numerous teleradiology applications, some of which are:

- Providing central reading in the hospital of exams acquired in community clinics.
- Providing radiologist coverage for off-hours operation of emergency rooms in satellite hospitals.
- Providing better service to referring physicians, presumably increasing referrals.
- Establishing the electronic equivalent of the circuit rider, linking rural hospitals to a central reading site for faster service.
- Linking an on-call radiologist's home to the radiology department to provide faster response for calls in the middle of the night.

Communication performance requirements vary widely with the application. Where speed is important and volume is substantial, communication costs can be quite high, so careful attention must be paid to the usage of the link and to compression of the image data. Today, alternative communication providers are beginning to compete with the traditional telecommunication carriers. Cable modems permit standard cable television circuits to carry digital data at up to 40 Mbps for reasonable monthly fees. This technology has even been applied to satellite-based television channels, although the high bandwith links in this case are asymmetric (40 Mbps one way, 64 Kbps phone line for the return).

If the preliminary investigation suggests there is a cost-effective application, the customer should write requirements for data volume and speed. Before writing any other operational requirements, the customer needs to define the various circumstances for initiating transfers (i.e., when the remote user should do so and when the central site should). Here are some considerations:

- If a teleradiology image distribution system is being planned in which the images are acquired in the central PACS, one approach is to have the remote workstations connect to the system and act like local workstations, pulling the images from the system. This might work well for the referring physician case, if the physician does not care to see the images for all the cases he referred.
- Another approach to the distribution system is to have the central PACS push the images to the remote workstation without intervention at the remote end. This might be better for the on-call radiologist case.

- If images are being transmitted from the acquisition location to a central PACS for interpretation, a reasonable approach is to require the remote site to push the images to the central PACS. A subsidiary issue is whether the action must be automatically initiated and, if so, what would be the trigger. It is possible that the volume from any remote site may be low enough to allow manual initiation.

In large PACS with teleradiology components serving multiple sites with different information systems, the RIS interface problem can become very complex and must be analyzed carefully.

System Integration: RFP Section 3

This section defines requirements at the system level.

Operations: Section 3.1

It is desirable to abstract certain specific requirements from the operational scenarios in the description that opens the document and include them here. Again, the requirements should be framed as operational issues, not as design definitions. The vendor should be required to provide a complete description of the proposed system's operation. This should include descriptions of key internal processes like image distribution, automatic image routing, database access, handshaking with external information systems, and so on. The vendor might also be required to include descriptions of the system's operation for some or all of the scenarios. Finally, the RFP should require a description of the staff required to operate the system, their necessary qualifications, and the tasks the staff will perform.

Performance: Section 3.2

System performance requirements were defined in several places in Section 2.

Reliability: Section 3.3

A full-hospital PACS total system failure is an unpleasant experience in the best of times. Even component failures that do not take out the entire system can be painful. The vendor should be required to provide reliability history for each key component in the system and a reliability analysis of the system as a whole. Even more important, the vendor should be required to describe the failover strategies to be employed when each system component fails, including interfaces to external information systems. A failover strategy cannot be one-sentence fluff; it should be a reasoned, detailed description of the following:

- How the failure will be detected.
- How much of the system will remain operational during the failure.
- How the function of the failed component will be performed during the failure.
- How the system will be restored after the failure has been corrected.

The last point is especially important after a total system failure or an external information system failure because the hospital continues to operate during the outage and the various systems have to resynchronize with the hospital and with each other afterward.

Purchased Components: RFP Section 4

The subsections of this section are where the specific configuration to be purchased is defined (see Table 3.3). To minimize the possibility of introducing self-contradictions in the RFP on such an important issue, no normative statements that define the purchased configuration should be included anywhere else in the RFP.

Configuration: Section 4.1

One of the first things a vendor must do in costing a proposal is to make a spreadsheet listing each component required by the RFP, along with its planned location. This spreadsheet should be included in the RFP as the normative configuration definition. Table 3.3 is an example of such a spreadsheet. For readability, the appendix defines a set of generic names for components as well as a location nomenclature. Here are some suggestions:

4.1.1. The vendor shall supply and install the equipment listed in Table 3.3 at the indicated locations.

Usually, hospitals want the vendor to supply workstation desks or other furniture for certain locations only. For that reason, requirements should be added in Section 2 defining optional furniture for the relevant components and using a column in Table 3.3 to indicate locations where furniture is required.

4.1.2. The vendor shall supply the furniture listed in Table 3.3.

Because the network is not specifically listed in Table 3.3, it should be separately required for completeness. Similarly, any telecommunication links should also be specified here.

4.1.3. The vendor shall supply and install a communication network as required to support the equipment listed in Table 3.3.

4.1.4. The vendor shall supply and install a telecommunication link between the main hospital and the satellite clinic as required to support the equipment listed in Table 3.3.

Startup Kits and Supplies: Section 4.2

To avoid confusion, requirements should specify who supplies expendable materials necessary for system startup. Here are some template requirements:

4.2.1. The vendor shall supply all necessary media to completely fill the online portion of the archive system.
4.2.2. Following successful completion of the acceptance test, the vendor shall supply 200 sheets of 14 x 17 film for each laser printer listed in Table 3.3.
4.2.3. Following successful completion of the acceptance test, the vendor shall refresh the chemicals in all film processors attached to the laser printers in Table 3.3.
4.2.4. The vendor shall supply the following CR cassettes and plates.

If the vendor will supply multiple kinds of computed radiography units and they do not have compatible plates and cassettes, multiple requirements like 4.2.4 should be written to cover each kind.

Shipping: RFP Section 5

Shipping Requirements: Section 5.1

Any special constraints on shipping should be defined as requirements here. For example, some procurements require shipment by a specific carrier; some require a specific nationality of carrier.

Delivery Schedule: Section 5.2

All delivery schedule requirements should be defined here and nowhere else. As in Section 4, the idea is to avoid any self-contradictions in the RFP that could lead to project delays. If there will be phased deliveries, the delivery schedule for each of the phases should be defined and the contents of each phase as defined in Table 3.3 should be referenced.

Installation: RFP Section 6

This section specifies who does what during the installation phase of the project. Like any significant project, it must be thought through carefully and written down to avoid as many unplanned expenses as possible. The subsections here are intended as reminders of the kinds of issues to confront.

TABLE 3.3. Table of components and locations.

This table serves, with Sections 4, 6, and 8, as the normative definition of the components that are being purchased. It also serves as part of the punchlist for acceptance of the physical components of the system. A tabular form will help the vendor prepare the proposal accurately. The following paragraphs provide a template which can be expanded to specify other kinds of equipment in the procurement or to divide the project into multiple phases.

The following component names and definitions are used below.

ARC	Archive System
CR-H	High Performance CR Reader
CR-L	Low Performance CR Reader
CR-M	Medium Performance CR Reader
CR-P	Dedicated CR Laser Printer
CW	Clinical Workstation
DB	Database Computer
DW	Diagnostic Workstation
EIS	External Information System Interface
FD	Film Digitizer
LP	Laser Printer
M	Modality Interface
STS	Short Term Storage System
TRI	Teleradiology Interface

Monitor types are defined as

A	2560 × 2048, monochrome, portrait mode
B	1280 × 1024, monochrome, portrait mode
C	1024 × 1280, monochrome, landscape mode

Workstations are defined by the nomenclature
    <names> - <number of monitors> <type of monitor>
For example, a diagnostic workstation with four 2.5K · 2K monitors is denoted, DW-4A.

The following building names and definitions are used below.

A	The Main Hospital
B	The ABC Pavilion
C	The XYZ Annex
D	The Satellite Clinic

Location are identified in III.4 using the nomenclature:
    <building> : <floor> . <room>

The approximate locations of network drops within rooms are identified in III.4 by compass point.

Location	Location Name	Component	Network	Furniture	Phase
A:B.100	MIS Computer Room	DB	TBD	Y	1
A:B.100	MIS Computer Room	STS	TBD	Y	1
A:B.100	MIS Computer Room	ARC	TBD	Y	1
A:B.100	MIS Computer Room	EIS – HIS	TBD	Y	1
A:B.100	MIS Computer Room	TRI	TBD	Y	2
A:2.101	Radiology Reading Room - 1	DW-4A	W	Y	2
A:2.101	Radiology Reading Room - 1	DW-4A	N	Y	2

TABLE 3.3. *(continued)*.

A:2.101	Radiology Reading Room - 1	DW-4A	S	Y	2
A:2.101	Radiology Reading Room - 1	DW-4A	E	Y	2
A:2.101	Radiology Reading Room - 1	DW-2B	NE	Y	2
A:2.107	Radiology Reading Room - 2	DW-4A	W	Y	1
A:2.107	Radiology Reading Room - 2	DW-4B	N	Y	2
A:2.115	Radiology Chairman's Office	CW-1C	N	N	1
A:2.116	Dr. ABC's Office	CW-1C	N	N	1
A:2.117	Dr. DEF's Office	CW-1C	N	N	1
A:2.300	Main Radiology	CR-H	W	N	1
A:2.300	Main Radiology	CR-P	W	N	1
A:2.300	Main Radiology	CR-H	W	N	1
A:2.300	Main Radiology	CR-P	W	N	1
A:4.222	Medical Media	CW-2C	E	Y	2
B:1.100	CT - Company A model 1	M	N		1
B:1.101	CT - Company B model 2	M	N		1
B:1.102	CT - Company C model 3	M	N		1
B:1.103	CT - Company D model 4	M	N		1
B:1.223	MR - Company E model 5	M	W		1
B:1.224	MR - Company F model 6	M	W		1
B:1.302	DSA - Company G model 7	M	SE		1
B:2.300	Pediatric Clinic	CR-M	SW	N	2
C:B.105	Film Library	FD	W	Y	1
C:B.105	Film Library	FD	W	Y	1
C:B.105	Film Library	LP	W	Y	1
D:1.123	Satellite Clinic	TRI	S	Y	2
D:1.123	Satellite Clinic	FD	S	Y	2

Customer-Furnished Equipment and Services: Section 6.1

If the hospital plans to supply certain components of the PACS, it should be made clear in this subsection. These are not written as normative requirements statements, but they should nevertheless be precise.

In a large PACS installation, one approach is to locate the core system components (database, storage system, archive, teleradiology communication equipment, and so on) in a central computer room. If the hospital has an information services (IS) department, they might be well positioned to take responsibility for the system management. If so, placing the core system components in the IS computer room will probably work best. This works particularly well if IS has around-the-clock operators who can service requests for mounting off-line archival media.

If the hospital plans to supply the computer room, the hospital may also decide to supply any additional air conditioning required. If so, that should be made clear.

The advantages and disadvantages of supplying network components were addressed briefly in Section 2.1. Again, if the hospital has a network backbone that is not currently in use, perhaps dark fiber which was pulled in anticipation of a PACS at the same time fiber was installed for another purpose, then it should be offered, but its use should not be required. Also as noted above, PACS traffic should not be added to a network that is used for another purpose.

If the project requires bridging the HIS network to the PACS network and the hospital plans to supply the bridge, those facts should be made clear. If the hospital plans to contract with a telecommunications vendor directly for links to satellite teleradiology locations, the vendor and the service to be provided should be defined here. Unless the hospital already has a link in place, it is probably best to let the vendor do the work. If there are operational constraints against having other groups modify the hospital building, it follows that the hospital should plan to do that work and so state in this section.

Supplier-Furnished Equipment and Services: Section 6.2

Section 4.1 covers the specific components and communication equipment required, but there are often other services required in the installation of a PACS. If the vendor is required to renovate space for a computer room or expand the current room, the requirements should be written in this subsection. Some considerations for the computer room are:

- The vendor is responsible for any required additional air conditioning and ventilation.
- The vendor is responsible for any required additional power.
- The vendor is responsible for any required fire suppression system.
- The vendor is responsible for any required plumbing.
- The vendor is responsible for any required raised flooring.
- If a plenum floor already exists in the space planned for use as a computer room and there are constraints about running cables under the floor, make that clear.
- If installation of a raised floor in the computer room space is not allowed, make that clear.
- If there are aesthetic requirements, make them clear.

If the vendor is required to perform any other site modifications (e.g., install plumbing, exhaust, and power for film processors), the requirements should be defined here. If the hospital will supply part of the network, this section should define the installation and test tasks for which the vendor will be responsible. This is another reason why it is best to let the vendor decide what components to use—then, there is no question that the vendor is responsible for everything. Note that 4.1.3 is written as if the vendor does it all, including pulling the cables. These comments apply to any required telecommunication links as well.

Interfacing to modalities should be the PACS vendor's problem. Given that all the information noted in Section 2.6 is included for each modality, nothing else should be required in this requirement. The external information system interface could be a modality-like problem as well. The internal HIS group may have to get more involved in this case, but again it is best to leave the integration as the complete responsibility of the PACS vendor.

The hospital may want the PACS vendor to provide operational support of the system during the warranty period. If so, this section should specify the kind of personnel and the coverage desired. For example, the vendor might supply an in-house trainer, a CR specialist, and a system administrator, all with coverage during the normal workday, in addition to any service personnel who would be part of the warranty support, around the clock. If a system administrator will be required for a few weeks or months while the hospital's internal specialist learns the system, this section should make that clear, but the vendor should be consulted to be sure that the time allowed is appropriate to the complexity of the system.

Environmental Requirements: Section 6.3

For planning purposes, the vendor should be required to specify the space, structural, and utility requirements for the proposed system. The requirement might be:

6.3.1. The vendor shall supply as part of the proposal a table specifying for each component in Table 3.3 the following utility requirements:

- Physical dimensions.
- Physical space required for operation.
- Weight.
- Building structural requirements.
- Power requirements.
- Air-conditioning requirements.
- Exhaust requirements.
- Water requirements.
- Chemical requirements.

Installation Facilities: Section 6.4

During the system installation, the vendor will require space to store material and to prepare components for installation. The requirement might be:

6.4.1. The vendor shall include in the proposal a list of the facilities required for installation support, including:

- Loading dock.
- Material storage.
- Workshop space.
- Office space.
- Communications (telephone, fax, and so on).

- Shipping and receiving department support.
- Anything else.

Another approach is to specify what facilities the hospital can supply and require the vendor to obtain any other facilities he needs externally. If there are constraints on the use of hospital facilities like the loading dock during packing and unpacking of equipment, include the requirements in this section.

System Acceptance: RFP Section 7

The key to a successful acceptance process lies in ensuring that the vendor's product and the customer's expectations are consonant. If the customer's expectations are accurately represented in the RFP, if the customer carefully weeded out those vendors who did not take the RFP seriously, and if the customer performs a benchmark test of the proposed system before committing to the vendor, then everything will be fine (famous last words). The time to avoid acceptance problems is before the contract is awarded.

To formalize the acceptance process, requirements like these should be included:

7.0.1. Acceptance of the system shall consist of verifying that all required equipment and services have been provided and that the equipment and services meet the RFP requirements.
7.0.2. Verification that the required equipment and services have been provided shall be accomplished by comparing the vendor's performance to the Equipment and Services Punchlist.
7.0.3. Verification that the required equipment and services meet the RFP requirements shall be accomplished through an Acceptance Test.

Equipment and Service Punchlist: Section 7.1

The requirements in Section 4, 6, and 8 define the set of equipment and services to be delivered before the beginning of the acceptance procedure. Most of the equipment is itemized in Table 3.3, which is referenced in Section 4. If the requirements are written clearly, checking that everything has been received is pretty hard to get wrong. A simple requirement might be:

7.1.1. The Equipment and Services Punchlist shall consist of the normative requirements of Sections 4, 6, and 8.

Acceptance Test Procedure: Section 7.2

The meat of the acceptance process is the acceptance test. The acceptance test consists of a series of validation steps for each normative statement. For example, each step should include the following in its specification:

- Normative requirement identification.
- Materials to be used: Films, exams from modalities.
- System population: The number of patients and exams in the database; the fraction of the storage system in use; the number of exams in the archive; the amount of local storage in use.
- System load: The number of active workstations and what they are doing; the number of requests queued for the archive; the number of messages queued from the external information system.
- Measurement technique: What to do to perform the test; how to make the measurement; the start and end points for timing measurements.
- Expected results.

There are two basic kinds of requirements: functionality and performance. Generally, functionality can be tested independent of system load. Performance, however, must be tested with the system running under its required load as specified in 2.3.2. This is critical to proper measurement, as performance is not a simple function of load in some systems. Performance tests usually require that personnel operate many workstations in a controlled fashion while the measurements are made. Sometimes the vendor will have special applications that run autonomously on workstations to provide the load. If these applications will be used, care must be taken to confirm that the system is loaded as in 2.3.2.

Note that when testing the performance of the archive, 2.4.9 and 2.4.10 do not specify the fraction of the archive that is full. This intentional omission is because the cost of archival media is such as to make a test on a nearly full archive very expensive. The vendor may be able to supply preloaded media for the test. Alternately, the customer may agree to verify the media changer speed with a test program, measure the archive time in a simple case, and analytically verify that the requirements in 2.4.9 and 2.4.10 will be met when the archive is nearly full.

The question arises as to how to write the acceptance test. At the time of the RFP, the acceptance test cannot be specified in detail because the structure of the system that will be proposed is not known. One option is to require the vendor to supply a draft acceptance test with the proposal:

7.2.1. The vendor shall submit with the proposal a complete draft acceptance test addressing every normative requirement in the RFP. The customer and the vendor will negotiate a final version of the acceptance test before the contract is awarded.

If the proposed test does not professionally address every normative statement (with whatever exceptions are noted in Requirement 11.2), the vendor should be dropped from consideration. This may appear harsh, but it is important. To be credible, a full-hospital PACS vendor must know how his system performs. If he does not, he is not worth the risk, no matter how attractive the price. And if he does not know how to test his system, he does not know how it performs.

It is important to reach agreement on the acceptance test before contract award. That is the time when both the customer and the vendor have leverage, so it is a fair negotiation. The customer can disqualify the vendor, and the vendor can withdraw, with minimal organizational fall-out in either case. There is no advantage to either side in deferring the definition. Doing so results in acrimonious debates when neither the customer nor the vendor has many options left.

Frequently, customers want some kind of unstructured or random test included in the acceptance test procedure. The rationale is understandable, but it is probably a bad idea during acceptance testing because it makes the test indeterminate. The acceptance test is not a contest; both sides want the customer to be happy, and there is no advantage to concealing any part of the acceptance test. One way to provide at least a limited random test is to formally define the length of time for unstructured testing. A reasonable limit, for example, might be two or three days for a large system. The customer should also define the categories of findings that will constitute failure, such as system or component crashes or false results like incorrectly assigned data or incorrect workstation output.

Training: RFP Section 8

Every system should come with manuals, but most people do not learn to use a PACS from manuals. For a full-hospital PACS, the customer usually requires training courses from the vendor to teach a core of the hospital's staff. After that, experience shows that most new users learn from experienced users. The following paragraphs describe some of the training issues for which requirements should be written.

Manuals

This section should specify how many manuals are required. One approach is to keep one manual with each component; another is to keep only one for each area. In any case, a few complete sets should be required for the library and one for the system administrator. In addition to manuals for the obvious components, a specialized system administrator's manual should be required.

Whether included in separate manuals or consolidated in a single volume, the vendor should supply documented quality control (QC) procedures for each component. For example, for workstations, the procedures might be the following:

- Clean the monitor screens with ABC screen cleaner.
- Vacuum all dust off the keyboard, monitors, and processor.

- Clean the mouse ball.
- Verify all cable connections are tight.
- Verify that all cabinet ventilation ducts are clear.
- Clean all filters.
- Measure the monitor brightness with test image DEF and photometer GHI according to procedure JKL.
- Measure the monitor focus with test image MNO according to procedure PQR.

For components like film digitizers, CR systems, laser cameras, and film processors, the procedures can be more complex. The vendor should be required to supply all of the necessary test materials (test images, and so on) as well as the test equipment (photometers, and so on).

If the hospital will do any of the maintenance on the system, requirements for all of the necessary service manuals should be included.

Courses

There are numerous categories of users. Some examples are:

- Department administrator.
- System administrator.
- Receptionist.
- Transcriptionist.
- Radiologist.
- Clinician.
- Referring physician.
- Radiologic technician.
- Nurse.
- ER staff.
- ICU staff.
- Physicist.
- Equipment service staff.

The proposal should be required to contain a training plan that covers all the categories relevant to the project. The RFP should specify the number of students in each category. At least two sets of course training materials should be required for the library as well. In addition, if the hospital will do any of the maintenance, requirements for service training should be included.

System Warranty and Maintenance: RFP Section 9

The RFP needs to define the kind of warranty and maintenance service required for the two kinds of service required on a PACS. The first, failure correction, consists of doing whatever is necessary to fix a broken component.

Its schedule cannot be predicted, but a response time should be specified. For large systems, RFPs may require that the vendor have service staff and a spare parts depot on-site. The second kind of service is scheduled preventative or operational maintenance. It consists of normal system management tasks like database backups, installation of new archive media and software releases, and quality control (QC) procedures to assure that the equipment is operating correctly. The RFP should define the extent to which the hospital will be responsible for these tasks. Some customers elect to have the vendor provide operational maintenance during and even after the warranty period. It is not uncommon for an RFP to specify that scheduled service be done during off-hours. Although this is not a bad approach, the real requirement is that the system remains available when needed. If the vendor can keep the system up (and meeting its performance and functionality requirements) while doing scheduled maintenance work during the day, off-hours service should not be an issue.

Typically the warranty period is one year. Many RFPs include a requirement that the warranty period be extended whenever the system fails to meet its required performance or functionality during a specified interval. Some RFPs require that if downtime hours in a month exceed a specified number, the warranty period is extended by one month. This leads to a need to define downtime. This is a complicated problem because different components affect the availability of the system differently and availability at some times during the week is more critical than at others. A little thought, along with discussions with vendors, can produce a reasonable approach. In addition to warranty extension, some kind of lemon-replacement requirement should be included.

One special concern during warranty and maintenance is the video monitors. As noted in the discussion of Requirement 2.7, monitors degrade over time. One approach is to buy monitors directly from the original manufacturer when failures occur, but most customers want that the PACS supplier to maintain the monitors because they are physically part of the workstation. Although it is difficult to write a definitive specification, discussion can produce a reasonable approach as to when to replace a monitor.

CR plates are another special concern, but as they are basically expendables, it is more cost-effective and no more risky to deal with the original plate manufacturer.

For both the warranty and maintenance sections, the vendor should be required to identify the space and communication facilities that the hospital will have to supply.

Warranty: Section 9.1

This subsection covers only the warranty period. Here are some template requirements:

9.1.1. The warranty period shall be deemed to start on the earlier of successful completion of the acceptance test or first clinical use of the system by the customer.

9.1.2. The warranty period shall last 12 months.

9.1.3. The warranty period shall be extended by one month whenever. . . .

9.1.4. The warranty shall cover parts and labor.

9.1.5. During the warranty period, the customer shall have the option of requiring replacement of any component that does not maintain at least 80 percent availability during the 0500 to 1800 time period on weekdays for any one-month period.

9.1.6. During the warranty period, the vendor shall provide the following operations support: . . .

9.1.7. The vendor shall identify in the proposal the space and other facilities that the hospital will have to make available during the warranty period.

Maintenance: Section 9.2

This subsection covers only the maintenance contract. Here are some template requirements:

9.2.1. The vendor shall include in the contract an offer of a one-year maintenance contract, specifying the ordering and payment terms.

9.2.2. The vendor shall include in the contract an offer of a five-year maintenance contract, specifying the ordering and payment terms.

9.2.3. The maintenance contract shall be extended by one month whenever. . . .

9.2.4. The maintenance contract shall cover parts and labor.

9.2.5. During the maintenance period, the customer shall have the option of requiring replacement of any component that does not maintain at least 80 percent availability during the 0500 to 1800 time period on weekdays for any one-month period.

9.2.6. During the maintenance period, the customer shall have the option of replacing without cause one third of the monitors in the system in any one-year interval.

9.2.7. The maintenance contract shall cover the following operations support: . . .

9.2.8. The vendor shall identify in the proposal the space and other facilities that the hospital will have to make available during the warranty period.

System Supplies: Section 9.3

9.3.1. The vendor shall provide a list of approved vendors of any required system supplies. Such supplies include archive media, CR plates and cassettes, laser printer film, and processor chemicals.

Spare Parts: Section 9.4

9.4.1. The vendor shall describe in the proposal the spare parts stocking strategy that he will employ during the warranty period, including on-site spares and any company depots to be maintained.

If the hospital will do its own maintenance, a requirement should be included like:

9.4.2. The vendor shall provide a guarantee that the customer will be able to purchase any required spare parts from the vendor for five years.

Contract Administration: RFP Section 10

This section should define any special requirements for communication between the customer and the vendor on contract matters. A single administrative point of contact should be defined for the entire procurement effort in the customer's organization. This person must be the final authority on financial and contract issues during the negotiation. The vendor should be required to define a single point of contact on his side.

The RFP should specify how communication between the two contract administrators should take place (phone, fax, letter, e-mail, and so on) along with telephone numbers and addresses. This should be formal enough that there can be no ambiguity whether a particular change in the requirements (as often happens) has been made or not. Some customers require that, other than between the two contract administrators, there be no contact between customer and vendor personnel during the time leading up to contract award. If there are any constraints like these to impose, they should be included here.

Special Contract Requirements: RFP Section 11

This section is intended to specify any special procurement requirements or other global project requirements.

Proposal Structure: Section 11.1

To facilitate the comparison of proposals from multiple vendors, it is reasonable to define the format the proposals must take. Among the things which might be specified are:

- The proposal sections (one approach is to have the proposal sections parallel the sections in the RFP).
- The inclusion of a requirements traceability matrix (the RTM can make verification that all requirements are met much easier).

- The inclusion of manufacturers' data sheets for all OEM components.
- The separation of the technical response from the pricing and payment terms (if visibility of the project cost is to be controlled).
- The provision of the proposal in softcopy as well as hardcopy (to facilitate the proposal review process).
- The maximum number of pages allowed in a proposal (although this requirement adds no real value, it is sometimes included).

Exceptions: Section 11.2

The RFP should allow for the possibility that a vendor will be unable to meet some of the normative requirements in the RFP. It is probably better to look at a vendor's best effort than simply not to receive a proposal at all. Therefore, the RFP should allow the vendor to list every exception explicitly, along with any reasons he may wish to offer for why the exception should be allowed. This makes the proposal review process more complex, but it provides the best chance of getting the best system possible.

Benchmark Test: Section 11.3

There is no way to know for sure what the vendor is supplying without seeing it in operation. To be sure the product is real, a site visit to a hospital with a clinically operational system is required. If the project involves primary diagnosis on softcopy, then the visit should provide time to work with the local staff as they perform their diagnostic duties.

A site visit will not usually allow verification of all the technical claims in the proposal. After reviewing the proposals received in response to the RFP, the two or three best should be tested in a setting where careful measurements can be made and proposal claims verified. This section should write a requirement that the vendor agrees to such a test. The benchmark test team must prepare and organize their test carefully or the effort is a waste of time. Test scripts should be written for all the components and for the system as a whole, and individual test responsibilities should be assigned to the team members. The test team should use its own images for the test, rather than those supplied by the vendor.

The benchmark test is like an acceptance test. A good way to start writing a test script is to review each normative requirement and decide whether, and if so, how, it should be tested during the benchmark. Image quality tests should be included for every image acquisition and output system (CR, FD, video acquisition, diagnostic workstation, clinical workstation, and laser printer). The key performance requirements should be tested, paying attention to the comments in Section 7.2 about system loading during performance measurements. Database queries and external information system message handling operations should be included in the performance measurements.

Payment Terms and Conditions: Section 11.4

Customers often insert boilerplate here. Because vendors usually want some kind of progress payments, the customer should expect to negotiate terms and conditions before the contract is awarded. It is prudent to assume at least one change between the contract award and system acceptance, either on the customer's side (e.g., modalities included, rooms networked, workstation configurations) or on the vendor's side (e.g., a component unexpectedly becomes unavailable). There should be agreement on how to handle the financial consequences of such changes before contract award. At the very least, the RFP should require the vendor to propose a way to handle such changes in his response.

Required Insurance: Section 11.5

Because the vendor will have equipment and staff in the hospital's facility, the RFP should require the vendor to observe the hospital's rules and to maintain insurance that protects the hospital from any problems caused by the vendor. As equipment, particularly workstations, can "grow legs," this section should define the responsibility for losses of equipment which occur before installation, before acceptance, and so on.

Licenses, Permits, and Building Codes: Section 11.6

This section should make clear that the vendor has the responsibility for all licenses and permits necessary to fulfill his commitments. It should also require the vendor to meet all applicable building codes, including any special ones imposed by the institution.

Project Control: RFP Section 12

A section on project control is intended to define how the sides will work together on the program after contract award. It is probably best to leave these issues out of the RFP and jointly define them with the selected vendor during the contract negotiation. They are mentioned here as a reminder of an important issue for consideration during the planning of the project.

Project Management: Section 12.1

Sometimes the contract administrator is not involved with the project on an operational basis. When this occurs, the customer must define a person who has the technical project management authority to make decisions on implementation details. The vendor should be required to do the same.

Project Correspondence: Section 12.2

Just as in the case of the contract administrator, a formal means of communicating changes between the project management organizations on the two sides should be defined. This is not to imply that only the formal channels can be used, only to say that after informal communication has resulted in an agreement on an issue, it must be formalized or it does not count.

Change Control: Section 12.3

Section 10 dealt with the financial consequences of the changes that seem inevitably to arise in the implementation phase of system projects. This section should define how to agree on the changes themselves. Changes can occur in anything:

- System configuration.
- Building or campus.
- Vendor-supplied services.
- Schedule.
- Functionality.
- Performance.

One approach is for the project managers to discuss the problem and agree on a solution that is then ratified by the contract administrators. In the best of all worlds, the financial consequences of the solution are clearly covered by Section 10.

Conclusion

Large institutions are shaped by their information systems. As an important part of the information system complex of a hospital, a PACS that alters the access to information throughout the hospital will inevitably change the hospital itself. The commitment to such a change is prudently done after careful analysis. The most effective way that has been found to structure this analysis is in the form of a requirements specification.

This chapter has provided a format and language for such a specification as well as a catalog of issues that PACS experience has shown to be significant. While structured as an RFP, a document defining a customer's expectations of a supplier, the chapter demonstrates that construction of the requirements specification is an effective way to guide the internal analysis itself.

References

Cho PS, Huang HK, Tillisch J. Centralized vs. distributed PACS for intensive care units. In: Schneider, Dwyer SJ, Jost RG, eds. Medical Imaging III: PACS System Design and Evaluation. Proc SPIE 1989, 387–391.

Institute of Electrical and Electronic Engineers. ANSI-IEEE Standard 830-1984. New York: IEEE, 1984.

Kuzmak PM, Norton GS, Dayhoff RE. Using experience with bidirectional HL7-ACR-NEMA interfaces between the federal government HIS/RIS and commercial PACS to plan for DICOM. In: Proc SPIE, 1992.

Meredith G, Anderson KR, Wirsz E et al. Modeling and simulation of a high performance PACS based on a shared file system architecture. In: Dwyer SJ, Jost RG, eds. Medical Imaging VI: PACS Design and Evaluation, Proc SPIE 1992, 169–179.

Prior FW, Nabijee KH. Information management for data retrieval in a picture archive and communication system. J Digital Imaging 1989, 2(3), 170–176.

Wilson DL, Prior FW, Glicksman RA. Virtual PACS, Open Systems, and the National Information Infrastructure. In: Jost RG, ed. Medical Imaging 1995: PACS design and evaluation, Proc SPIE 1995, 553–563.

Section 2

4

The Impact of Medical–Legal Issues in Strategic Planning for PACS and Teleradiology Implementation

SCOTT B. BERGER AND BARRY B. CEPELEWICZ

The shift from traditional film-based to filmless radiology promises to dramatically change the mechanism for interpreting radiologic images and the traditional relationships between radiologists and patients and referring physicians. Picture Archiving and Communications Systems (PACS) and other digital imaging technologies have been available as research tools for many years, but only recently has the technology become available with sufficient reliability, capability, and cost-effectiveness to bring these into wide use. As a result, many radiology providers are seeking to shift from traditional film-based to filmless departments. The infrastructure of PACS also provides the necessary technology to permit the widespread use of teleradiology. This rapid change in technology has introduced issues that were previously untested in the legal forum. This chapter discusses the current status of medical-legal issues pertaining to image retention and fraud, privacy, malpractice liability, licensing and credentialing, and contracts for PACS and teleradiology. Special emphasis is placed on the technical factors that may result in differences in image properties, and consequently affect radiologic diagnosis, with the potential for liability.

Image Ownership and Retention

Radiographs are a form of medical record and are the subject of much legislation and regulation. Although the patient has paid both technical fees for production of an image and physician fees for interpretation, the radiograph itself remains the property of the hospital or physician, and may not be removed from the premises except for court purposes. Traditionally, the rationale for this has been that the radiograph is indispensable to the physician or hospital to care for the patient, but that it is generally of little meaning to the layperson.

The retention of radiologic images is defined by state and federal laws (for a review of legal issues with respect to medical records, the reader is

referred to Roach, Younger, Conner, and Cartwright, 1994). In general, retention of images is required for approximately seven years after the most
recent examination. For minors, this is extended to seven years after they
reach adult age. The retention time is quite variable because many states
impose different retention requirements. For example, in Connecticut (CT
Agencies Regs. § 19-13-D3), patient hospital records must be preserved for
a minimum of 25 years. An important issue for PACS and teleradiology is to
determine which copy of the image is considered the "original" and must be
retained. The American College of Radiology (ACR) has created a Standard
for Teleradiology ("Standard"), which recommends that storage of the images at the transmitting and receiving sites should meet the jurisdictional
requirements of the transmitting site. The Standard further states that images need not be stored at the interpretation site if stored at the transmitting
site; however, should the receiving site choose to retain the images, the receiving site should meet the jurisdictional requirements of the receiving site
as well (ACR, 1996).

Storage Format

At the time this chapter was prepared, several states, including California,
Hawaii, Idaho, Louisiana, Massachusetts, New Jersey, and Virginia (CA
Health and Safety Code § 123149, et al.), authorized the use of microfilming or other photographic reproduction of records provided that "the method
used creates an unalterable record" and that these would be furnished to the
patient or such representative "without unreasonable delay." This issue is
one of the most central to the use of PACS. Most radiologists seeking to use
PACS will ask, "Can I eliminate film copies of radiologic images?" The
answer to this question will impact on the cost analysis of a PACS system
because a major incentive for the use of PACS is elimination of film copies
and film management personnel.

One aspect of this question is whether radiographs are treated as any other
part of a patient medical record, or whether they are subject to specific rules
and regulations. Furthermore, if images have been archived electronically
and the provider intends to destroy the original films, then several states
control the method of medical record destruction (for example, TN Code
Ann § 68-11-305; ID Code § 39-1394).

Images originally acquired in different formats may require separate consideration. For images acquired using digital technology, such as computed
radiography (CR), computed tomography (CT), or magnetic resonance imaging (MRI), where the original acquisition was in the form of a digital
matrix, the use of digital storage is an inherent part of the image production.
However, for film-screen radiographs, electronic storage introduces significant questions concerning the digitization methods, storage format, and use
of image compression technology. As a hypothetical example, if a patient is

suing for failure to diagnose a lung nodule (carcinoma) and the original film-screen radiograph has been replaced by a digitized, compressed record, then the plaintiff may claim that the health care provider has, in essence, failed to retain the original radiograph (Rogers v St. Mary's Hospital). Until some of these issues have been resolved, it may be advisable to retain film-screen images, despite having digitized copies on electronic (permanent) storage media.

Privacy and Access Issues

The transmission, storage, and retrieval of electronic medical information create issues involving privacy protection and confidentiality (Eid, 1995; Schwartz, 1995). Unauthorized access to computer systems by "hackers" and sabotage because of "viruses" has been widely publicized, and the public is acutely aware of the vulnerability of even the most sophisticated computer systems. Patients have the right to the privacy of their medical records, and the increasing use of electronic medical records systems has prompted widespread concern (Kolata, 1995; Love, 1996). Despite the claim that electronic systems offer improved security, even the most sophisticated electronic system cannot be expected to provide a perfect security system. We must therefore look to the privacy laws that are available.

Privacy laws vary from state to state, and as a result, the privacy protection offered by interstate networks will be limited to the minimal level of privacy afforded by any one of the states. Some authors have suggested creating a Uniform State Medical Information Code, which would provide a minimal level of privacy protection for interstate telemedicine, yet allow states to supplement it with additional protections (Eid, 1995). This concern has culminated in the requirements of the 1996 Health Insurance Portability and Accountability Act, which requires health plans and providers that transmit health information to maintain reasonable and appropriate administrative, technical, and physical safeguards to ensure the integrity and confidentiality of information and protect health information from any reasonably anticipated threats to its security (P.L. 104-191).

An additional problem is the Digital Telephony Act of 1994, which requires telecommunications systems to be accessible to wiretaps by law enforcement agencies (Sanders and Bashshur, 1995). This law further increases the risk of privacy invasion by unauthorized individuals. Furthermore, in addition to the patient or a representative, access to medical records is provided to hospital personnel involved in the care of the patient and personnel in the hospital billing center or a designated third-party billing agency. Access to medical records (and radiographs) is also often granted to peer review organizations (PROs) and to those involved in utilization review and quality assurance. In the era of managed care, access of records and radiographs for utilization review has become problematic. At present, it remains the responsibility of the healthcare provider to maintain and enforce a network security system that may include passwords, encryption, security cards, and surveillance software.

Authentication and Security

The increased use of digital imaging systems introduces new opportunities for errors in image identification, authentication, and integrity. Furthermore, the availability of highly sophisticated digital image editing systems may permit new means of image tampering. With film-screen radiography, the patient's name and identification number are exposed ("flashed") directly onto the film. Rarely, a film might be mislabeled, and this is considered a grave error. However, it is generally difficult to tamper with the images once they have been exposed and placed in a film archive. In the PACS era, however, there may be increased opportunity for image fraud. Systems for authentication of an image and the determination of whether any unauthorized image manipulation has taken place are necessary. The DICOM 3.0 electronic standard, adopted by the ACR, permits a more open means of communications between devices, but does not contain specific features for image security (Prior, 1993).

With regard to system security, it is the responsibility of the licensed healthcare provider to ensure that there is no unauthorized access to images. To access images, it can be expected that a personal identification and user verification will be required. Furthermore, it may be advisable to maintain a detailed log of access for each image. For example, any time an image is retrieved, a log entry should record the name of the person accessing the image, the date and time of access, and whether they also accessed any ancillary data, such as the interpretation report. Many systems permit the radiologist to "sign" reports using a unique and secure signature code. Recently, a publication described an approach for security in teleradiology based on legal considerations in Germany (Baur, Engelmann, Saurbier et al., 1997). However, the use of electronic signatures has not been addressed in many states.

Teleradiology

The incorporation of PACS systems into the practice of radiology provides the infrastructure to permit the widespread use of teleradiology, the transmission of images from a local (transmitting) to a remote (receiving) site for interpretation at the remote site.

In its simplest form, teleradiology may involve a radiologist previewing studies on a monitor at home after hours (on-call) and then making a final interpretation from the original films several hours later. However, potential applications of teleradiology promise to dramatically change the mechanism for interpreting radiologic studies, and the traditional relationships radiologists have with patients and other physicians. We have recently reviewed the medical–legal issues for teleradiology (Berger and Cepelewicz, 1996).

Malpractice Liability Issues

Because PACS and teleradiology in most states are in the demonstration phase, there currently is no reported malpractice case involving telemedicine, including teleradiology. A significant issue with respect to malpractice liability is whether there has been any "information loss" in the image data viewed by the radiology consultant. New standards may be required to establish what will be the minimally acceptable level of image transmission, and whether some form of image data (e.g., digitized images) will become part of the patient's medical record. The lack of a hands-on examination by the provider may also become an important issue. Finally, there is the question of whether a local physician's failure to consult a teleradiology specialist who is known to be available may constitute negligence.

There are many advantages of PACS and teleradiology systems that may improve the radiologists' ability to interpret images. For example, having access to a patient's prior examinations at other sites via a PACS/teleradiology network will reduce the number of TIMES a radiologist is asked to interpret films without the aid of prior studies. Furthermore, access to a PACS/teleradiology system has been shown to reduce the time needed to obtain and interpret a film in an intensive care unit setting (Humphrey, Fitzpatrick, Atallah et al., 1993). A study of 116 neurosurgical patients showed that access to teleradiology system significantly shortened the time required for transfer, and was associated with a significantly reduced number of adverse events that occurred prior to transfer (Goh, Lam, and Poon, 1997). These issues are relatively intangible, however, and the focus of malpractice liability will almost certainly be missed diagnoses. In the context of PACS/teleradiology, the question raised is whether a radiologist may be more likely to miss a clinically important finding on an image interpreted via a network than in the local environment.

Image Characteristics and Comparison Studies

There are important differences between traditional film-screen radiographs (FSR) and those that are used in a PACS/teleradiology network. These include: (1) spatial resolution; (2) intensity response and dynamic range; (3) image digitization; (4) display device (computer monitor versus viewbox); and (5) image compression. The latter is of intense interest, and utilizes an algorithm to create a digital representation of an image that is smaller (in bytes) than the original image. Image compression algorithms operate by reducing the data on the basis of inherent properties of the image and involve a wide range of strategies that can yield compression ratios (original:compressed) of greater than 20:1. The compressed form of the image can then be restored to the original image by "uncompressing."

There are compression algorithms that result in no loss of image information (lossless) and others that result in some loss of information (lossy), and the effects of small amounts of image loss and new approaches to compression are subjects of active investigation. A central issue is whether these physical differences in teleradiology images introduce a loss of image information that affects clinical image interpretation. To date, these have not been the subject of a liability case, but it is expected that these issues will be raised in any liability case directed against PACS/teleradiology equipment manufacturers and users, including physicians and hospitals.

Most studies comparing the interpretation of images via digital or teleradiology systems, when compared with FSR, have been limited by three factors: (1) lack of sufficient cases with subtle findings; (2) lack of system spatial resolution; and (3) inadequate structure of the interpretation setting. In a typical medical setting, a significant number of images are normal. Of the remaining fraction that are abnormal, most contain findings that are not very subtle. Only a small fraction of cases contain sufficiently subtle findings to test a system adequately.

Chest radiographs have been the subject of much investigation. In a study of 30 chest radiographs (posteroanterior (PA) projection only), compressed using a discrete cosine transform (DCT) algorithm, the sensitivity and specificity for detecting pulmonary nodules or linear shadows were measured (Ishigaki, Sakuma, Ikeda et al., 1990). At 10:1 compression, there were no significant differences in sensitivity or specificity between the compressed and original images. In a larger study, 122 chest radiographs depicting a variety of pathology, including lung nodules, interstitial disease and mediastinal masses, were interpreted with or without compression, using a 2048 × 2048 matrix system (Aberle, Gleeson, Sayre et al., 1993). The receiving-operator-characteristic (ROC) for detection of interstitial disease or nodules were not significantly different between the original digitized images and images compressed at a ratio of approximately 20:1. A study of 310 PA radiographs of the chest compared the ROC curves for nine experienced radiologists for traditional FSR images, digitized images displayed as hardcopy, and digital images displayed on a computer monitor (Thaete, Fuhrman, Oliver et al., 1994). Observer performance was significantly lower for interstitial disease and pneumothorax when evaluated in digital radiographs displayed on a monitor. A small study of 20 abnormal (and 20 normal) chest radiographs, compared computed radiography (CR) with conventional FSR images, for evaluation of subtle interstitial disease. Even at high resolution (2048 × 2048), 11 radiologists detected significantly less disease in CR images than FSR images (Kondoh, Ikezoe, Inamura et al., 1994). Finally, a study of 23 chest radiographs with subtle pneumothoraces was performed, and the ROC curves were compared for five radiologists interpreting images as either conventional FSR, or small or large format CR images, the latter either as hardcopy or on a monitor (Elam, Rehm, Hillman et al., 1992). The ROC curves ranged from 0.87 for the digital monitor to 0.92 for FSR. The sensitivity for detecting pneumothoraces on a monitor (0.65) was significantly less than that for FSR (0.82). A recent study of portable chest radiographs obtained in 252 critically ill patients showed that there was a significant benefit in a thoracic radiologist viewing the studies via a home teleradiology system, when compared with the readings provided by first-year radiology residents on-call at the hospital (Steckel, Batra, Johnson et al., 1997).

Radiologic evaluation of orthopedic trauma and diseases has also been a focus of comparative studies, but these have generally indicated that radiologists are less accurate with transmitted images than with the original plain radiographs. In a study comparing radiographs of 25 patients with cervical spine fractures and 25 with no fracture, images were digitized at 2048 × 2048 resolution, and four radiologists reviewed conventional images and transmitted (uncompressed) images (Yoshino, Carmody, Fajardo et al., 1992). The ROC curves for two of four radiologists were significantly lower for transmitted images (0.883, 0.840, respectively) compared with conventional images (0.964, 0.907, respectively).

Another study compared the performance of eight in-training radiologists in detecting subtle orthopedic fractures in 120 films rated as difficult by an experienced orthopedic radiologist (Scott, Rosenbaum, Ackerman et al., 1993). For those films considered to be moderately or highly difficult, the mean accuracy for detecting fractures was significantly lower for transmitted images (61 percent, 38 percent, respectively) than that of the original images (83 percent, 72 percent, respectively). A series of 71 compressed (DCT) radiographs of the hands were reviewed by five experienced musculoskeletal radiologists for detection of subperiosteal resorption and compared with the original images (Sayre, Ho, Boechat et al., 1992). There were no significant differences between the ROC curves for the original images and those for the compressed images. Interestingly, a recent comparison of conventional and storage phosphor radiography showed a statistically significant improvement in detection of cervical spine fractures for the digital images (Wilson, Mann, West et al., 1994).

A review of transmitted images from 100 urograms was performed by four radiologists. Although there was no significant difference in sensitivity for detecting any abnormality in transmitted images (86 percent) when compared with the original FSR images (89 percent), there was an increased number of false positive interpretations (44 versus 32, respectively) (Halpern, Newhouse, Amis et al., 1992). Another study of 25 abdominal plain films obtained in urologic patients showed that only one of 25 images transmitted via a teleradiology system was not interpreted correctly when compared with the original films (Averch, O'Sullivan, Breitenbach et al., 1997). A prospective analysis of 685 consecutive cases from an outpatient center was performed, and interpretations of transmitted images were compared with those of the original films (Goldberg, Rosenthal, Chew et al., 1993). In the 196 abnormal films, the sensitivity (96 percent) and specificity (99 percent) for detecting abnormalities were high in the transmitted images, and there was no significant difference when compared with the original images. A more recent study of 2,688 outpatient films, 628 of which were peer reviewed, demonstrated six (0.96 percent) major discrepancies in interpretations performed on transmitted images, when compared with the original films (Gale, Vincent, and Robbins, 1997). Another study of 120 cases, of which about half were considered "difficult cases," showed that a 1024×836 pixel teleradiology system was "clearly inferior" to film evaluation (Stormer, Bolle, Sund et al., 1997).

In mammography, very high resolution is required. One study has evaluated the effect of image compression on mammograms (Good, Maitz, and Gur, 1994), and two studies (Brettle, Ward, Parkin et al., 1994; Jarlman, Borg, Braw et al., 1994) have compared conventional and digital mammography and have found no significant difference in the interpretation of sets of digital and film-screen mammograms. The ACR Standard does not include explicit guidelines for the use of digital mammography.

These results are limited but encouraging, and additional studies are in progress. A major question is whether the data sets used contain sufficiently subtle abnormalities to thoroughly test a teleradiology system. In aggregate, these studies indicate that further progress is needed in technical quality of the transmitted images, and that additional studies will be required to conclusively show whether teleradiology systems provide radiology diagnoses at the same level of quality as the original plain radiographs.

One of the most dramatic differences between FSRs and digital images is the mechanism of display. For FSRs, the film was viewed on viewboxes with relatively high brightness, and a "bright-light" was available for underexposed portions of the film. The mechanism for viewing a digital image is quite different, and involves the use of monitors, most of which are far less bright than traditional viewboxes. Digital images can be printed onto a hardcopy film and viewed on a viewbox, but this negates the many benefits of digital technology. Radiologists are shifting from viewboxes to digital monitors for image interpretation and using digital image display settings, such as window and level, and image processing to perform diagnosis. An important question arises as to the need for image manipulation for diagnosis. For example, if a radiologist fails to adjust the window and level settings, certain image features may not be visible on the monitor. In such a case, an important finding could be missed, and may become the subject of a lawsuit. (This situation is analogous to CT imaging with various tissue density settings, e.g., "bone windows.") It may become necessary to maintain an audit trail not only of who viewed each image, but what window and level settings were used for viewing.

Duty of Care and Jurisdiction

To successfully litigate a malpractice lawsuit, the plaintiff must prove that a physician–patient relationship existed between the teleradiologist and patient; that the consultant breached the applicable standard of care; and that the breach caused the injury. As a medical malpractice lawsuit cannot be brought if no physician–patient relationship existed, this is a very important issue confronting the teleradiology arrangement.

The teleradiologist will argue that there was no physician–patient relationship because services were rendered to the referring physician and not the patient. Case law involving consultants and patients currently supports the conclusion that a physician–patient relationship may exist between a telemedicine consultant and the patient sufficient to form the basis for a malpractice suit. The elements which establish a traditional physician–patient relationship between the consultant and patient are: (1) if the consultant examined the patient's record (Upsey v Sacchetti); (2) if the consultant has met or knows the name of the patient (Hill v Kokosky); (3) if the consultant examined the patient (Hill v Kokosky); (4) if the consultant expected a fee (Clarke v Hoek); or (5) if others have contracted with the physician on the patient's behalf (Dougherty v Gifford).

In contrast, a teleradiologist, who only offers advice to the referring physician and has no direct contact with the patient, may be immune from malpractice liability. In Hill v Kokosky, the Michigan Court of Appeals found that because the consultant directed advice only to the physician treating the patient, who in turn was able to use the advice in any reasonable manner, and because no advice was offered directly to the patient, the relationship between the referring and consulting physician did not create a relationship between the latter and the patient. This holding may lend support to the argument that a teleradiologist who consults only with the local physician, and not the patient, may have reduced exposure to liability. However, the radiologist–patient relationship has traditionally lacked direct contact with the patient, and one can therefore argue that a teleradiology consultation with the referring physician only does constitute a relationship. Clearly, a teleradiologist who interacts directly with a patient will be within a physician–patient relationship.

In a misdiagnosis, plaintiffs may argue that the consulting physician should not have relied on the technology and that the computer companies, including PACS vendors, should be held strictly liable for selling defective products. The consulting physician may, in turn, allege that the network service providers and PACS vendors provided assurances that their products would perform accurately and that they relied on the referring physician. Finally, the computer vendors may argue that their technology was state of the art and that the physician customers were aware of the risks.

Several important issues arise concerning teleradiology. One is when remote consultants with great expertise are available via teleradiology and can benefit the patient. At that time, courts may find that failure to utilize a consultant's services is evidence of negligence. In one case, for example, a physician (nonradiologist) was found to be negligent by failing to diagnose a hemothorax in a patient who sustained trauma, and specifically for failing to consult the radiologist on-call (Upsey v Sacchetti). When teleradiology networks are fully functioning, it can be expected that radiologists of all specialties will be virtually on-call at any time, in any location.

There are also jurisdiction and choice of law issues. The plaintiff patient may claim that the consultant did business in the patient's state, whereas the consultant may argue that all services were provided in the consultant's jurisdiction. Depending on the jurisdiction, a court may find that a teleradiology consultant who rendered advice which was used in a specific state will be subject to the jurisdiction of that state because the teleradiologist practiced in that state and that is where the alleged injury occurred (Rosenblum, 1995).

Theoretically, a plaintiff can sue a teleradiologist in every state or in any state that the teleradiologist practiced teleradiology. Different states have different laws, for example, regarding standard of care and damages, which can affect the potential recovery by the plaintiff. Thus, each party will look to the state that would be the most advantageous. These factors may result in "venue shopping" by parties in malpractice suits. Parties can attempt to limit this type of activity by inserting choice of law provisions in their telemedicine contracts, or potentially by the use of patient waivers with appropriate informed consent.

Teleradiology consultants must be aware of these issues because their malpractice insurance may not cover liability in the patients' states. The ACR's Standard has advised teleradiologists to "consult with their professional liability carrier to ensure coverage in both the sending and receiving sites" (ACR, 1996). Recently, some states have extended statutory malpractice liability limitation statutes to include out-of-state practitioners, which would also presumably discourage venue shopping.

Licensure and Credentialing

With regard to teleradiology, there are several important issues concerning licensure and credentialing (Berger and Cepelewicz, 1996). States possess the power given to them by the Tenth Amendment to protect the health and safety of their citizens. In health care, states fulfill their duty by regulating licensure and the practice of medicine. Based on the current state licensure system, physicians utilizing teleradiology for consultative purposes would have to be licensed in multiple states.

Does the law consider the patient as being electronically transported to the consulting physician who is already licensed in his or her particular state, thus negating the need for the consulting physician to be licensed in the state where the patient resides? Is the teleradiology consultation regarded as recommendations only with the referring physician retaining responsibility for the care of the patient? Is the teleradiologist practicing, and therefore should he or she be licensed, at the receiving site or at the transmitting site (where the patient resides)?

In many states, there are exceptions to the rule requiring a physician to be licensed in the state of practice. A "consultation exception" permits out-of-state physicians to enter the state in order to consult with a locally licensed physician regarding a local patient. California has a very liberal consultation exception, and out-of-state physicians are exempted from licensure requirements "when in actual consultation . . . with a licensed practitioner of this state" (CA Business and Professional Code § 2060). Several states have broad consultation exceptions that do not place any limitation on the consultation exception, outside of the requirement for a local physician to be involved (DE Code § 1726 (a) (1996), et al.).

However, a significant number of other states have a limited consultation exception. Under the limited form, these states will permit an out-of-state physician to consult with local physicians, but only for a specific number of days or months, or only for exceptional circumstances, or allow only physicians in bordering states to enter the state for consulting purposes. For example, South Dakota's consultation exception is so narrow that an out-of-state practitioner may only provide "[a] one time consultation . . . for a period of not more than twenty-four hours" (SD Codified Law § 36-4-39).

In 1995, the Federation of State Medical Boards proposed a Model Act that would create a limited license for physicians who possess full unrestricted licenses to practice telemedicine in another state and avoid the usual requirements of obtaining state licensure. The Model Act did not permit out-of-state physicians to practice medicine physically within the states granting the limited license, the states retained the power to deny or revoke the limited license for appropriate reasons, and telemedicine physicians remained accountable to the state board.

In 1996, the American Medical Association's House of Delegates recommended that physicians be licensed in every state where their patients are located. Similarly, the ACR's Standard recommends that physicians who provide official interpretation of teleradiology images maintain licensure that is appropriate to the delivery of radiologic services at the transmitting and receiving sites (ACR, 1996).

The utilization of telemedicine, and in particular teleradiology, has created a fear that managed care plans may use teleradiology to establish networks that shut out local physicians or that a hospital may replace its local radiologists by using a system connected with an out-of-state radiology group. This has already happened in Melbourne, Florida, where Harris Corporation, a worldwide electronics firm, requires its employees and dependents to use a teleradiology network for nonemergency outpatient imaging. Medical Technology Transfer Corporation, and its subsidary, University Center Imaging, Inc., established a teleradiology facility in Florida that transmits images to the University of California at Los Angeles (UCLA) Medical Center. Images are initially read in the Florida facility and are then sent to UCLA for an overread. Harris entered this agreement because it concluded that it would be more economical and would offer a higher quality of care when compared with local Florida radiologists (Smith, 1995).

Since then, over the past two years, telemedicine has received greater funding, more services are becoming reimbursable, and potential benefits have received more attention in the media. As a result, many states have perceived teleradiology as a threat to their local radiologists and other providers and have moved to narrow their consultation exceptions or, in many cases, require the out-of-state telemedicine consultant to be fully licensed in the local state. South Dakota prevents out-of-state physicians from providing diagnostic or treatment services "under contract" to individuals in South Dakota via "electronic means," unless the out-of-state physician is licensed to practice in South Dakota (SD Codified Laws § 36-4-41). Kansas has a regulation stipulating that out-of-state physicians who practice "the healing arts" on Kansas citizens must first obtain a Kansas license (KS Regulation § 100-26-1). Texas permits episodic telemedicine consultations by a specialist only if the request for the consultation is made by a physician licensed in Texas who practices in the same medical specialty (Tex. Rev. Civ. Stat. Art. 4495b). Connecticut requires any out-of-state telemedicine physician whose practice is ongoing or regular, or based upon a "contractual arrangement" to be licensed in Connecticut (CT General Statutes § 20-9). The act has exemptions including telemedicine consultations with medical schools for educational or training purposes.

Although the majority of states created licensure laws adverse to the expansion of interstate telemedicine, California passed a law that authorizes its medical board to create a registration program that would enable out-of-state physicians who are licensed in the state in which they reside to practice telemedicine in California, provided they comply with various educational and training requirements. As with the Federation's Model Act, California's medical board can deny an application for registration and the out-of-state physicians accepted are still subject to the review and disciplinary powers of the board.

Credentialing is a problem similar to licensing that applies to out-of-state and in-state physicians who do not have privileges at the hospital in which the patient is located. Hospitals have an obligation to ensure their patients that members of their staff are competent in the practice of medicine. Furthermore, in many jurisdictions, under the doctrine of "ostensible agency," if a plaintiff can successfully argue that as a reasonable patient he or she believed that the telemedicine consultant was an agent of the hospital, the plaintiff may be able to recover from the hospital for the consultant's negligence. The ACR's Standard recommended that the interpreting radiologist be credentialed by the medical staff of the sending hospital consistent with its bylaws and obtain appropriate privileges at that institution (ACR Standard, 1996).

It is therefore crucial for providers to understand the licensure laws of the local state and what impact they may have on their telemedicine network since a violation of these laws can result in civil and/or criminal penalties as well as suspension or revocation of the consultant's license.

Contracts

The use of PACS/teleradiology systems creates numerous issues and potential exposures to liability that can be addressed by the creation of contracts between the interested parties. As the purchase of a PACS system is a large capital expenditure, most facilities utilize detailed contracts as a means of ensuring that the system provides the capabilities promised by the manufacturer. Many other arrangements will be best addressed by contractual agreement, including the agreement between a teleradiology provider and his or her clients (Cepelewicz and Berger, 1996). As hospital mergers continue, there will be incentive for more than one provider to utilize all or part of a PACS system of another entity. For example, it may be cost effective for a smaller hospital to lease space on a large archive system from a larger hospital or network, rather than investing in and maintaining a separate but smaller archive. However, such an arrangement would require carefully constructed contracts to specify the terms of agreement.

We have recently reviewed numerous contracts for business ventures involving electronic data interchange and have developed a model for a teleradiology contract based on the "request for consultation" or RFC (Cepelewicz and Berger, 1996). The model contract includes an explanation of intent, the responsibilities of each party in detail, and the technical requirements and communications procedures for teleradiology consultations. The contract must set forth the equipment to be used, as well as the owner and party responsible for maintenance. A standard format for image transmission must be agreed upon, as well as a standard format and mechanism for reporting results. Some agreements may outline a format for interface with the RIS/HIS system.

The central interchange is the RFC, which triggers a specific sequence of clearly defined events. In our model, the RFC is first acknowledged with a record of the date and time. The image for interpretation is verified and checked for errors using commercially available error checking systems. This step should also include some means of authentication of the sender and source, as well as authorization for the RFC. This may rely on passwords or on a transmission via a separate means (i.e., fax, voice) to verify the authenticity of the request.

Transmission rates are very important to speed the time for clinical decision making and to determine the cost of transmission. For teleradiology providers that agree to pay the cost of telecommunications, there is great incentive to transmit the images at high speed. Meeting the requirements of transmission speed may involve significant costs; and this should be clearly outlined in the contract.

In the event of a failed or garbled transmission, there should be a well-defined procedure for transmission. These may include alternate means of electronic transfer, such as download onto magnetic tape. Parties must also assign responsibility of confirming receipt of the transmission, verifying that there are no errors or omissions in the transmission or conversion of the data.

A busy teleradiology system could generate a large number of megabytes of image data per day. If so, this could require significant system administration and maintenance, and these duties and responsibilities should be clearly defined. If dedicated personnel are required, then the responsibility for approving and hiring should be mutually agreed upon. Other issues that must be addressed in the teleradiology contract include confidentiality and security, data storage (retention), and nondisclosure.

Conclusions

The shift from traditional film-based to filmless radiology promises to provide higher quality health care with significant cost savings, and may allow more efficient access to patient medical records by authorized individuals. However, these technologies also introduce a wide range of issues that are largely untested in the legal forum and pose additional risks to the practicing radiologist. There are strategies by which the risk of liability can be reduced. Above all, it remains the responsibility of interpreting radiologists to determine whether the images communicated to them are sufficient to make a diagnosis.

References

Aberle D, Gleeson F, Sayre J et al. The effect of irreversible image compression on diagnostic accuracy in thoracic imaging. Invest Radiol 1993, 28, 398–403.

American College of Radiology (ACR). Standard for teleradiology, Res. 26, 1996.

Averch TD, O'Sullivan D, Breitenbach C et al. Digital radiographic imaging transfer: comparison with plain radiographs, J Endourol 1997, 11, 99–101.

Baur HJ, Engelmann U, Saurbier F et al. How to deal with security issues in teleradiology. Comp Meth Prog Biomed 1997, 53, 1–8.

Berger SB, Cepelewicz BB. Medical–legal issues for teleradiology. AJR 1996, 166, 505–510.

Brettle D, Ward S, Parkin G et al. A clinical comparison between conventional and digital mammography utilizing computer radiography. Br J Radiol 1994, 67, 464–468.

CA Business and Professional Code § 2060 (1996).

CA Health and Safety Code § 123149 (1996); HI Rev Stat § 622-58(a) (1996); ID Code § 39-1394(a) (1997); LA Rev Stat § 40:2144(F) (1997); MA Ann Laws ch 111, § 70 (1997); NJ Stat § 26:8-5 (1997); VA Code Ann § 32.1-127.1:01 (1997).

Cepelewicz BB, Berger SB. Contracts minimize risk for teleradiology services. Diagnostic Imaging, 1996 (April), 23–25.

Clarke v Hoek, 219 Cal. Rptr. 845 (1st Dist. Ct. App. 1985).

CT Agencies Regs. § 19–13–D3(d)(6).

CT General Statutes § 20-9 (1997).

DE Code § 1726(a) (1996); FL Statutes Annotated § 458.303(1)(b) (1996); GA Code Annotated § 43-34-26(b)(6) (1997); OR Revised Statutes § 677.060(2) (1996).

Dougherty v Gifford, 826 S.W. 2d 668 (Tex. Ct. App. Texarkana 1992).

Eid TA. Privacy protection for patient-identifiable medical information. In: Action Report, Western Governors Association, 1995a (June), 42–47.

Eid TA. Roadblocks on the information superhighway: removing the legal and policy barriers to telemedicine. J National Information Testbed 1995b, 1, 46–54.

Elam E, Rehm K, Hillman B et al. Efficacy of digital radiography for the detection of pneumothorax: Comparison with conventional chest radiography. AJR 1992, 158, 509–514.

Gale ME, Vincent ME, Robbins AH. Teleradiology for remote diagnosis: a prospective multiyear evaluation. J Dig Imag 1997, 10, 47–50.

Goh KY, Lam CK, Poon WS. The impact of teleradiology of the inter-hospital transfer of neurosurgical patients. Br J Neurosurg 1997, 11, 52–56.

Goldberg M, Rosenthal D, Chew F et al. New high-resolution teleradiology system: prospective study of diagnostic accuracy in 685 transmitted clinical cases. Radiology 1993, 186, 429–434.

Good WF, Maitz G, Gur D. JPEG compatible compression of mammograms. J Dig Imag 1994, 7, 123–132.

Halpern E, Newhouse J, Amis S et al. Evaluation of teleradiology for interpretation of intravenous urograms. J Dig Imag 1992, 5, 101–106.

Hill v Kokosky, 463 N.W. 2d 265 (Mich. App. 1990), appeal denied, 438 Mich. 873 (1991).

Humphrey LM, Fitzpatrick K, Atallah N et al. Time comparison of intensive care units with and without digital viewing systems. J Dig Imag 1993, 6, 37–41.

Ishigaki T, Sakuma S, Ikeda M et al. Clinical evaluation of irreversible image compression: analysis of chest imaging versus computed radiography. Radiology 1990, 175, 739–743.

Jarlman O, Borg A, Braw M et al. Breast imaging: a comparison of digital luminescence radiographs displayed on TV monitor and film screen mammography. Canc Detect Prev 1994, 18, 375–381.

Kolata G. When patients' records are for sale. New York Times, 1995 (Nov. 15), P. B1.

Kondoh H, Ikezoe J, Inamura K et al. A comparison of conventional film screen radiography and hard copy of computed radiography in full and two-thirds sizes in detection of interstitial lung disease. J Dig Imag 1994, 7, 193–195.

KS Regulation § 100-26-1 (1995).

Love J. Privacy protection or legalized prowling? Who should have access to your medical record? Business & Health 1996, 14(2), 59.

P.L. 104-191.

Prior FW. Specifying DICOM compliance for modality interfaces. Radiographics 1993, 13, 1381–1388.

Roach WH Jr, Younger P, Conner C, Cartwright KK. Medical records and the law. Gaithersburg, MD: Aspen Publications, 1994.

Rogers v St. Mary's Hospital, 556 NE 2d 913 (4th Dist. 1990); appeal granted, 564 NE 2d 847 (1990), and affirmed, 597 NE 2d 616 (1992).

Rosenblum J. Legal aspects of computerized medical records. Legal Med. 1995.

Sanders JH, Bashshur RL. Challenges to the implementation of telemedicine. Telemedicine Journal 1995, 1, 115–123.

Sayre J, Ho BKT, Boechat MI et al. Subperiosteal resorption: effect of full-frame image compression of hand radiographs on diagnostic accuracy. Radiology 1992, 185, 599–603.

Schwartz PM. The protection of privacy in health care reform. Vanderbilt Law Review 1995, 48, 295.

Scott W, Rosenbaum J, Ackerman S et al. Subtle orthopedic fractures: teleradiology workstation versus film interpretation. Radiology 1993, 187, 811–815.

SD Codified Law § 36-4-39 (1997).

SD Codified Laws § 36-4-41 (1997).

Smith R. Productivity coast to coast: teleradiology network links UCLA and Florida clinic. Imaging Economics, 1995 (July/August), 25–28.

Steckel RJ, Batra P, Johnson S et al. Chest teleradiology in a teaching hospital emergency practice. AJR 1997, 168, 1409–1413.

Stormer J, Bolle SR, Sund T et al. ROC-study of a teleradiology workstation versus film readings. Acta Radiologica 1997, 38, 176–180.

Tex. Rev. Civ. Stat. art. 4495b, § 3.06(i)(1) (1997).

Thaete FL, Fuhrman CR, Oliver JH et al. Digital radiography and conventional imaging of the chest: a comparison of observer performance. AJR 1994, 162, 575–581.

TN Code Ann § 68-11-305(c) (1997); ID Code § 39–1394(d) (1997).

Upsey v Sacchetti, LRP Publications, Jan 1991, available in LEXIS, Verdict Library, Case No. 6302.

Wilson A, Mann F, West O et al. Evaluation of the injured cervical spine: comparison of conventional and storage phosphor radiography with a hybrid cassette. Radiology 1994, 193, 419–422.

Yoshino M, Carmody R, Fajardo LL et al. Diagnostic performance of teleradiology in cervical spine fracture detection. Invest Radiology 1992, 27, 55–59.

5
PACS and Productivity

BRUCE I. REINER AND ELIOT L. SIEGEL

Timely management of medical imaging information is one of the greatest challenges facing medicine today. As imaging technology has grown more complex, the capacity of film-based systems has not kept up with the increasing demands of radiology departments.

Picture Archiving and Communication Systems (PACS) offer unique improvements in operational efficiency by providing economical storage, rapid image retrieval, access to images acquired with multiple modalities, and simultaneous image access at multiple sites (Choplin, Boehme, and Maynard, 1992).

The initial acceptance of this new technology was somewhat limited by concerns of capital costs, spatial resolution, image display time, and the need for system redundancy to provide backup in the event of component failure. As these challenges are addressed, the acceptance of PACS is expanding rapidly. This chapter focuses on many of the productivity issues facing PACS.

Practical Experience Using PACS

In the past five years of filmless operation at the Baltimore Veterans Affairs Medical Center (BVAMC), the following advantages of PACS have been demonstrated when compared with the conventional film-based alternative including (Siegel, Diaconis, Pomerantz et al, 1995):

- Better image management with fewer lost and unread studies.
- Use of computer enhancement to produce consistently higher quality images.
- Ability to provide real-time image interpretation.
- Greater image accessibility.

The overall improvement in image management is largely a function of fewer lost and unread exams, which has positive medico-legal and economic implications. After the transition to filmless operation, there has been a reduction in the lost examination rate from 8 percent to less than 0.7 percent.

In assessing image quality, radiologists consistently report preference for PACS over conventional film-screen images. This has been largely attributed to the greater dynamic range of computed radiology (CR), allowing for less variation in overall image quality when compared with film images. This reported improvement in image quality is particularly noticeable in the interpretation of portable exams, which are notoriously suboptimal on film-screen exams. The greater dynamic range of CR has the additional potential benefits of decreasing image retake rates, increasing the effective field of view on a typical radiograph, and providing the potential for radiation dose reductions.

Softcopy interpretation allows for utilization of several standard software tools, including window/level, zoom and magnify, distance and angular measurement, and pixel value display. Less standard, but common, tools include cine capability, area and perimeter measurement, edge enhancement, and histogram equalization.

The ability to provide real-time interpretation allows for much greater participation by radiologists in patient care. Radiological findings can be discovered quickly and promptly communicated to the appropriate clinician. This is of particular importance in the settings of the emergency room, operating room, and intensive care unit.

Increased image accessibility is one of the most frequently reported advantages of PACS. Outside the radiology department, monitors are located throughout the hospital in physician team rooms, the intensive care unit, operating rooms, and the emergency room. The presence of monitors in conference rooms, the auditorium, and medical media offer educational benefits not provided by film-based imaging.

Teleradiology in a PACS environment refers to the transmission of images to and from another site for evaluation. This is currently being performed at the BVAMC with two smaller satellite hospitals. The BVAMC serves as the image archival hub, with the capability of providing subspecialty, back-up, or primary image interpretation.

As future systems offer an increased number of connectivity options and enhanced speed, a user will have the ability to log in remotely and have the same functionality as he or she would using an in hospital workstation. Throughput can be further maximized by the use of image compression algorithms, which can also minimize costs.

To date these experiences have shown the unique benefits of a fully functional large-scale PACS system and the inherent productivity gains it offers.

PACS-Related Organizational Changes

Replacing conventional film-based imaging with PACS has a multitude of effects inside and outside of the radiology department. The major organizational effects within the radiology department can be classified into two categories (Warburton, 1992):

- Improved handling of clinical information, resulting in time savings in the performance and reporting of examinations.
- Net reductions in staffing, through the elimination of film-handling tasks and fewer lost films and reports.

Major organizational effects outside the radiology department center on the effects PACS has on overall patient care and include:

- Faster and more accurate diagnoses resulting in reduced time to initiate clinical action.
- Potential reduction in average length of patient stay.
- Potential improvements in overall health outcomes.

Several studies have attempted to demonstrate these organizational effects of PACS with varying degrees of success. Saarinen, Wilson, Iverson et al. (1990) performed time-motion analysis with activity sampling and interviews to estimate the savings in film handling times associated with PACS. The estimated time savings were achieved for film library staff (55 percent), technologists (10 percent), and radiologists (10 percent).

An interesting study (DeSimone, Kundel, Arenson et al., 1988) evaluated the impact of PACS on clinical practice in the setting of the ICU and showed statistically significant reductions in time to perform clinical actions following the diagnostic exam. Using PACS, significant alterations were demonstrated in the processes of obtaining radiological information, viewing exams, and consultations between ICU physicians and radiologists. The results of this study suggest that the use of a PACS affects both patient management and radiology department work flows in the ICU setting.

A recent study by Reiner, Siegel, Pomerantz et al. (1996) evaluated the impact of filmless radiology on the frequency of clinician consultations with radiologists. Results demonstrated a significant decrease of greater than 50 percent in the number of general radiography consultations following the transition to filmless operation. The diminution in consultation frequency was observed in CT, ultrasound, nuclear medicine, and MRI. The etiology of this decrease in radiological consultations is thought to be multifactorial. Contributing factors include the ease and reliability of image retrieval outside of the radiology department, along with improved report turnaround and availability using PACS. Report turnaround times have decreased from 24 to 2 hours during the weekdays. In addition, the bidirectional interface between PACS and the hospital/radiology information systems (HIS/RIS), has allowed for paperless in addition to filmless operation.

This overall decrease in consultations has the undesired effect of diminishing the radiologists' direct involvement with their clinical colleagues and their ability to participate in patient management decisions. "In-person" communications have been replaced by electronic communication using digital dictation with enterprise wide phone access, image annotation using PACS, electronic mail, and so on.

Radiologist Productivity

Following the conversion to filmless imaging at the BVAMC, the overall productivity of radiologists has increased by more than 50 percent. Although the actual reading time using PACS has been shown to be only slightly faster compared with radiographs displayed on a view box, the disproportionate increase in efficiency was found to be the result of several factors including:

- Easier, more rapid, and more reliable access to old exams and reports.
- Elimination of frequent interruptions by clinicians and file room staff searching for films.
- Improved workload distribution with less dependence on file room personnel.
- Addition of newer software enabling automatic retrieval of comparison studies.

Reports evaluating radiologist productivity using PACS in the interpretation of CT images have yielded conflicting data, largely dependent on workstation design and monitor resolution (Beard, Hemminger, Perry et al., 1993; Beard, Hemminger, Denelsbeck et al., 1994; Foley, Jacobson, Taylor et al., 1990; Hirota, Shimanota, Yamakawa et al., 1995; Itoh, Ishigaki, Sakuma et al., 1992). In the study by Itoh et al., for example, the increased reading time required when using PACS compared with film in CT interpretation was shown to be largely a function of prolonged image retrieval time and limitation in the number of images that could be simultaneously displayed.

Recent developments in software design have allowed for greater efficiency in image interpretation using PACS. One such development is an intelligent image arrangement algorithm referred to as *Default Display Protocol (DDP)*, which serves to automatically retrieve previous related exams and arrange them in logical order for comparison with the current examination. We found the use of this newer software has led to significant increase in radiologist productivity, on the order of 10 to 20 percent, depending upon the imaging modality being evaluated. Radiologists also report less fatigue with DDP's automation of repetitive tasks.

A recent study (Reiner, Siegel, Hooper et al., 1996) demonstrated a two- to three-fold time savings in image display time using PACS in the evaluation of chest and abdominal CT exams, when compared with conventional film-based images. The ability to rapidly display current and prior studies in unison along with appropriate patient data and old reports resulted in a substantial decrease in image display time, thereby accounting for reduction in the overall interpretation time. As the number of images to review and the complexity of the examination increases, the time savings using PACS is further accentuated.

Several of the functions available on the computer workstation further enhance radiologist productivity, most notably the ability to perform rapid window/level setting adjustments using presets. In addition to producing significant time savings, use of window/level presets has been shown to improve diagnostic accuracy in CT interpretation. Recent work (Pomerantz, Krebbs, White et al., 1996) demonstrated additional clinically significant findings in approximately 10 percent of thoracic and abdominal CT examinations. When all cases were reviewed with a greater number of window/level settings (e.g., bone settings).

In addition to the above mentioned quantitative advantage offered by PACS, several subjective advantages have been reported, resulting in improvements in radiologist satisfaction and job performance, as shown in Table 5.1. The greater dynamic range (ability to capture and display more levels of contrast) of computed radiography (CR) results in a greater consistency in image quality when compared with conventional film-screen images; this disparity is most noticeable with portable exams. The consistently higher image quality of PACS has been one of the major advantages of PACS cited by both radiologists and other clinicians on surveys conducted in the department (unpublished data).

The quality of work life has improved as well. PACS has allowed for greater flexibility in working hours for radiologists, with less dependence on file room personnel. Since the introduction of PACS at the BVAMC, the number of interruptions during read-out has dramatically decreased, largely because of the increased accessibility of images throughout the hospital and rapid availability via the telephone access to the digital dictation system or the hospital information system.

A frequently overlooked aspect of PACS that enhances radiologist productivity is the bidirectional interface between PACS and HIS/RIS. This provides the radiologist with a complete set of patient data at the time of image interpretation, which is frequently lacking in the interpretation of conventional film-based images. The data available includes patient demographics, physician identification, patient history, laboratory data, and previous radiology reports.

TABLE 5.1. Radiologists' productivity with PACS.

Increased Productivity	Decreased Productivity
1. Fewer interruptions.	1. More tools and options at workstation.
2. Increased availability of old exams and reports.	2. Learning curve required to develop proficiency.
3. Enhanced distribution of workload throughout the radiology department.	3. Increased fatigue (luminance, monitor flicker).
4. Increased flexibility in scheduling.	4. Potential for equipment breakdown.
5. No delay related to file room	
6. Overall reduction in report turnaround time	
7. Higher quality exams (greater dynamic range of computed radiography)	

Economic Issues Affecting Productivity

A number of issues are critical in the overall diagnostic efficacy of PACS including workstation monitor resolution, operability the number of monitors, workstation, monitor and room illumination, and operator fatigue.

The imaging workstation functions to retrieves images rapidly (<1.5 seconds) and permits rapid and intuitive navigation of the database to facilitate retrieval and comparison of relevant historical or related exams. Monitor resolution should be at least 1500 to 2000 pixels, with a display surface comparable in size to a conventional 14 to 17 inch film. The software for image display and manipulation should be intuitive and easy to use.

Laboratory observer studies indicate display brightness is an important parameter in the reading of radiological images (Britton, Sumkin, Curtin et al., 1990; Gur, Fuhrman, Thaete, 1993). The average luminance of a radiographic image displayed on a CRT monitor is lower than that of the same radiograph displayed on a view box. The retina is adapted to this lower luminance with some loss in sensitivity and this adaptation can be spoiled by extraneous light (Kundel, 1986).

There are competing effects of decreasing ambient light. An early study (Alter, Kargas, Kargas et al., 1982) showed small lesion detection is improved with lower ambient light. However, observer fatigue during prolonged observation time is increased at lower illuminance, thereby reducing visual performance.

There has been an observed increase in observer fatigue using existing PACS workstations. This increase in fatigue is caused by a combination of factors including:

- Relative decrease in monitor brightness when compared with film view box.
- Monitor flicker (related to the monitor refresh rate).
- Small cursors currently available on some workstations.
- More active role required of the radiologist in image manipulation.

An additional drawback that currently exists is the tendency for current high-resolution monitors to drift or change brightness over time. A careful quality control program is therefore essential for any large-scale PACS.

Radiology Staff/Technologist Productivity

The measurement of activities in the performance of diagnostic imaging examinations is divided into technical, support, and availability functions. Technical functions include image processing and quality assessment. Support functions include scheduling of exams, report filing, and administrative supervision. Ancillary functions include reception, darkroom maintenance, and statistical recording.

PACS has been shown to improve productivity in all three areas. Requirements for support functions have been minimized by the enhanced archival capabilities of PACS, allowing for short- and long-term image storage, along with corresponding reports. The bidirectional interface between PACS and HIS/RIS scheduling has reduced clerical steps and has resulted in near paperless operation at the Baltimore VA Medical Center. The net effect has been substantial a decrease in required radiology department staffing.

Several studies to date (Saarinen, Haynor, Loop et al., 1989; TMG, 1990; van der Loo and van Gennip, 1992) have performed cost-benefit analysis and predicted large personnel savings as a consequence of PACS implementation. Surprisingly, little has been done to quantify the actual time savings and improved technologist productivity expected with PACS. This is of crucial importance in assessing PACS productivity, because technologist working time represents the major portion or a radiology departments' controllable costs (Trisolini, Baswell, Johnson et al., 1988).

Before the advent of PACS, several studies (MacEwan, 1982; Schoppe, Hessel, and Adams, 1981; Trisolini et al., 1988) were performed calculating the average times to perform various radiological examinations. When subjected to multivariate analysis, these procedure times showed a range of up to 300 percent (Janower, 1988), largely as a result of a number of uncontrollable variables including:

- Uneven, unpredictable patient flow.
- Personal and fatigue time (technologist).
- Additional time requirements for administrative, supervisory, and educational activities.

Although difficult to objectively quantify, subjective perceptions suggest all three variables are enhanced with PACS utilization. Patient flow is enhanced by streamlined efficient scheduling, which is assisted by the interface between the PACS and HIS/RIS. Technologists report a decreased fatigue factor with PACS, largely because of decreased interruptions by clinicians looking for images and the elimination of filming and dark room responsibilities. Administrative time requirements are also reduced with PACS because of its ability to assess time management and productivity through objective means.

A recent study performed at the BVAMC evaluated differences in technologist productivity in CT imaging when comparing PACS with conventional film-based operation (Reiner, 1998). Using time-motion analysis, statistically significant differences were found in all aspects of CT image acquisition, with PACS far more productive than film. In the evaluation of total time required to scan and display CT images, PACS resulted in an average time savings of more than 50%, independent of technologist and CT scanner type.

Productivity Issues: Referring Physicians

Subjective assessments by radiology service users indicate there is a significant hidden cost as a result of delayed access to imaging information (Straub and Gur, 1990). Increasing access to images and reports, through either conventional or electronic means may prevent costly delays in patient management decisions and has the potential to improve overall patient care (Gur, Straub, Lieberman et al., 1992).

Extensive survey data has been collected during the five years of filmless operation at the BVAMC. During this time referring physicians were questioned as to their imaging preferences, comparing PACS with the conventional film-based alternative. The data shows a progressively strong preference for PACS over film over time. Data from a 1995 survey show a 92 percent physician preference for PACS, with only 3 percent of surveyed physicians preferring film (5 percent report no preferences).

The most commonly cited advantages of PACS were improved image quality and image availability. Almost all physicians reported improved time management following implementation of PACS, largely as a result of improved image accessibility throughout all locations of the hospital. This extends into the operating rooms where PACS workstations are utilized for intraoperative image evaluation, particularly in the practices of orthopedic and vascular surgery (Pomerantz, Siegel, Protopapas et al., 1996).

The presence of PACS workstations in clinics, hospital floors, intensive care units, and clinician work rooms results in rapid image retrieval and evaluation during the course of the patient evaluation. This has resulted in the perception of earlier diagnoses and treatment planning with increased patient throughput and reduction in hospital stay.

Quality Assurance

Through its bidirectional interface with the HIS/RIS, the PACS can be utilized for continuous monitoring of timeliness of reports, equipment down time, repeat exam analysis, retrievability of radiology records, and production volume indicators. The individual variables and data points within the reporting process can be analyzed on a continuing basis and studied as objects for improvements.

The ultimate result is an improvement in the overall imaging process with elimination of lost images, late reports, and unbilled services, so that the radiology practice can be complete, accurate, timely, and cost effective.

Future Advances in Productivity

The trend toward complete conversion to filmless imaging will be made possible as the technology advances. Hardware costs will decline, and cost effectiveness will be documented. All imaging modalities will become digital, including mammography with the advent of high-resolution, full-breast digital mammography and direct digital radiography (DR). Images will be acquired, stored, and displayed digitally and will be readily available to physicians across large hospital networks and accessible through personal computers. Software design advancements will result in more efficient imaging with enhanced ability to perform complex image enhancement along with computer assisted diagnosis.

References

Alter AJ, Kargas GA, Kargas SA, et al. The influence of ambient and view box light upon visual detection of low-contrast targets in a radiograph. Invest Radiol, 1992, 17, 402–406.

Beard DV, Hemminger BM, Denelsbeck KM, et al. How many screens does a CT workstation need? J Digit Imag 1994, 7, 69–76.

Beard DV, Hemminger BM, Perry JR, et al. Interpretation of CT studies: single-screen workstation versus film alternator. Radiology 1993, 187, 565–569.

Britton CA, Sumkin JH, Curtin HD, et al. Subjective perceptions of and attitudes toward primary interpretation of x-ray images in a PACS environment. Proc SPIE 1990, 1234, 94–97.

Choplin RH, Boehme JM, Maynard CD. Picture archiving and communications systems: an overview. Radiographics 1992, 12, 127–129.

DeSimone DN, Kundel HL, Arenson RL, et al. Effect of a digital imaging network on physician behavior in an intensive care unit. Radiology 1988, 169, 41–44.

Foley WD, Jacobson DR, Taylor AJ, et al. Display of CT studies on a two-screen electronic workstation versus a film panel alternator: sensitivity and efficiency among radiologists. Radiology 1990, 174, 769–773.

Gur D, Fuhrman CR, Thaete FL. Requirements for PACS: users' perspective. Radiographics 1993, 13, 457–460.

Gur D, Straub WH, Lieberman RH, et al. Clinicians' access to diagnostic imaging information at an academic center: perceived impact on patient management. AJR 1992, 158, 893–896.

Hirota H, Shimanota K, Yamakawa K, et al. Clinical evaluation of newly developed CRT viewing station: CT reading and observers performance. Comput Med Imag and Graph 1995, 19, 281–285.

Itoh Y, Ishigaki T, Sakuma S, et al. Influence of CRT workstation on observers' performance. Comput Method Program Biomed 1992, 37, 253–258.

Janower ML. Productivity standards for technologists: How to use them. Radiology 1988, 166, 276–277.

Kundel HL. Visual perception and image display terminals. Radiol Clin North Amer 1986, 24, 69–78.

MacEwan DW. Radiology workload system for diagnostic radiology: productivity enhancement studies. Radiology Manage 1982, 5, 24–38.

Pomerantz SM, Krebbs TL, White CS, et al. Efficacy of routine review of liver and bone window settings in thoracic and abdominal CT imaging in the PACS environment. American Roentgen Ray Society Annual Meeting, San Diego, CA, May 5-10, 1996.

Pomerantz SM, Siegel EL, Protopapas Z, et al. Experience and design recommendations for PACS in the surgical setting. J Digit Imag 1996, 9, 123–130.

Reiner BI, Siegel EL, Hooper F, et al. Effective productivity of PACS in the interpretion of CT exams. Proc SCAR Proceedings 1996, 399–402.

Reiner BI, Siegel EL, McLaurin T, et al. Evaluation of soft-tissue foreign bodies comparing conventional plain film radiograpy, computed radiography printed on film and computed radiography displayed on a computer workstation. AJR 1996, 167, 141–144.

Reiner BI, Siegel EL, Pomerantz SM, et al. The impact of filmless radiology on the frequency of clinician consultations with radiologists. American Roentgen Ray Society Annual Meeting, San Diego, CA May 5-10, 1996.

Reiner BI, Siegel EL. Effect of film based versus filmless operation on the productivity of CT technologists. Radiology 1998 May, 207(2), 481–485.

Saarinen AO, Haynor DR, Loop JW, et al. Modeling the economics of PACS: what is important? Proc Med Im III Conf 1989, 1093, 62–73.

Saarinen AO, Wilson MC, Iverson SC, et al. Potential time savings to radiology department personnel in a PACS-based environment. Proc SPIE 1990, 1234, 261–269.

Schoppe WD, Hessel SJ, Adams DF. Time requirements in performing body CT studies. JCAT 1981, 5, 513–515.

Siegel EL, Diaconis JN, Pomerantz S, et al. Making filmless radiology work. J Digital Imag 1995, 8, 151–155.

Straub WH, Gur D. The hidden costs of delayed access to diagnostic imaging information: impact on PACS implementation. AJR 1990, 155, 613–616.

TMG: Executive Summary of Ten-Year Cost Projections of the Operation of PACS Radiology Image Management, Des Plains, Illinois, 1990.

Trisolini MG, Baswell SB, Johnson SK, et al. Radiology work-load measurements reflecting variables specific to hospital, patient, and examination: results of a collaborative study. Radiology 1988, 166, 247–253.

van der Loo RP, van Gennip EMSJ. Evaluation of personnel savings through PACS: a modeling approach. Int J Biomed Comput 1992, 30, 235–241.

Warburton RN. Evaluation of PACS-induced organizational change. Int J Biomed Comput 1992, 30, 243–248.

6
Economic Analysis of Filmless Radiology

CHARLES D. FLAGLE

The economic implications of innovations in diagnostic radiological services have been of major concern for health policy analysts and health service administrators for several decades. Areas of concern include:

- High costs of digital imaging equipment in an environment of attempted cost containment.
- Developmental problems of image quality and acceptance by radiologists and clinicians.
- Unknowns about the impact on the organization and financing of radiological services.
- Questions about the ultimate effects on content and outcomes of patient care.

However, outside the arena of healthcare policy, practical successes in digital imaging for diagnostic radiology have challenged the advancing state of the art in computer/communications technology and have offered strong economic incentives to advance in an area and era of global competition.

The interplay of forces within the policy making apparatus of health services and forces representing government's role in the development and promotion of the industrial economy gave rise to the first fully operational filmless Picture Archiving and Communication System (PACS) for diagnostic radiology at the new Baltimore Veterans Administration Medical Center (BVAMC) in 1993, which is the central object of analysis here. Some history of the evolution of national policy in setting priorities for assessment and support of technological development will be helpful in understanding the background of economic analysis of the Baltimore VAMC experience with this prototype technology in a public sector healthcare setting.

Policy Evolution

In 1990, a report of the Council on Health Care Technology of the National Academy of Sciences listed 20 highest priority areas of medical technology and practice in need of assessment (IOM, 1990). Selected from a set of 496 candidate topics, 14 of those given high priority were for medical practice related to specific health conditions; six were equipment-embodied technologies applicable to a broad range of medical conditions and health services. Diagnostic imaging ranked among the six, with the term covering x-ray, the cross sectional modalities, PACS, and teleradiology. Criteria for selection of high-priority technologies were based on immediate focus on efficacy, safety, and appropriateness, as well as on the traditional concerns of health technology assessment for long-range health, social, and economic consequences. Priority-setting criteria for assessment included the potential of the candidate technology to improve patient care outcomes, to affect a large patient population, to reduce unit or aggregate cost, and to affect policy decisions for healthcare financing, resource allocations, and formulation of regulatory and reimbursement strategies.

Diagnostic imaging technologies scored high on all the criteria used by the Council to establish national priorities for assessment. In the matter of improvement of outcomes of care, new imaging modalities were seen to lessen the need for invasive diagnostic procedures, with increased opportunity for early detection of disease. As to the population affected, the Council cited a national survey on diagnostic imaging services, estimating an annual total of more than 170 million procedures (American Health Care Radiology Administrators, 1987), with more than one fourth of the $8.3 billion spent annually by hospitals on capital equipment accounted for by diagnostic imaging devices. In a later survey (Sunshine et al., 1991), diagnostic procedures in 1990 were estimated at 257 million.

With respect to national health policy decisions, the Council noted with concern the high capital and maintenance costs of the newer imaging technologies and the need to develop purchasing and reimbursement policies to justify and control the diffusion of imaging facilities. Despite its high priority, useful technology assessment of a total system of digital diagnostic radiology has been elusive, handicapped by lack of a working system that included digital radiography, PACS, and distributed workstations for clinical access to images.

The work of the Council on Health Care Technology was preceded a decade earlier by a related effort of an ad hoc Committee on Technology and Health Care, organized within the National Research Council (Wagner, 1979). This Committee addressed policy issues related to the diffusion of high-cost, equipment-embodied technology. Here, too, the voice of caution reigned, citing the impact of medical technology on total health care costs and the uncertainty of benefits. These concerns posed particular problems for economic justification of computer based medical information systems, including digital imaging, whose application spans the universe of clinical conditions and services.

However, in an appendix to the Committee's report, another voice was heard—that of the engineering and physician community. These groups were most knowledgeable about the fundamentals and details of computer/communications technology. They understood its direction of development and had a vision of its potential. Their view of government's role argued that large investment in a technology predicted to be of significant public benefit should be based not on piecemeal cost justification, but on achievement of the potential benefit as a matter of "national intent" (Lindberg, 1979). The economic rationale for government and industry collaboration in this view is more closely related to the imperatives of technology in Galbraith's new industrial state than to the restricted roles of government posed long ago by Adam Smith. In that earlier view, market forces were guided by "the unseen hand," and government intervention for public benefit was justified only when there was insufficient profit to be gained by one or a few to attract risky investment.

Although the Committee's final report did recognize federal funding of large scale technological development of medical information systems as a "reasonable approach," the cautious atmosphere of the times was reflected in a contemporary shift of research funds from development of new technologies to evaluation of current and tangible applications. Dedicated support of research and development of digital radiology had to come from other sources than the healthcare establishment. Fortunately the voice of development by "national intent" found expression in the move toward the national information infrastructure (NII). A decade after the report of the Committee on Technology and Health Care, the study director, Judith Wagner, gave an assessment of the status of digital imaging:

> In the past 10 years, the American Health Care System has been influenced by two independent forces, one driven by economics and the other by technology. The first is the force of cost containment; the second is the imperative of computer technology in medicine. To some extent, these forces have come from outside the health care system: the pressure to contain costs emanates from employers, insurers, and governments, not health care professionals, and the new computer-driven capabilities in medicine are riding the coattails of the information processing revolution underway in other industries. (Wagner, 1987)

Wagner went on to forecast that the ultimate test of digital imaging "will be to replace traditional film-based radiography," and that

> Digital x-ray will therefore be evaluated in comparison to an existing modality that already provides high resolution images at reasonable cost. Thus, the ability of digital radiography to produce images of comparable quality to those of x-ray at a cost that is less than current methods will be the key to future acceptance of this new technology. . . . The goal of such a system would be to develop an integral digital imaging department.

Almost at the time Wagner's paper appeared, breakthroughs in high-resolution image acquisition and high-speed data transmission had been made. Further, "riding the coattails of the information revolution," investment in health technology had shifted to a nationwide emphasis on large scale development of computer/communications technologies.

This leap of faith appeared to spring from visible and foreseeable trends—that is, ever-increasing capacity for information storage and transmission with continuous lowering of capital costs and improved functionality—along with the ability to capture images of sufficient spatial and contrast resolution to meet diagnostic quality standards. However infeasible the dream may have seemed, the pursuit of its fulfillment as a matter of national intent is the view that has prevailed. Simultaneously it was recognized that the technical demands were not to be satisfied within the medical–industrial community, but would need transfer of capabilities across scientific areas and agencies. Gradually the notion of an NII took shape, brought about by formal federal interagency and industrial collaboration, coming to fruition in the early 1990s with the creation of the National Coordination Office for High Performance Computing and Communications (HPCC, 1995).

Baltimore VAMC Experience

Paralleling the development of the NII, the capabilities of direct digital imaging in radiology reached satisfactory levels of image quality and functionality. Progress was sufficiently encouraging for the Department of Veterans Affairs (VA) to plan its new Baltimore Medical Center, scheduled to open in 1993, for high technology applications, with a fully digital imaging radiological service. At the time, from a cost/effectiveness point of view, the decision to make a near $10 million capital investment in a computed radiography/PACS in a radiology service producing a little over 30,000 examinations per year seemed absurd.

However, by 1997, capital costs for a similar system had fallen to one third of the original and demand for radiological services in the filmless environment had nearly doubled. Inherent and achieved productivity gains had been revealed and, in combination with film-based costs that were averted, were great enough to make the cost/effectiveness of filmless PACS plausible. In the spirit of development by national intent (that is, act now and evaluate later), cost studies of the BVAMC filmless PACS were deferred until the system was up and running, with issues of radiologist and clinician acceptance resolved and with routine operations in the filmless mode. The cost related analysis described here examines the experiences of the BVAMC in filmless radiology. Now producing approximately 60,000 examinations per year, the BVAMC's volume of diagnostic radiology services is a 1 percent microcosm of the VA's total production, which is in turn approximately a 2 percent microcosm of radiological services nationwide. If implemented throughout the VA, the BVAMC experience would translate to a capital investment of approximately $300 million, over 100 terabytes of information storage capacity, and transfer of $50 million in annual radiology department staff wages to the products and services of the computer and communication industries.

To date, efforts to assess the economic significance of PACS have been limited by the absence of a complete working system with computed radiography (Baaker, Greberman & van Gennip, 1992; Hailey & McDonald, 1996; Huda, Honeyman, Frost, Staab, 1996; Kuzmak & Dayhoff, 1996; Langlotz & Seshadri, 1996; van Gennip, 1995). The BVAMC experience offers the opportunity through direct observation of a pioneering application of filmless PACS, through access to the well-documented administrative records, and studies made during the period of transition to formulate and implement an approach to evaluation, guided by earlier evaluation efforts.

The analysis has been performed in two steps:

1. Study of the impact of filmless radiology at the BVAMC through comparative analysis of operations and costs before and after the transition from film-based procedures and with comparison during the same period to costs and productivity in the film-based operations of the Philadelphia VAMC.
2. Continuing study aimed at generalization of findings to determine the ranges of volume and mix of services for which filmless radiology can be appropriate in other settings.

Transition to Filmless Radiology

The new BVAMC was designed to include interstitial spaces for flexibility in introducing and upgrading cabled services. The justification was an awareness that a stream of advances in medical technology, including filmless PACS, would become increasingly feasible. The VA had developed its own information system, known as the Decentralized Hospital Computer Program (DHCP), over many years (VA, 1992). The goal of DHCP (now named V*IST*A) is the integration of digital images with electronic medical records through a strenuous program of in-house development, including its own PACS with state-of-the-art commercial components, and the creation of a set of "hybrid" systems of commercial products interfaced to DHCP. The implementation of filmless radiology through the program known as Hybrid Open Systems Technology (HOST) has been an important element of the VA systemwide expansion of its hospital information systems (HIS) and radiology information systems (RIS) to an Integrated Imaging System (VA, 1996/1997).

The introduction of filmless PACS in the BVAMC took place in four phases:

1. Film-based operations (by force of circumstance).
2. Transition to filmless PACS.
3. The current and continuing filmless mode.
4. The transition to merged operations for multiple VA facilities.

From the outset, radiology services and facilities at the BVAMC were planned to be filmless. However, as the time approached for opening of the new hospital in January 1993, it became apparent that the commercial PACS would not be ready for installation. The system had three major elements. Two of these, image acquisition (computed radiography, or CR) and display workstations, were available. A delay of several months was anticipated for the third, the information storage units at the heart of the PACS, responsible for creating and delivering filmless capability. This forced the radiology service to operate initially in a film-based mode. Although the delay in PACS installation was disappointing, it proved to be a blessing in disguise. It offered both a baseline period of film-based operation and an unpressured transitional period. The experience stands as a model for successful introduction of radically new technologies.

Fortunately, the image acquisition components for CR lent themselves readily to production of digitally captured, high-quality filmed images. In fact, the CR scanners were designed for that purpose. Still, the delay necessitated continued provision of a traditional film library for several months in the long-established mode of film creation, interpretation, and reporting. Fortunately again, for comparative evaluation, the delayed PACS delivery permitted an onsite accumulation of baseline data for a before and after design of operational cost analysis. With arrival and installation of PACS in mid-1993, a transitional phase of operation began. Images acquired by CR were still printed on film, but were also stored in the PACS unit for retrieval in diagnostic and clinical workstations. The commercial vendor provided an onsite representative for training in the use of PACS and monitors. To ease the transition, radiologists were free to choose between the digital image display or film images accessible in the traditional manner and stored in the file room. Within several months, the call for film images in active diagnostic procedures diminished to the vanishing point. By September 1993, films were no longer produced automatically, but only on demand.

At that point, the transition phase ended. All general radiographic images, except mammography, were captured by CR, and all were stored and displayed in digital form. A residual film capability was retained as backup and to produce hard copy for export to non-PACS sites or for research and other special purposes. By the beginning of Fiscal Year (FY) 1995, 92 percent of radiologists had experienced preference for PACS over film (Siegel, Pomerantz, and Protopapas, 1995), and the time had arrived to begin empirical studies of cost feasibility.

Phase 3, typified by operations in FY 1995 and 1996, forms the basis for cost comparison with Phase 1; it also serves as basis for projections to Phase 4. This last phase follows the merger of VAMCs at 40-mile-distant Perry Point and nearby Fort Howard into a single Maryland VAMC (MDVAMC), with radiological services administered from Baltimore.

During the transition to filmless radiology, dramatic changes took place in nearly every aspect of provisions of radiological services in the BVAMC. From the 1993 opening of the new VA hospital to the end of FY 1996, outpatient clinic visits rose 31 percent, while outpatient radiological examinations rose 73 percent (107 percent in weighted units). Over the same period, inpatient admissions rose 27 percent, while radiological examination for inpatients increased 17.4 percent (46 percent in weighted examinations). These increased demands were absorbed by radiologist and technologist staffing with rises of 17 and 13 percent, respectively, in full time equivalent (FTE) positions.

Cost Comparisons

The first analysis is one of monetary tradeoffs. This compares operations of Phase 1 (1993) and Phase 3 (1995) to determine the extent to which the cost of investment in filmless PACS is offset by the elimination of elements of cost inherent in film-based systems, costs that would have been incurred had operations continued in the film-based mode. This is followed by comparison of BVAMC in Phase 3 with an equivalent film-based installation, the Philadelphia VAMC. Several cost analyses are feasible, given the phased nature of the implementation. First is the comparison of Phase 1 and Phase 3 operations, estimating changes that would have been necessary for the film-based system to meet the volume of service demands currently being met by the PACS. There are threats to internal validity of inference from a prechange/postchange design for evaluation, stemming primarily from the confounding of attributes of interest in the two technologies with influential factors uniquely related to the two periods of operations (Flagle, 1989). For example, the observed characteristics of film-based operation are confounded with events surrounding the opening of the hospital, such as changes in the patient population during the early period of the hospital's opening and possible overstaffing of the services. Filmless operation is confounded with effects of the learning curve of a new technology, continuing updates to the evolving new technology itself, and a changed volume and pattern of demand for service modalities.

There are means of testing and adjusting for effects of confounding variables in each phase. This has been done by comparing actual productivities in Phases 1 and 3 with expected productivities drawn from the American Health Care Radiology Administrator's (AHRA) large-scale staff productivity survey of computed radiography (CR), computed tomography (CT), magnetic resonance imaging (MRI), ultrasound (US), and angiography (Hanwell and Conway, 1996). For radiologist productivity, guidelines given in VHA Directive 10-94-087 (September, 1994) set upper and lower bounds of expected number of procedures per year for diagnostic x-ray, CT, US, MRI, and interventional procedures (VA, 1994). In the calculations below, the upper bound (i.e., the highest level of expected radiologist productivity for each modality) has been used as the standard of comparison.

The availability of norms of productivity for major radiological service modalities for both technologists and radiologists enables the construction of composite measures of expected productivity for comparison with actual performance determined from radiology service fiscal year workload reports. Results are shown in Tables 6.1 through 6.4 for technologists, film librarians, and darkroom personnel, and in Tables 6.5 through 6.7 for radiologists in Phases 1 and 3 and for the Philadelphia VAMC.

The difficulty of direct comparison of Phases 1 and 3 at BVAMC is immediately apparent. A 42 percent increase in the number of procedures (from 36,563 in FY 1993 to 51,770 in FY 1995) was accompanied by a drop in radiography from 76 percent of total to 65 percent, the introduction of MRI, and an increase in the category "other" from 4 percent to 8.5 percent. Expected productivity for the "other" category, given a weight of 5 units in the VA radiology workload reports, where the unit weight is an administrative measure approximately eight minutes of technologist time, was interpolated from correlations of weights for service modalities with their norms of performance.

Some interpretations of Tables 6.1 through 6.7 bear on the comparison of productivities before and after implementation of the filmless PACS. Table 6.1 indicates a smaller than expected need for technologists than actually staffed in FY 1993. In FY 1995, the reverse is true post PACS when, as shown in Table 6.2, actual technologist staffing is 6.5 FTE less than would have been expected in film-based operation. The favorable comparison for

TABLE 6.1. Expected full-time equivalent staff: Baltimore VAMC, fiscal year 1993.

Modality	#Exams	%Total	Technologist[1]		Librarian[1]		Darkroom	
			Exams/ FTE	FTE	Exams/ FTE	FTE	Exams/ FTE	FTE
Radiography	27,960	76.5	2,760	10.1	25,437	1.08	49,551	.56
Tomography	4,393	12.0	1,690	2.6	11,425	.38	14,016	.31
Ultrasound	1,889	5.2	1,311	1.4	11,593	.16	17,545	.11
Angiography	769	2.1	354	2.2	2,268	.34	3,299	.23
Other	1,552	4.2	2,200[2]	0.7	17,500	.09	29,175	.05
Total	3,563	100	2,271[3]	17.0		2.05		1.26

Expected technologist FTE = 17.0

$$\text{Actual technologist FTE} = \frac{36,808 \text{ paid hrs}}{2,087} = 17.6$$

$$\text{Actual productivity} = \frac{36,563}{17.6} = 2,077 \text{ exams/FTE}$$

$$\text{Expected productivity} = \frac{36,563}{17.0} = 2,151 \text{ exams/FTE}$$

[1] Based on AHRA survey data.
[2] Exams/FTE interpolated from weights assigned in workload reports.
[3] Composite expected productivity = weighted sum of exams/FTE over all modalities.

technologist productivity is attributable in part to a 30 to 50 percent reduction in the amount of time required to perform a CT examinations (Reiner, Siegel, Hooper et al., 1998). Tables 6.3 and 6.4 shows the experience of the film-based operations in the Philadelphia VAMC, with actual technologist FTEs exceeding the expected number.

A similar picture emerges from Tables 6.5, 6.6, and 6.7, in which radiology staffing exceeded the norms in FY 1993 by 1.5 FTE, but was less by 1.64 FTE in FY 1995. Note that FTEs for expected and actual radiologist staffing in the Philadelphia VAMC are similar, supporting the use of the VA Directive upper bound of performance expectation as a criterion.

Using the difference between actual staffing and the composite expectation, expressed as FTE staff, and the costs of film and chemicals, an estimate can be made of the degree to which averted operating costs offset the annualized capital and operating costs of PACS technology.

TABLE 6.2. Expected full-time equivalent staff: Baltimore VAMC, fiscal year 1995 (hypothetical film-based operation).

Modality	#Exams	%Total	Technologist[1]		Librarian[1]		Darkroom Technologist	
			Exams/FTE	FTE	Exams/FTE	FTE	Exams/FTE	FTE
Radiography	34,129	65.9	2,760	12.36	25,347	1.35	49,551	0.69
Tomography	6,066	11.7	1,632	3.71	11,425	0.53	14,016	0.43
Ultrasound	3,341	6.5	1,603	2.08	11,593	0.29	17,545	0.19
MRI	2,309	4.5	855	2.70	5,129	0.44	4,831	0.48
Ang/Int	1,510	2.9	429	3.52	22,680	0.67	3,299	0.67
Other	4,415	8.5	2,200[2]	2.01	17,500	0.38	29,175	0.38
Total	51,770	100	1,961[3]	26.4		3.66		2.84

Expected technologist FTE = 26.4

Actual technologist FTE = $\dfrac{\text{paid hrs} = 19.9}{}$

$$\dfrac{41,539}{2,087} = 1,961 \text{ exams/FTE}$$

Expected productivity =

$$\dfrac{51,770}{26.4} = 2,602 \text{ exams/FTE}$$

Actual productivity =

$$\dfrac{51,770}{19.9}$$

[1] Based on AHRA survey data.
[2] Interpolated.
[3] Composite expected productivity = weighted sum of exams/FTE over all modalities.

TABLE 6.3. Expected full-time equivalent staff: Philadelphia VAMC, fiscal year 1996.

Modality	#Exams	%Total	Technologist[1]		Librarian[1]		Dark Room	
			Exams/ FTE	FTE	Exams/ FTE	FTE	Exams/ FTE	FTE
Radiography	33,932	79.1	2,760	12.29	25,437	1.33	49,551	0.68
Tomography	4,485	9.8	1,632	2.75	11,425	0.39	14,016	0.32
Ultrasound	2,429	5.3	1,603	1.52	11,593	0.21	17,545	0.14
Ang/Int	1,254	2.7	354	3.54	2,268	0.55	3,299	0.38
Other	3,707	8.1	2,200[2]	1.69	17,500	0.21	29,175	0.13
Total	45,807	100	2,102[3]	21.79		2.69		1.65

Expected technologists FTE = 21.79

$$\text{Actual technologist FTE} = \frac{62,580}{2,087} \text{ paid hrs} = 30.00$$

$$\text{Expected productivity} = \frac{45,807}{21.79} = 2,102 \text{ exams/FTE}$$

$$\text{Actual productivity} = \frac{45,807}{30.00} = 1,527 \text{ exams/FTE}$$

Expected librarian & darkroom = 4.23 FTE

Actual librarian & darkroom = 7 FTE

[1] Based on AHRA survey data.
[2] Exams/FTE interpolated.
[3] Composite expected productivity = weighted sum of exams/FTE over all modalities.

Cost Offsets to the Investment in Filmless Radiology

The investment in filmless radiology calls for a large expenditure in capital equipment. Current vendor quotations for the filmless system at the BVAMC total $2.8 million for equipment. Current quotations are less than half the cost in 1993 and are subject to further decline through competitive technological development, including the potential contribution of the VA's own DHCP integrated imaging system and its potential for reduced reliance on commerical sources.

Current service contracts, as quoted by the vendor, would carry an annual cost of $280,000 and include software updates to defer obsolescence. Current VA budgeting and accounting procedures treat depreciation with life expectancy of 8.8 years; they are used here to derive a lower bound of annualized capital and fixed cost. For comparison, calculations of annual fixed costs for hardware are repeated for a 5-year lifecycle. Combining annual share of depreciation and annual maintenance cost gives a range of capital and fixed cost attributable to filmless PACS. This is the target for seeking offsetting cost reductions through elimination of film-based operations.

TABLE 6.4. Expected full time equivalent staff: Philadelphia VAMC, fiscal year 1993.

Modality	#Exams	%Total	Exams/FTE[1]	FTE
Radiography	28,842	80.2	2,760	10.45
Tomography	3,395	9.4	1,690	2.01
Ultrasound	2,152	6.0	1,311	1.64
Ang/Int	868	2.4	354	2.45
Other	718	2.0	2,200[2]	0.32
Total	35,975	100	2,132[3]	16.37

Expected technologist FTE = 16.9

$$\text{Acutal technologist FTE} = \frac{41,867}{2,087} \text{ paid hrs} = 20.1$$

$$\text{Acutal productivity} = \frac{35,975}{20.1} = 1,790 \text{ exams/FTE}$$

$$\text{Expected productivity} = \frac{35,975}{16.9} = 2,129 \text{ exams/FTE}$$

[1] Based on AHRA data.
[2] Interpolated.
[3] Composite expected productivity = weighted sum of exams/FTE over all modalities.

The traditional meanings of the terms "depreciation" and "maintenance" are challenged by the nature of computer/communications technology. Change is continuous and the life of major components can be prolonged by internal modifications and updated elements. For analysis and planning, it is

TABLE 6.5. Radiologist productivity: Comparison of actual to expected (VA directive upper bound), Baltimore VAMC, fiscal year 1995.

Modality	#Exams	%Total	Exams/FTE[1]	FTE
Radiography	27,960	76.5	13,000	2.15
Tomography	4,393	12.0	3,500	1.26
Ultrasound	1,889	5.2	3,500	.54
Ang/Int	769	2.1	1,200	.64
Other	1,552	4.2	5,000[2]	.31
Total	36,563	100	7,462[3]	4.90

$$\text{Composite/expected exams} = \frac{36,563}{4.9} = 7,462$$

Acutal radiologist FTE = 6.4

$$\text{Acutal productivity} = \frac{36,563}{6.4} = 5,713$$

[1] From VHA directive 10-94-087.
[2] Interpolated.
[3] Composite expected procedures/FTE/year = weighted sum of the expected procedures over all modalities.

TABLE 6.6. Radiologist productivity: Comparison of actual to expected (VA directive upper bound), Baltimore VAMC, fiscal year 1995.

Modality	#Exams	%Total	Expected Exams/FTE[1]	Expected FTE
Radiography	34,129	65.0	13,000	2.63
Tomography	6,066	11.7	3,500	1.74
Ultrasound	3,341	6.5	3,500	.95
MRI	2,309	4.5	2,500	.92
Ang/Int	1,510	2.9	1,200	1.26
Other	4,415	8.5	5,000[2]	.89
Total	51,770	100	6,170[3]	8.39

Expected radiologist FTE = 8.39

Actual radiologist FTE = 6.75

$$\text{Expected productivity} = \frac{51,770}{8.39} = 6,170$$

$$\text{Actual productivity} = \frac{51,770}{6.75} = 7,669$$

[1] From VHA directive 10-94-087.
[2] Interpolated.
[3] Composite expected procedures/FTE/year = weighted sum of the expected procedures over all modalities.

TABLE 6.7. Radiologist productivity: Comparison of actual to expected (VA directive upper bound), Philadelphia VAMC, fiscal year 1996.

Modality	#Exams	%Total	Expected Exams/FTE[1]	Expected FTE
Radiography	33,932	74.1	13,000	2.61
Tomography	4,485	9.8	3,500	1.28
Ultrasound	2,429	5.3	3,500	.69
Ang/Int	1,254	2.7	1,200	1.05
Other	3,707	8.1	1,500[2]	.74
Total	45,807	100	7,191[3]	6.37

Expected radiologist FTE = 6.37

Actual radiologist FTE = 6.7

$$\text{Expected productivity} = \frac{45,807}{6.37} = 7,191$$

[1] From VHA directive 10-94-087.
[2] Interpolated.
[3] Composite expected procedures/FTE/year = weighted sum of the expected procedures over all modalities.

more useful to consider operational cost reductions as returns to capital investment and to determine the extent to which the stream of operational cost offsets can support the technology that produces it. Operational costs averted are of three types:

1. Elimination of capital costs uniquely related to use of film.
2. Operating costs averted through elimination of routine film-based technology, with increased productivity of radiology service personnel.
3. Economies of scale of operations achieved through enhanced productivity with larger volume and merger of outlying services into a single centralized department.

Capital costs averted are also of three types—those related to image acquisition, storage, and display. Estimates of the components of averted costs are given here for the specific experience of BVAMC, with some discussion of how they may be affected by trends in technology development, or special characteristics of the BVAMC installation.

The three aspects of capital investment, image acquisition, storage, and workstations are examined separately, since each has potentially different trends in technical performance, cost of manufacture, and rate of obsolescence. Progress in one may place demands in another. For example, the availability of higher resolution scanners will increase the information storage requirements, whose costs may in turn be reduced by acceptable techniques for image compression.

Capital Cost Offsets

Image Acquisition

Capital cost offsets credited to image acquisition are limited by the need to maintain a residual film-based capacity for a variety of reasons such as the generation of hard copy images for services external to PACS that are unable to receive digital images. Scanners used for computed radiography were in place for Phase 1 and have not been charged to the film-based system in this analysis. Given the need to maintain film producing capability, we are left without significant capital cost offsets in hardware for image acquisition.

Image Archiving

The 2,560 square feet of space in the BVAMC hospital designed for film-based operation and used for temporary film storage since 1993 was divided between PACS equipment/staff offices and a film file room during Phases 1 and 2. The current film library space of 1,280 square feet is a little over the median size reported by AHRA for services in the 80,000 to 100,000 per year range and should have been adequate for onsite storage. However, had a 6-year retention been hypothesized, offsite storage of 1,000 square feet would have been required, at an annual cost of approximately $20/square foot, or $20,000. In several years, films produced before mid-1993 will have been retired and the 1,280 square feet of film file room space made available for other use. At a construction cost of $180/square foot, with a 40-year life cycle for building and 10 years for renovations, the annualized value of the space is $28,280, which combined with elimination of offsite storage, yields a total of $48,280.

Retrieval and Image Display

Had the operation continued in the film-based mode, an array of viewboxes and alternators would have been required for viewing interpretation of old or imported films or research. Viewboxes are still needed for research or for reading hard copy from the residual film library or other sites. However, costs of alternators to handle high-volume film operations, 6 at $30,000 each, can be eliminated for a total of $180,000. If an annual 10 percent maintenance cost of $18,000 is added, the total offset is $38,000 to $59,000 per year.

Operating Cost Offsets

Film and Chemicals

Annualized film and chemical costs during the period in which all images were printed to film, Phase 1 and 2 of operations, totaled $125,000. Had fully film-based operation been in effect in Phase 3, during which the radiology workload increased more than 40 percent, from 36,563 to 51,770 examinations per year, total film and chemical costs would have risen to $217,000. Actual costs during the first year of filmless PACS totaled $54,000, thus averting direct costs of $163,000.

Technologist Productivity

The productivity of diagnostic technologists improved during the transition to filmless radiology at the BVAMC. Between 1993 and 1995, a 40 percent increase in examinations (70 percent in weighted examinations) was accommodated without an increase in the number of technologists handling the modalities in use during Phase 1, although one FTE was added with the addition of MRI. The apparent increase in productivity experienced can be partially explained by research studies in progress. These show 30 to 50 percent increases in inherent productivity in CR and 50 to 100 percent increases in inherent productivity in CT. The possibility that an additional factor was temporary overstaffing (or underloading) in FY 1993 is demonstrated in Table 6.1, with evidence from Table 6.2 that an expected staff of 25.4 FTE is comparable to an actual staff 19.9 FTE. In short, the perceived ability of the BVAMC to absorb an increased workload can be attributed to small early overstaffing followed by the inherently more productive filmless acquisition, storage, and interpretation of images.

Radiologist Productivity

Tables 6.5, 6.6 and 6.7give similar comparisons of actual to composite expected radiologist productivity in the three scenarios. The greater operational productivity of radiologists in filmless PACS is demonstrated, although
related to a much more complex process involving radiologist–clinician interactions. From the point of view of operational cost offsets, the reduction
in radiologist FTE is approximately $246,000 per year.

A summary of annual capital and operating cost offsets to the investment
in filmless radiology for the configuration of equipment and the volume and
mix of workload experienced at BVAMC before and after filmless PACS
operation is as follows:

Capital Investment Offset		
Elimination of alternators {8.8 yr–5 yr depreciation}		$38,545 to $54,000
with 10 percent annual service contract cost		
Recovery of film library space		
40-year building life		
10-year renovation intervals		$48,280
Operating Cost Reduction		
Reduction in film and chemicals		$163,000
Reduction in diagnostic technologists	5.5 FTE	$154,000
(from expected 25.4 to 19.9 FTE)		
Reduction in darkroom and library personnel	5.0 FTE	$130,000
(from 6.0 to 1.0 FTE)		
Reduction in radiologist FTE	1.64 FTE	$246,000
Total Cost Reduction		$779,825 to $795,280

The sum of cost offsets calculated above can be regarded as an annual
return to capital to cover depreciation, upgrades, and finance changes. It
falls near the upper bound of annual capital and maintenance costs of
$840,000 for 5-year depreciation, with a workload of 51,770 examinations
per year. The question arises, "What would volume of production have to be
for the capital costs of filmless costs to be completely offset by replacement
of film-based procedures?" To answer the question, we need to estimate comparative unit costs as a function of volume of examinations per year.

Unit Cost Analysis

On first examination, the economic aspects of filmless radiology display the
familiar characteristics of much technological innovation in human enterprise. With a large capital expenditure, a new technology is introduced, one
with potential for increasing productivity to an extent that justifies the investment made in it. Typically, justification of a new technology on the ba-

sis of costs alone requires either increased production to spread the increased capital or reduced unit variable costs attributable to the new technology. A comparative analysis of unit costs as a function of volume of production reveals the range of volume over which each of the compared technologies is cost beneficial. In the event the new technology does not achieve a lower unit cost over the meaningful practical range of production volume, the gap between unit costs is a monetary measure of the costs of achieving the qualitative benefits offered by the new technology.

A typical relationship of unit cost as a function of volume of production has the form:

$$\text{Unit cost} = \frac{\text{Annualized Capital Investment} + \text{Annual Fixed Cost}}{\text{Annual Volume of Production}} + \text{unit variable cost}$$

The unit cost function is used here for construction of Table 6.8, which is a comparison of unit costs for film versus filmless technologies over a range of an annual number of examination, N, from 20,000 to 100,000 year. Unit variable cost is estimated as the sum of unit costs of personnel inputs plus unit costs of consumable inputs. For estimation of unit cost for each category of personnel, expected or actual number of exams per year is divided into typical annual wage. Film and chemical costs for film based operations are derived from the Baltimore VAMC experience in FY 1993.

Capital and fixed costs used here are those specific to the introduction of filmless PACS, and do not include fixed costs similar for both technologies (e.g., administration, overhead and general services). Interest charges or possible effects of inflation or deflation on current costs have not been taken into account.

The elements of unit costs are shown in Table 6.9 at breakeven volume, denoted N^*, where unit costs are identical, the point at which the savings in variable or operating costs offset the difference in annual capital and other fixed costs.

The rate of decline in unit cost with increasing volume is made up of several factors—first the broad sharing of capital and fixed cost; second, the internal operating economies of scale observed in increasing productivity in each service modality with rising production volume. The internal operating economies of scale in image production are evident in the AHRA staffing studies. For example, gains in technologist output between the smallest and largest annual volumes are 60 percent in conventional radiography, 38 percent in computed tomography, and nearly 400 percent in interventional angiography over the range of total production. The phenomenon is less significantly related to the inherent productivity of technologists in the service modality than to the inherent instability of workloads in small service units.

In addition to volume of operations, the mix of service modalities is a significant variable in overall unit cost of production of radiological examinations. This is evident in Tables 6.1 through 6.6. Used earlier to estimate staffing requirements, these tables can be used again to estimate the contributions to overall unit cost of types of imaging staff. Unit costs are calculated for two scenarios, updating figures to reflect added gains in productivity and increased wage scales in FY 1997.

- First, expected performance of a film-based system with 1997 workloads, service mix, and productivity.
- Second, observed performance of a filmless system with similar workload and service mix. Reduction of costs of film and chemicals, darkroom and library personnel, and adjusting expected imaging staff and radiologist productivity to reflect experience at BVAMC after filmless PACS installation.

Capital and fixed costs used in the analysis are those related to the two technologies compared. They are direct costs and do not include general overhead costs incurred independently of the imaging technologies or expenses common to both modalities.

Table 6.8 gives unit costs across a range of annual volume from 20,000 to 100,000, comparing film to filmless systems for the two depreciation periods. For 8.8-year depreciation, crossover or breakeven occurs between 20,000 and 30,000 exams per year; for a 5 year lifecycle, the crossover occurs between 30,000 and 40,000. To be more precise about crossover points, we can equate the expression for film and filmless unit costs and solve for the unknown volume at which equality occurs. This is carried out in Table 6.9 in which the crossover point, designated N^*, is seen as 26,918 and 38,827, for 8.8-year and 5-year depreciations respectively. These values are approximated in other studies, one that places breakeven near 50,000 examinations per year (Langer & Wang, 1996), another that places breakeven at 4 years (Braunschweig, Pistich & Nissen-Meyer, 1996),

Table 6.9 tells an interesting story about the economics of filmless radiology. By definition the direct unit costs of both technologies at the cross-

TABLE 6.8. Comparative unit cost[1] per examination versus total examinations per year.

Examinations per year	Unit cost (dollars) for 8.8-year depreciation		Unit cost (dollars) for 5-year depreciation	
	Film	Filmless	Film	Filmless
20,000	62.14	68.71	62.93	80.81
30,000	60.70	58.76	61.22	66.81
40,000	59.97	53.76	60.31	59.87
50,000	59.54	50.77	59.85	55.61
60,000	59.26	48.76	59.52	52.81
80,000	58.89	46.28	59.09	49.37
100,000	58.64	44.79	58.83	47.21

[1] Unit costs contain the annualized capital costs applicable to CR and PACS and film technology, but do not include other equipment, e.g. CT and MRI. Unit operating costs do not include overhead or operating costs similar for both technologies.

TABLE 6.9. Components of unit costs at crossover point N^*.

Depreciation rate (in years)	8.8		5.0	
Component of unit/cost	Filmless	Film-based	Filmless	Film-based
Capital & maintenance				
Net annualized cost	598,181	86,734	840,000	102,280
Unit capital cost	22.22	3.22	21.63	2.63
unit operating costs				
technologist	17.60	27.37	17.60	27.37
Librarian & dark room[1]	0.60	3.26	0.60	3.26
Film & chemical[1]	1.06	2.90	1.06	2.90
Radiologist	19.55	24.28	19.55	24.28
Total unit cost	61.03	61.03	60.40	60.40

$$N^*_{8.8} = \frac{598,181 - 86,734}{(27.37+3.26+2.90+24.28)-(17.60+.60+1.06+19.55)} = \frac{511,44}{19.00} = 26,918$$

$$N^*_5 = \frac{840,000-102,280}{(27.37+3.26+2.90+24.28)-(17.60+.60+1.06+19.55)} = \frac{737,720}{19.00} = 38,827$$

over point are the same, but their components are very different. To bring the filmless unit cost down to the level of the essentially constant unit cost for the film-based system, the annualized capital cost has to be offset by reductions credited to elimination of film and film related personnel and to increases in productivity of radiologists and diagnostic technologists. For example, at the breakeven point for the 5 year depreciation cycle, the portion of unit cost transferred to capital cost from personnel and film costs is $19.00, roughly a third of the total unit variable or operating cost. In broader terms, what we are seeing is a transfer of costs from wages for health services personnel, and automation of the film library to products and services of the computer/communications industries, totaling almost $700,000 per year for the 38,827 examinations at breakeven.

Examination of the equation (Table 6.9) for volume of examinations at breakeven reveals the sensitivity of breakeven points to the validity of estimation of the variables involved. The denominator is essentially the difference in the variable operating costs of the technologies compared. It is a relatively small difference between large numbers, which accentuates the influence of errors of estimation of any of its components; in a denominator, it has strong influence on the breakeven point. However, all its components are objective and subject to measurement. The numerator, on the other hand, is a product of several administrative assumptions and policies: rates of obsolescence and depreciation, cost of maintenance and upgrades, salvage values, and workload levels at which discrete increments of capacity increase must be made. In the absence of clearcut guidelines for handling depreciation and financing, it is useful to speak in terms of potential returns to capital requirements as a function of scale of operations and reductions in unit variable costs.

Effects of Scale of Operations

Tables 6.8 and 6.9 give comparative unit cost's of radiological procedures across a range of annual volume from 20,000 to 100,000 examinations per year. In the computations, the annualized capital cost of PACS is based on the BVAMC configuration of equipment and its prices as quoted in fall 1997 across the entire range. This assumption penalizes the unit cost of PACS at lower levels of volume where a less costly configuration would be adequate. Conversely, the assumption underestimates unit cost of PACS at higher levels of demand, where additions to acquisition and storage capabilities would be required.

To examine the effect on unit annualized capital cost of configurations appropriate for the higher and lower levels of demand, 1997 prices for ongoing PACS installations in five VAMCs have been obtained, covering a range of planned volume from 30,000 to 100,000 examinations per year:

Planned volume (exams per year)	Cost	Cost of workstations
30,000	$1,969,950	28 %
55,000	$2,822,400	48%
70,000	$3,619,000	38%
100,000	$4,500,238	46%
100,000	$5,212,640	60%

The annual cost of a full service contract, including software upgrades, averages 10 percent of purchase price. The relationship between capital investment, and designed capacity, can be approximated by a linear relationship of the form:

$$I = aN + b,$$

where a is the marginal capital investment required for an additional annual unit of production, and b is the intercept on the zero demand axis.

When fitted to the data above, expected initial capital investment, I, as a function of planned annual volume, N, can be approximated by the relationship

$$I = 41.2\,N + 734{,}000$$

The annual dollar return to capital requirements, including upgrades, depreciation, and interest (RTC) is the product of N and the unit cost saving, S, less service contract cost, taken as 10 percent of the initial investment, I

$$RTC = N \cdot S - .1\,I = N \cdot S - .1\,(41.2N + 734{,}000)$$

The return on investment (ROI) is RTC as a percentage of initial investment, I,

$$ROI = \frac{N \cdot S - .1\,I}{I}$$

a quantity which, using earlier data that places S near $19.00 per exam, gives annual return on capital investment ranging from 19 percent for 30,000 examinations per year to 32 percent for a planned 100,000 examinations per year installation.

For the BVAMC quotations, where I is $2,800,000

$RTC = 19.0 \times 55,000$ *exams per year* $- \$ 280,000 = \$ 765,000$

$$ROI = .273$$

These returns can be enhanced by any offsets to the price of filmless PACS through avoidance of purchase or salvage value of equipment and space specific to film-based operations.

An example of such offsets appears in earlier estimates for the BVAMC. The calculated RTC and ROI investment attributable to increased productivity and elimination of film are only part of the total returns. Depending on local circumstances, some capital or fixed cost eliminations can be deducted from the first cost of filmless PACS equipment, either as cost averted or salvage value. Examples are costs of film handling equipment (e.g., alternators, and film library space).

The philosophy of the HOST project within the DHCP program has been first to achieve a working implementation of a commercial product, then to examine feasibility of incorporating elements of the product into the DHCP system or substituting DHCP elements for commercial ones. The filmless PACS installation at BVAMC was purchased as a complete system to enhance the likelihood of a smooth transition, by delegating to the vendor responsibility for interfacing components and providing installation, service, and training. Although purchase costs have declined substantially since the original contract, all three of the major elements are subject to further decline.

The most critical elements of initial cost are computed radiography systems. Their cost is high, quoted at $200,000 to $300,000, calling for 5,000 to 8,000 additional examinations per year to justify an additional scanner and to hold total capital costs within the norm. Competition is expected to force lower costs in the near future, but this component, essential to filmless radiology, remains an obstacle to economic merger of small outlying services into central services.

The cost of information storage is also subject to lowering either by continuing advances in technology or through acceptance of data compression (SCAR, 1997).

Most likely to experience sharp decreases in cost are the image display units. As noted in the table of quotes, workstations account for 40 to 60 percent of total cost.

Summary and Conclusions

The introduction of CR and PACS in the radiological services of the BVAMC in FY 1993 has been followed by substantial increases in personnel productivity and in utilization of radiological services by clinicians, particularly in outpatient services. The increases in both productivity and utilization appearing in FY 1995 continued to increase in FY 1996 and FY 1997 and into FY 1998. The gains in personnel productivity can be seen in administrative statistics since FY 1993. An increase in total examinations from 36,353 to 51,770, a 42 percent rise, was absorbed with a 13 percent increase in technologist staff. Weighted work units of production have increased 68 percent, indicating a shift toward more complex modalities. Weighted work units of production per paid hour had increased from 3.9 to 5.3 between 1993 and 1997.

To make a valid comparison of performances before and after PACS, standards of expected productivity for technologist and radiologists were developed, using a national survey of radiology staff productivity over the range of service modalities and a VA guideline for radiologist productivity. From comparisons, using the standards, of expected productivity applied to the workloads in FY 1993 and FY 1995 with actual productivity in BVAMC, it is estimated that the increased personnel productivity and elimination of film related activities result in average savings over film-based operations $19.00 per examinations which, for current performance of 55,000 examinations per year in BVAMC returns about $1,000,000 annually to apply to capital and service costs of filmless PACS.

Since 1993, the prices of filmless PACS equipment have fallen markedly; and annual service contracts, at 10 percent of the purchase price, have become more comprehensive, including software upgrades. Prices are sensitive to scale of operations. An analysis of the set of current (1997) quotations for filmless PACS systems in the VA, ranging in planned capacity from 30,000 to 100,000 examinations per year, gives:

Expected Initial Investment =
$41.2 × number of planned evaluation × $734,000

Under this relationship, annual return to capital equipment needs ranges from 0 for a planned capacity around 9,000 to 32 percent for a planned capacity of 100,000 examination per year. The picture is improved by deducting averted capital costs of film related space and equipment. The capital investment required for filmless PACS is expected to decline further. Competition is entering the market for digital image acquisition units, and information storage capacity is increasing at the same time data compression techniques are lowering storage needs. Moreover, image display monitors of adequate resolution to serve all the needs of the V*IST*A Integrated Imaging System are becoming available. The prototype PACS and workstations in the Wilmington VAMC were assembled for half the expected cost of a commercial system.

At present, however, the high costs of scanners for digital radiography, at $200,000 to $300,000 per unit, remain an obstacle to merging outlying small services into a large central system. At a marginal cost of $41.20 per additional planned annual examination, economic justification requires a minimum of an additional 5,000 to 7,000 examinations per year.

Return to annual capital and service cost is proportional to the savings in variable cost. The values used here are derived from experiences in Baltimore. Another VAMC considering the transition to filmless radiology can determine its baseline and predicted productivity by replicating the calculations used to produce Tables 6.1 to 6.7, using its own radiology workload and staffing reports.

The BVAMC experience with filmless radiology has revealed a profound change in practice patterns of physicians and radiologists with the introduction of filmless PACS, particularly in outpatient services. Between 1993 and 1996, outpatient radiology examinations increased 73 percent, with weighted units up 107 percent. A trend to increased utilization has been observed also in the Philadelphia VAMC, but the effect is less pronounced.

As VA policy emphasizes the shift from inpatient to outpatient services, the phenomenon of increasing orders for radiological services per outpatient visit calls for examination. Within radiology, a few explanatory variables can be recognized (e.g., the effect of greater accessibility of images or the shortened reporting time and enhanced opportunity for direct or asynchronous communication between radiologists and clinicians. Whatever the explanation of increased demand for services, the fact of the increase has implications for cost, content, and quality of care.

It is evident by this time that filmless radiology can be justified economically anywhere, as in the case of the BVAMC, where the cost savings inherent in PACS can be realized and the scale of operations is sufficient to meet capital requirements.

Although the analysis here has focused on the costs of diagnostic radiological services, other areas needing further economic analysis have been revealed, particularly to assess the consequences of increased clinician demand for radiological services elicited by ready availability of images on clinical workstations. The situation will likely be intensified as other imaging is incorporated into an integrated multispecialty system.

Concerns for security and confidentiality have ramifications for administration as telemedicine and merger with outlying services increase image communication outside the central imaging service.

Beyond aspects of delivery of imaging services, there are economic implications for the health care organization and for the community at large, as the implementation of filmless PACS transfers a significant portion of operating budgets from the traditional health service workforce to products and services of the computer/communications industries.

References

American Health Care Radiology Administrators (AHRA). Statistical survey. Sudbury, MA: AHRA, 1987.

Baaker AR, Greberman M, van Gennip EMSJ, eds. Technology assessment of PACS. Int J Biomed Computing 1992, 30 (34).

Braunschweig R, Pistich C, Nissen-Meyer S. Digitale radiographie = Kosten-nutzenanalyse. Radiologie 1996, 306–314.

Flagle CD. Pitfalls in evaluation. Proc First International Conference on Image Management and Communication. Washington DC: IEEE Computer Society Press, 1989.

van Gennip EMSJ, Talmond JL, eds. Assessment and evaluation of information technologies in medicine. Amsterdam: IOS Press 1995.

Hailey D, McDonald I. The assessment of diagnostic imaging technologies: A policy perspective. Health Policy, 1996, 36, 185–197.

Hanwell LL, Conway JM. Utilization of Imaging Staffs Measuring Productivity: Sudbury, MA: American Healthcare Radiology Administrators, 1996.

High Performance Computing and Communication (HPCC). America in the age of information. A report of the committee on information and communications. Bethesda, MD: HPCC, 1995.

Huda W, Honeyman JC, Frost MM, Staab EV. A cost analysis of computed radiography and picture archiving and communication systems in portable radiography. J Digit Imaging, 1996, 9(1), 39–44.

Institute of Medicine (IOM). National priorities for the assessment of clinical conditions and medical technologies, ME Lara & C Goodman, eds. Washington DC: National Academy Press, 1990.

Kuzmak PM, Dayhoff RE. DHCP VISN-Level Teleradiology and PACS, VA Washington Information Management Field Office, Draft for comment, June 1996.

Langer S, Wang J. User and system interface issues in the purchase of imaging and information system. J Digit Imaging, 1996, 9(3).

Langlotz CP, Seshadri S. Technology assessment methods for radiology systems. Radiol Clin North Am 1996 (May)3.

Lindberg DAB. The development and diffusion of a medical technology. In: JL Wagner, ed, Medical technology and the health care system: A study of the diffusions of equipment-embodied technology, Washington DC: National Academy Press, 1979.

Reiner BI, Siegel EL, Hooper FJ, et al. Effect of film-based versus filmless operation of the productivity of CT technologists. Radiology 1998, 207, 481–485.

Siegel EL, Pomerantz SM, Protopapas Z. PACS in a "digital hospital": Preliminary data from the phase III evaluation of the experience with filmless operation of the Baltimore VA Medical Center. Proc IMAC, 1995.

Society for Computer Applications in Radiology (SCAR). SCAR technology forum: Understanding compression. Reston, VA, SCAR, 1997.

Sunshine JH, Marby MR, Bansal S. The volume and cost of radiological services in the United States in 1990. Am J Rev, 1991, 157, 609-618.

Veterans Affairs (VA). Decentralized hospital computer program. Washington DC: VA, 1992.

Veterans Affairs (VA). Veterans health information systems and technology architecture. Washington DC: VA, 1996/7.

Veterans Affairs (VA). FTE based staffing guidelines for evaluating radiologists, VHA directive 10-94-087. Washington DC: VA, 1994.

Wagner JL. Cost containment and computerized medical imaging. Int J Technology Assessment in Health Care 1987, 3(3), 343–354.

Wagner JL, ed. Medical technology and the health care system: A study of the diffusions of equipment-embodied technology. A report by the committee on technology and health care. Washington DC: National Academy Press, 1979.

7
Computed Radiographic Imaging and Artifacts

CHARLES E. WILLIS

Computed radiography (CR) is the only practical method available today that is capable of acquiring in digital form and diagnostic quality all the ordinary radiography exams produced by a moderately sized hospital. There are other devices being developed for direct digital capture of large field radiographic projections, but none with the combination of acceptable radiographic speed and diagnostic image quality that CR boasts. Thus, for now, without CR, there can be no filmless radiology.

CR has existed as a means of radiographic imaging in laboratories since 1975, when the premier Luckey patent for the apparatus was issued.[1] Fuji introduced the first commercial CR, the Model 101, into clinical practice in Japan in 1983 (Sonoda, Tanaka, Miyahara et al., 1983). The first clinical use of CR in the United States occurred in that same year, but CR has only been in routine practice in the United States since 1992.

Currently, as shown in Figure 7.1, there are three major manufacturers (Fuji, Kodak, and AGFA) and many original equipment manufacturers (OEM) that supply devices from the primary vendors. Fuji CR continues to be the most widely used, with multiple generations and models of scanners, including dedicated chest units and table units. The discussion that follows is intended to be applicable to all CR without regard to manufacturer. For terminology and features that are manufacturer specific, the manufacturer's literature is the best reference.

Physical Basis of CR

CR is founded on the physical process of photostimulable luminescence. Although this process has been known for some time, details of the mechanism, as shown in Figure 7.2, are still only theoretical (von Seggern, Voight, Knupfer, and Lang, 1988). Material that exhibits photostimulable lumines-

---

[1] Luckey G. Apparatus and methods for producing images corresponding to patterns of high energy radiation. US Patent 3,859,527; January 7, 1975. Revised No. 31847; March 12, 1985.

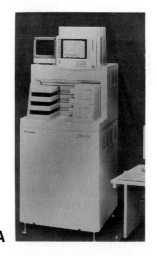

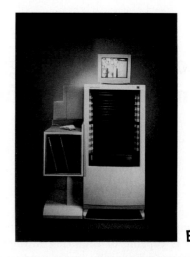

A

B

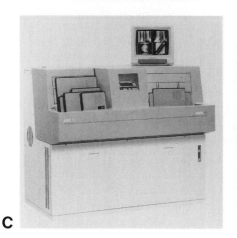

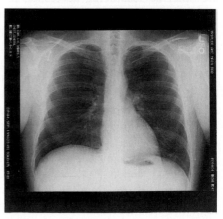

C

D

FIGURE 7.1. Three commercial CR scanners and a clinical CR image. (A) Fuji AC3S (courtesy Fuji Medical Systems U.S.A., Inc.). (B) Kodak Model 400 (courtesy Eastman Kodak Company). (C) Agfa ADC-70 (courtesy Agfa-Gevaert N.V.). D. A diagnostic quality CR chest radiograph of the author.

cence, that is, the photostimulable phosphor (PSP), is similar to intensification screens in conventional radiography, but with a subtle difference. When x-rays strike the PSP, valence band electrons are excited into the conduction band by photoelectric interactions. These electrons de-excite by producing fluorescence, so much so that it is possible to expose conventional film inside a CR cassette (Chotas, Dobbins, Floyd et al., 1981). Because the PSP has local potential energy traps caused by impurities in its crystalline structure, some of the excited electrons are trapped in an excited state. The trapped electrons constitute CR's latent image. Exposing the PSP to the proper wave-

Conduction Band

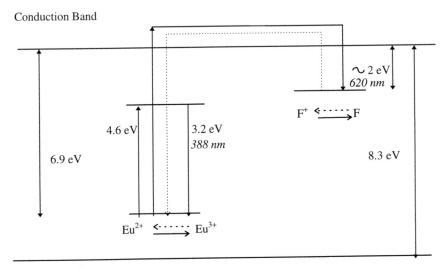

Valence Band

FIGURE 7.2. Quantum diagram of presumed mechanism of photostimulable lumines-cence. When radiation is absorbed by the phosphor, electrons are excited from the valence band into the conduction band. Absorbed radiation can also ionize an elec-tron from europium forming a stable "electron hole." Electrons in the conduction band are free to de-excite back into a vacancy in the valence band or into a eu-ropium hole by emitting light. An "F-center," a halogen vacancy in the crystal lat-tice, forms another energy level that conduction band electrons can occupy by emitting light. Electrons in the F-center constitute the CR latent image. Laser light excites the electrons into the conduction band where they can de-excite into eu-ropium electron holes by emitting light which is collected by the CR scanner.

length of light can free the trapped electrons and allow them to de-excite. The light that is emitted by the freed electrons is termed photostimulable luminescence.

Electrons will not stay trapped indefinitely. On their own, by random ther-mal mechanisms, the electrons will gain enough energy to escape the traps and de-excite by phosphorescence. This implies that the CR latent image will fade over time, so it is important that the halftime for decay of the trapped electrons is relatively long. The halftime for fading is about 19 hours for typical imaging plates. It is also important that the halftime for decay of the stimulated luminescence is short; if not, the material would not accom-modate rapid scanning. Any trapped electrons that remain after scanning are removed or erased by bathing the material in high intensity light.

The chemical composition of the PSP in its most common clinical use is barium fluoro halide: europeum, where the halide could be bromine or io-dine; or a mixture of the two, where europeum is the impurity. The chemical composition, primarily barium, determines the x-ray absorption characteris-

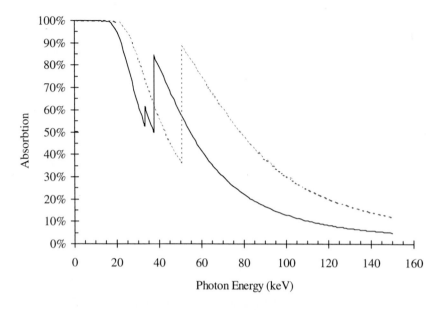

FIGURE 7.3. Energy absorption diagram for BaFB*X*:Eu imaging plates. Solid line is for Kodak GP-25 imaging plates. Broken line is for Kodak Lanex Regular screens. Note that the k-edge for the imaging plate is 37.4 keV, which is lower than that for this rare earth intensification screen, which is 50 keV (courtesy of Eastman Kodak Company).

tics of the PSP. The AGFA plates substitute strontium for fluorine. As shown in Figure 7.3, the k-edge of the PSP is about 37 keV, which is different from (lower than) rare earth screens in routine clinical use (Boguki, Trauernicht, and Kocher, 1995). CR's greater sensitivity to scattered radiation has been ascribed to this lower k-edge. Perhaps another observation is that the appropriate technique for CR might utilize a different accelerating potential (kVp) than the conventional screen/film used previously in a department.

As shown in Figure 7.4, the amount of light that can be harvested from the PSP increases linearly with radiation dose over a wide range, perhaps five decades (Takahashi, Kohda, Miyahara et al., 1984). Although the signal from the CR imaging plate is linear over a wide range, the scanner may have more modest performance.

Engineering Aspects of CR Image Acquisition

Construction of Imaging Plates and Cassettes

As shown in Figure 7.5, the structure of the imaging plate is not unlike that of a conventional intensification screen. The PSP is a ceramic material incapable of self-support, so it is mixed with a binder material and coated onto some sort of

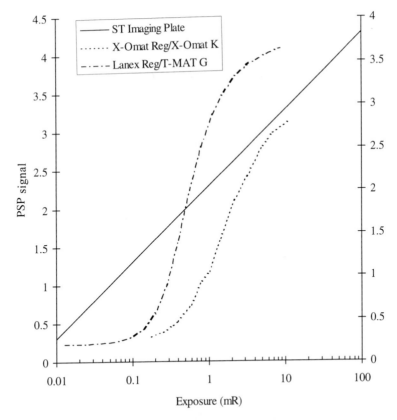

FIGURE 7.4. Graph of linear signal response function for CR. The signal obtained from the imaging plate after log amplification is linear with the log of exposure over four decades in exposure. For comparison, the linear region of screen/film response is approximately one decade, with the useful range of exposures of about one-and-one-half decades (Lanex Regular/T-MAT G data courtesy of Eastman Kodak Company).

support structure. Fuji uses polyester, because their scanner requires flexibility of the imaging plate, while Kodak uses lead and an aluminum honeycomb panel. The phosphor layer is also sealed with a protective layer that must be transparent to both the laser light and the stimulated emissions.

Imaging plates are constructed in two varieties. Standard resolution plates have a thick phosphor layer (230 μm) in order to increase x-ray absorption. High resolution plates are made with a thinner phosphor layer (100 μm). This means that, during scanning, the laser beam will spread less, providing more sharpness, but the plate will have a slower radiographic speed, similar to conventional extremity cassettes. This improved sharpness is realized without an increase in the sampling rate. Some scanners will not accommodate both standard and high resolution plates.

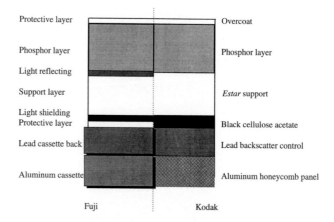

Fuji

Kodak

Protective layer — Overcoat
Phosphor layer — Phosphor layer
Light reflecting
Support layer — *Estar* support
Light shielding
Protective layer — Black cellulose acetate
Lead cassette back — Lead backscatter control
Aluminum cassette — Aluminum honeycomb panel

FIGURE 7.5. Structure of the imaging plate. The imaging plate consists of layers, not unlike conventional intensification screens. The thickness of the layers affects the properties of the imaging plate. Although Fuji plates do not incorporate the lead and aluminum honeycomb layers of the Kodak plate, the lead backing and aluminum cassette material are functionally equivalent.

There have been different manufacturing generations of imaging plates— six for Fuji and at least two for Kodak. These different generations have different compositions and conversion efficiencies. Some are appropriate for use only in specific models of scanners. Operation with mixed generations of plates introduces undesired variation. The fact that a particular generation of plate is no longer manufactured is no guarantee that one will not show up in any given facility.

CR cassettes are designed to have the same form factor as conventional screen/ film cassettes, although some common conventional sizes are absent, notably 9 × 9 in. Because the composition and thus x-ray transmission and backscatter characteristics of the cassettes and plates differ from conventional cassettes, photodetectors should be recalibrated. Fuji has added lead backing to its CR cassettes after experiencing backscatter artifacts (Tucker, Souto, and Barnes, 1993). Recent improvements have been made in cassette sturdiness.

Laser Scanning and Detection of the CR Latent Image

After the radiographic examination, the imaging cassette is introduced into a device that removes the imaging plate from the cassette. (In a dedicated chest or tabletop unit, this step is not necessary.) The imaging plate is exposed to laser light to stimulate the trapped electrons and develop the latent image. Helium-neon lasers (633 nm) and solid state lasers (680 nm) produce light that is capable of harvesting the trapped electrons (Matsuda, Arakawa, Kohda et al., 1993). The laser beam is deflected across the imaging plate by a galvanometer-driven or rotating polygon mirror, as shown in Figure 7.6.

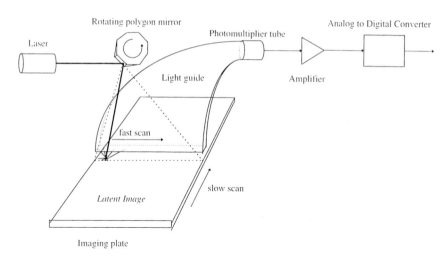

FIGURE 7.6. Diagram of the CR laser scanning mechanism.

This is the fast-scan or scan axis. The plate is advanced mechanically along the slow-scan or subscan axis to expose more of the plate to the beam.

The color of the emitted light (violet) is quite different from the laser light (red), so stray laser light can be filtered out. The stimulated light is collected and directed to one or more photomultiplier tubes, so that the tiny light signal can be converted into a useful electrical current. The electric current is converted either by a logarithmic, linear, or square root amplifier into a usable analog voltage. The voltage is sampled by an analog-to-digital converter (ADC) to produce a 10-, 12-, or 16-bit digital code value. The timing of the ADC is coordinated with the motion of the laser beam and imaging plate to determine the dimensions of the digital picture elements, or pixels, and hence the sampling matrix for the image. The ADC code values stored in a computer file constitute the raw digital image.

CR systems use approximately the same number of pixels to represent an image, that is, a 2000 × 2000 pixel matrix, regardless of the size of the cassette (with the exception of Fuji's HQ option, a 4000 × 4000 pixel matrix, and very asymmetrical cassettes). That means that the pixel dimensions are smaller for smaller cassettes. The pixel dimensions determine the smallest features that can be represented in the digital image with perfect registration, or the Nyquist limit. The actual limiting spatial resolution is always less. For this reason, many CR practitioners recommend using the smallest cassette size that will capture the projected anatomy. However, for the same radiation exposure, the smaller the pixel dimensions, the fewer x-ray quanta that contribute to the signal from each pixel. The quantum noise in each pixel increases as the pixel dimensions decrease. This adversely affects the

TABLE 7.1. Effect of cassette size on spatial resolution and quantum noise.

Cassette size	Nyquist limit (lp/mm)	Quantum noise (est.)
14 × 17 in.	2.5 – 3.0	1.5%
10 × 12 in.	3.3 – 4.3	2.1%
8 × 10 in.	4.2 – 5.0	3.1%

ability to distinguish features that differ little in radiographic contrast; and the low contrast detectability suffers.

Table 7.1 shows the effects of matrix size on spatial resolution and quantum noise. The Nyquist limit reported is a range for all manufacturers. The quantum noise at 1 mR is estimated by assuming 50 percent absorption of x-rays by the imaging plate (Barnes, 1993) and approximating the beam as monochromatic 40 keV photons. The quantum noise is about one-third of the total system noise at this exposure level for the smallest pixel size (Kato, 1994).

Processing the Digitized Image

In all CR systems, the raw digital image is processed to improve its appearance. It is important to understand the steps in processing the image, as illustrated in Figure 7.7, because errors at each stage give rise to different types of artifacts.

Preacquisition Processing

This category of processing carries a historical name that today is perhaps a misnomer. In early CR devices, this processing was performed on a low intensity prescan of the imaging plate to determine the appropriate photomultiplier gain setting for the main scan. Present systems use this set of processes to normalize the image for further processing, so acquisition processing might be a better title (Nakajima, Takeo, Ishda et al., 1993).

The first step in acquisition processing is made by the operator, who tells the scanner which examination and view the imaging plate contains. Many subsequent steps rely on the correct identification of view by the operator.

The first task for the CR machine is to determine number and orientation of views in the raw digital data. This is called partitioned pattern recognition. Each view can then be analyzed independently. Although offering multiple views on a single cassette is good practice in conventional radiography, it is a complication for CR.

Within an exposure field, it is important for the CR to distinguish the useful region of the image by locating the edges of collimation. This is called exposure field recognition, or collimation detection. Some CR systems further segment the image by defining of the edges of the anatomic region.

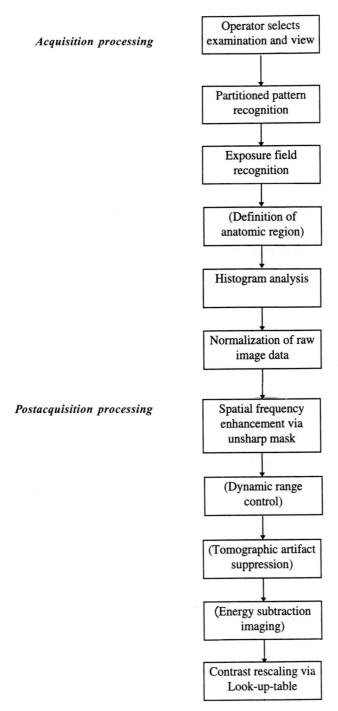

FIGURE 7.7. Flow chart of CR preacquisition and postacquisition processing.

Once the useful image is located, the CR can disregard the image information beyond the collimator boundaries when performing further analysis.

The default method for determining the useful signal for most CR scanners requires the construction of a gray-scale histogram of the image, which is a graph with signal value on the x-axis and relative occurrence on the y-axis (i.e., a spectrum of pixel values; see Figure 7.8). By identifying peaks and valleys in this histogram, the analysis algorithm attempts to distinguish among the parts of the histogram which are contrast media, bone, soft tissue, skin, and unattenuated x-rays. If not excluded from the histogram, the signal from the parts of the imaging plate beyond the edges of the collimators produces a low signal tail on the histogram that can interfere with histogram analysis.

The result of histogram analysis is a set of instructions for the normalization of raw image data for standard conditions of speed, contrast, and latitude. Rescaling is optimized for the specific anatomic examination. Newer systems employ neural networks that have been trained to analyze a broad range of histogram shapes for a specific anatomic view. An effective histogram analysis program produces images of consistent quality over a wide range of variations in mAs and kVp.

Two other methods for normalizing the raw data do not depend on histogram analysis. In area sensing or semiautomatic mode, an average pixel value is cal-

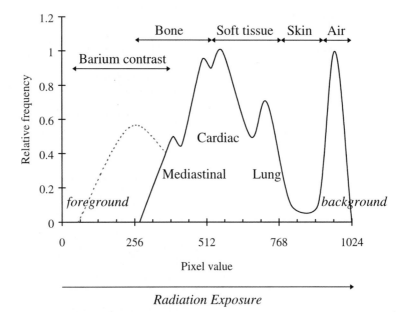

FIGURE 7.8. Image histogram. Regions from left to right, that is from low exposure to high exposure, are bone, soft tissue, skin, and air. The broken line indicates the presence of contrast media. The shape of the histogram depends on the anatomy imaged. The extent of the histogram before rescaling depicts the subject contrast and depends on the accelerating potential. The location of the histogram along the x-axis before rescaling depends on the dose to the imaging plate.

culated from a specific area or areas of the data. The raw data is then rescaled according to the expected average value. Like phototimed technique, the position of the patient relative to the sample area is critical. In fixed mode, the CR functions at a fixed radiographic speed much like a conventional screen/film system without rescaling. The results thus depend on appropriate radiographic technique. Acquisition processing determines how the raw data is to be modified to prepare for subsequent processing, so errors here tend to be irreversible.

Postacquisition Processing

A major advantage of CR over conventional film/screen radiography is that, once acquired, the digital image data is readily manipulated to produce alternative renderings (Boguki, Trauernicht, and Kocher, 1995; Ishida, 1993). A great deal of effort has been directed toward determining the optimum image processing for the wide variety of anatomic views.

By contrast rescaling (also known as contrast processing, gradation processing, tone scaling, and contrast enhancement), the normalized CR pixel values can be rapidly rescaled by means of a look-up table (LUT). The intent of the rescaling is to optimize contrast and density, either to enhance the conspicuity of clinical features or simply to mimic the appearance of a conventional film/screen radiograph. Typically a variety of LUTs can be selected, including linear and nonlinear transformations, as well as inverse (black-bone) transforms. In Fuji CR, this LUT is controlled by the values selected for four parameters, namely contrast (curve) type, rotation amount, rotation center, density shift. Although described here first, contrast rescaling is the last application of postacquisition processing.

By frequency processing, also known as Unsharp Masking and Edge Enhancement, the appearance of the CR digital image can be modified to accentuate or suppress details according to their spatial frequency. The unsharp mask technique takes the original image, applies a low pass filter to generate a blurred image, and subtracts the blurred version from the original image to yield a difference image that contains only the high spatial frequency components of the original. This difference image can be amplified and then added back to the original image to create an image in which the contrast of high frequency details such as edges, small objects, and noise is increased. Specific frequency ranges or object sizes can be selected through control of the kernal size (frequency rank) of the unsharp mask, the characteristic of the low pass filter. The degree of enhancement is controlled by selection of the boost factor (frequency enhancement), the amount of amplification of the difference image. The amount of amplification can be applied negatively or according a nonlinear function (frequency type) of spatial frequency. While frequency processing has been shown to be especially useful for increasing conspicuity of lines and tubes, it can also give rise to artifacts.

A variation of the unsharp mask technique is used to modify the global contrast of the image while preserving the local contrast in either the low signal region (mediastinum or subdiaphragmatic) or the high signal regions (air contrast or skin margin). In Dynamic Range Control (DRC), the boost is applied according to a nonlinear function of gray-scale; the result is that all important clinical details can be displayed on a medium with limited latitude or dynamic range, such as a laser printer or CRT.

Another application of the unsharp mask technique provides suppression of streaking artifacts in conventional rectilinear tomography. In this case, the enhancement is applied in one dimension only.

Agfa's global contrast enhancement is an integral part of MUlti Scale Image Contrast Amplification (MUSICA®). MUSICA® decomposes the image into a set of coefficients corresponding to image features in twelve specific frequency subbands. The image is decomposed according to a Laplacian pyramid transform (Burt, Adelson, 1983). During acquisition, rather than via histogram analysis described above, both global contrast enhancement and normalization are accomplished by automatic modification of the coefficients of subbands of the Laplacian pyramid.

Energy Subtraction Imaging, also called Dual Energy Subtraction, is performed using two images, either acquired sequentially or simultaneously with different filtration. These images are used to reconstruct a soft tissue-only image and a bone-only image. This technique is used in chest imaging to improve the conspicuity of pulmonary nodules.

It is important to recognize that depending on the CR interface, sometimes only the normalized data may be available to the workstation in a filmless radiology system. Most workstations provide features to perform gradation processing (typically window and level adjustments), but other forms of postacquisition processing are typically available only on specialized workstations or on the laser printed image. Most workstations do provide other real-time image manipulation features, such as zoom, that are advantageous over a static rendering. Some workstations provide capabilities for individualized nonlinear LUTs to correct for monitor gamma variation.

Control of Exposure Factor Selection

Toleration of Overexposure

CR's tolerance of inappropriate exposure factor is a double-edged sword: underexposure and overexposure are not obvious from the appearance of the normalized CR image (Freedman, Pe, Mun et al., 1993). Instead of a light or dark film, derived indices of exposure based on the results of the normalization process are used to monitor patient radiation exposure. These indices differ among manufacturers. From a radiation management prospective, it is critical to insure that the index is reported along with the image in any clinical practice of CR (Willis, Leckie, Carter et al., 1995).

The process of normalization feature of the raw digital data, as described above, provides a feature of CR known as autoranging. After normalization, the overall appearance of an image acquired at one-tenth of the usual radiographic technique and an image acquired at ten times the usual technique are almost indistinguishable from the properly exposed exam. The noise characteristics of each of these images is, however, quite different, as is the radiation dose to the subject. The quantum mottle in the underexposed image may mask significant low contrast clinical features. Beyond delivering more radiation than necessary to the subject, features in the overexposed image may be clipped if the CR scanner lacks sufficient dynamic range to capture them.

Because of auto-ranging, changing the x-ray beam current (mAs) has little effect on the overall appearance of the image. Unfortunately, this is the primary method used by technologists to modify the appearance of conventional screen/film radiographs. Changing the accelerating potential (kVp), however, changes the subject contrast and can have a dramatic effect on the CR image.

Derived Indices of Exposure

To facilitate exposure factor control, each CR manufacturer has provided a numerical parameter that yields information about the amount of signal harvested from the imaging plate. The parameter, therefore, also provides some indirect information about the quantity of radiation that exposed the plate. To make meaningful comparisons among CR scanners, the calibration of these parameters, called Sensitivity (Fuji), Exposure index (Kodak), and "lgM" (AGFA) is critical (Willis, Weiser, Leckie et al, 1994).

In Fuji CR, the Sensitivity or S-number is calibrated so that an exposure of 1 mR from an 80 kVp x-ray beam to a standard type imaging plate will yield $S=200$, when the plate is scanned using a test menu in semiautomatic mode. The same plate would be expected to yield $S=2000$ for a 0.1 mR exposure and $S=20$ for a 10.0 mR exposure. In normal operating mode, the S number follows a similar dose response: one-half the exposure results in double the S number using the same anatomic examination. Comparisons of S numbers acquired using different anatomic exams are not typically quantitative. Anecdotal evidence suggests that observers will reject images that have S numbers between 800 and 1000, because of perceived graininess. An image with a latitude of 2.0 (i.e., two decades of subject contrast), will be clipped if its central value is at 10 mR, or $S=20$. Images with greater latitude are common, and these will encounter problems at higher S numbers. For these reasons, hospitals monitor the S number as a quality assurance indicator. It is important to understand that the S number is affected by many technical factors, especially collimation, and should not be regarded a perfect dosimeter. The visibility of clinical landmarks and the clinical question to be addressed should be the determinants in decisions to reject or repeat an exam.

In Kodak CR, the exposure index is the average pixel value calculated within the defined anatomic region. The exposure index is calibrated so that for a general purpose screen, a 1 mR exposure from an 80 kVp beam filtered by 1.5 mm Al and 0.5 mm Cu will yield a value of 2000. An exposure of 0.1 mR results in an exposure index of 1000 and an exposure of 10 mR results in a value of 3000. A doubling of exposure will cause an increase in the value exposure index of 301; halving the exposure causes a drop in exposure index of 301.

The exposure index reported in AGFA CR is the log of the median of the image histogram, or lgM. The index is reported for the useful histogram, that is, after elimination of features outside the collimators. The scanner is calibrated with a beam of 75 kVp with 1.5 mm added Cu filtration for a 20 uGy dose to the plate. The plate is scanned using a speed class setting of 100 to yield a Scan Average Level (SAL) of 1800, where SAL is the average of all pixel values in the image. For a given speed class setting, the value of lgM varies according to the log of radiation dose to the imaging plate. A doubling of exposure should result in an increase in the value of lgM by 0.301; halving the exposure should reduce the lgM value by 0.301.

Although the change in the values of these exposure indices with changes in exposure is clear, neither the appropriate target values nor the range of acceptable values is well established in the literature. These values are likely to depend on the specific radiologic projection.

Adjustment of Phototimers

The primary method of exposure factor control is phototimed technique. It is important to recognize that the composition of CR cassettes and imaging plates is different than conventional cassettes and that phototimers can not be expected to deliver the same dose to the receptor. Phototimer adjustment is not straightforward with CR because in normal operating modes, CR delivers a uniform density regardless of phototimer setting. Phototimers could be set to yield a specific Skin Entrance Exposure, a specific value of exposure index, or a specific density using conventional screen/film and then used with CR. Because of histogram analysis, phantoms that worked well with screen/film may not produce appropriate results with CR.

Artifacts

Artifacts are features in an image that mask or mimic clinical features. Every practitioner of CR should appreciate that artifacts will occur and should be able to recognize their sources, as shown in Figure 7.9. Specific CR artifacts occur in addition to artifacts encountered in the practice of conventional screen/film radiography, such as mispositioning, patient motion, and inappropriate technique selection (Oestmann, Prokop, Schaefer et al., 1991; Solomon, Jost, Glazer et al., 1991). Although artifacts are well documented for Fuji CR, it would be unwise to assume that these artifacts are not encountered with the systems from other manufacturers. One approach to the classification of artifacts is to divide

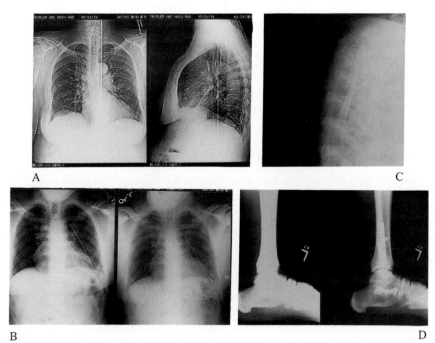

FIGURE 7.9. Four examples of CR artifacts. (A) The vertical lines are from dust on light collection optics. Short horizontal lines are cracks in the imaging plate. (B) Acquisition processing failure secondary to mispositioning of patient. (C) Grainy images because of underexposure. Both are underexposed images of left hilum of same patient: left 1/5, right 1/10. (D) Right image shows appropriate postacquisition image processing. Left image demonstrates incorrect processing.

them according to the culprit, whether hardware, software, or operator. For purposes of this discussion, they are categorized according to the mechanism of interference with image acquisition, processing, and display.

Interference with Projected X-Ray Beam

Anything of appreciable density that winds up between the focal spot of the x-ray tube and the phosphor layer of the imaging plate can cause an artifact. This includes loose parts of the collimator, jewelry worn by the patient, contrast media on patient support, foreign matter on the cassette, or debris on the imaging plate itself.

Defects in the Imaging Plate

Mechanical damage to the imaging plate, such as scuffs or cracks, can mimic fractures and signs of pneumothorax. Discoloration of the plate can also cause nonuniform harvesting of the latent image, resulting in splotches in the image.

Manifestations of Scatter

CR is reputed to be more sensitive to scatter than conventional screen/film. Before the addition of lead to Fuji cassettes, the "tombstone" artifact was common especially in bedside radiology. This was the image of a metal clip located on the reverse of the cassette. The "lightbulb" artifact, where central portions of the image appeared lighter than the periphery, was also attributed to backscatter.

Interference with Detection of the Stimulated Light

Dust and debris somehow find their way to the light collection optics. This results in one or more lines parallel to the subscan axis.

Digitization Errors

The CR image is a digital approximation of an analog radiographic projection in terms of both geometry and intensity. There are errors inherent in the pixelization process. These include contouring (quantization error) and stairstep effects on linear features that are diagonally oriented, which are usually only apparent under extreme values of contrast adjustment and zoom, respectively. Moire patterns can be encountered when using a fixed grid. Aliasing with fixed grid depends on pixel matrix and display zoom factor. As mentioned above, spatial resolution and noise characteristics vary with plate size.

Errors in Automatic Image Processing

These artifacts have attracted the most attention. Errors that confound pattern recognition and histogram analysis are usually unrecoverable. Failure of the algorithm to detect radiation field can be caused by nonparallel collimation, multiple fields, poor centering, the presence of implants, and failure to follow collimation rules. These errors cause inappropriate histogram analysis and result in images that have been incorrectly rescaled. Errors can also be caused by incorrect exam selection. Some exams are just technically difficult, even with screen/film, and some exams just do not seem to produce good images. A good deal of development has been directed to improving CR pattern recognition and histogram analysis algorithms.

Errors in postacquisition processing tend to be recoverable. Inappropriate parameter values can cause clinical features to be clipped. For example, too much contrast can cause the hilar region of some patients' lungs to disappear into blackness. Extreme values can cause a "rebound" effect along boundaries of light and dark borders. The dramatic effect of the parameter values and the ability to change them introduces a configuration management problem. It is important to verify what parameter values are resident in the CR scanner and to ensure that all machines have the same values. In some cases, improper exam selection only changes the postacquisition processing, so the appropriate image can be recovered.

Underexposure

As mentioned, underexposure results in a increase in quantum mottle and a loss of contrast in dense features. Observers usually complain about image quality at one-half to one-fourth of the appropriate exposure.

Overexposure

The results of overexposure include a loss of latitude, loss of dense features, and loss of thin features. An overexposed PA chest might include disappearance of one or both clavicles and dropout of the hilum.

Double Exposure

The source of double exposures can be the classic operator error or can be the result of computer error, for example, during a power interruption or communications failure, or erasure failure, which could be secondary to inadequate erasure or overexposure.

Display Errors

In a CR department that routinely prints hardcopy images, the entire repertoire of laser printer problems can cause artifacts. These include incorrect density calibration, chemistry problems, roller pickoff, light leaks, and laser misalignment. In an operation that depends on softcopy images, CRT monitors can introduce artifacts. The sources of CRT artifacts include calibration/matching, improper LUT, and software errors.

Data Dropout

Infrequently, the CR image may contain missing lines or missing pixels caused by memory problems, digitization problems, or communication errors.

Summary and Conclusions

CR is a marvelous technology that provides diagnostic quality images in digital form so that they can be readily modified, distributed throughout the hospital, and conveniently archived for future reference. The sickest patients in the hospital benefit from the improved consistency of autoranged CR images in bedside exams. However, the wonders of CR do not absolve practitioners from following conventional principles that govern the judicious application of radiation for diagnostic purposes. CR is not yet a "solved problem." Improvements in CR can only come from an understanding of the technology and a critical eye for clinical details.

References

Barnes GT. Digital x-ray image capture with image intensifier and storage phosphor plates: imaging principles, performance, and limitations. Digital Imaging. AAPM Monograph No. 22. Madison, WI: Medical Physics Publishing, 1993, pp. 25–48.

Boguki TM, Trauernicht DP, Kocher TE. Characteristics of a storage phosphor system for medical imaging. Technical and Scientific Monograph No. 6. Rochester, NY: Eastman Kodak Company, 1995.

Burt PJ, Adelson EH. The Laplacian pyramid as a compact image code. IEEE Trans on Comm 1983, 31(4): pp 532–540.

Chotas HG, Dobbins JTIII, Floyd CE et al. Single exposure conventional and computed radiography image acquisition. Invest Radiol 1981, 26, 438–445.

Freedman M, Pe E, Mun SK et al. The potential for unnecessary patient exposure from the use of storage phosphor imaging systems. Proc SPIE, 1993, 1897, 472–479.

Ishida, M. Digital image processing. Fuji Computed Radiography Technical Review No. 1. Tokyo: Fuji Photo Film Co., Ltd., 1993.

Kato H. Photostimulable phosphor radiography design considerations. In Seibert JA, Barnes GT, Gould RG, eds. Specification, acceptance testing and quality control of diagnostic x-ray imaging equipment. Medical Physics Monograph No. 20. Woodbury, NY: American Association of Physicists in Medicine, 1994, pp. 731–770.

Matsuda T, Arakawa S, Kohda K et al. New technological developments in the FCR9000. Fuji Computed Radiography Technical Review No. 2. Tokyo: Fuji Photo Film Co., Ltd., 1993.

Nakajima N, Takeo H, Ishida M et al. Automatic setting functions for image density and range in the FCR system. Fuji Computed Radiography Technical Review No. 3. Tokyo: Fuji Photo Film Co., Ltd., 1993.

Oestmann JW, Prokop M, Schaefer CM et al. Hardware and software artifacts in storage phosphor radiography. Radiographics 11, 795–805.

Solomon SL, Jost RG, Glazer HS et al. Artifacts in computed radiography. AJR 1991, 157(1), 181–185.

Sonoda M, Tanaka M, Miyahara J et al. Computed radiography utilizing scanning laser stimulated luminescence. Radiology 1983, 148, 833–838.

Tucker DM, Souto M, Barnes GT. Scatter in computed radiography. Radiology 1993, 188, 271–274.

von Seggern H, Voight T, Knupfer W, Lang G. Physical model of photostimulated luminescence of x-irradiated BsFBr:EuZ$^+$. J. Appl. Phys. 64(3), 1988, pp. 1405–1412.

Willis CE, Leckie RG, Carter J et al. Objective measures of quality assurance in a computed radiography-based radiology department. Proc SPIE 1995, 2432, 588–599.

Willis CE, Weiser JC, Leckie RG et al. Optimization and quality control of computed radiography. Proc SPIE 1994, 2164, 178–185.

Section 3

8
Digital Radiography

MATTHEW T. FREEDMAN AND DOROTHY STELLER ARTZ

This chapter is divided into two sections: An introduction to the basic principles of digital radiography and a discussion of its clinical applications.

Basic Principles of Digital Radiography

Digital radiography is an essential component of filmless radiology. It is used to provide a digital input of radiological information from chest, bone, abdominal, and other conventional radiography. The alternative method of entering these standard forms of radiographs into a digital imaging system is to digitize the film obtained in a conventional way. The direct digital capture of digital information provides specific advantages both for worker efficiency and image quality. Improved worker efficiency occurs because of time savings that result from not having to manually feed the standard film into the film digitizer. It is possible to simultaneously create a film (if one is desired) and produce the digital information for storage and soft copy display. Digital radiography also allows for distributed acquisition and processing of images. Because the film need not be transported back to the central radiology facility, digital radiographic devices can be placed close to the intensive care units or other high volume users and can transmit the digital information to both the radiology and special care units.

Image quality is improved because the digital recorder has a wider range of exposure information that can be captured. This additional exposure information allows the radiologist to adjust the window level through the full range of exposure information, thereby improving the visibility of regions of the image that on conventional radiographs would be under- or overexposed, such as the retrocardiac region on a chest radiograph, the up side of the decubitus view of the colon in an air contrast barium enema, or the soft tissues of an extremity. Alternatively, images can be created that use lookup tables, making it possible to bring the lightly exposed and heavily exposed regions into better optical density balance using different forms of histogram equalization.

This wider exposure range and the image processing software allow the system to accommodate incorrect exposures. This has major value in bed-

157

side radiography. Radiographs tend to maintain a near optimal optical density regardless of the amount of exposure used (Freedman, Lo, Nelson et al., 1992; Schaefer, Greene, Oestmann et al., 1989).

Much work has been done by the manufacturers of digital radiographic systems to make them easy to use, and successive generations of this equipment have resulted in progressive improvement of image quality and ease of operation. The images that will be shown in this chapter have been created on the Fuji AC-3 and Fuji 9000 systems. These systems are based on storage phosphor technology. AGFA and Kodak also produce digital radiography systems based on storage phosphor technology, and there are digital systems based on other technological approaches that are in preclinical trial. These competing systems are likely to have certain features that overlap those of the Fuji system and features that are unique.

Advantages and Disadvantages

The main advantages of digital radiography result from the separation of the four components of a radiograph: image acquisition, image processing, image storage, and image display. This differs markedly from conventional screen film radiography, where acquisition is based on a combination of the screen and film; image processing is based on the screen, film, and chemical processing; and storage and display are film based. The main disadvantages of digital radiography are its lower spatial resolution for certain high resolution examinations and the difficulty of learning how to use digital radiography equipment correctly. Some digital radiographic systems print their images smaller than life size. This, in most cases, has not been shown to affect the conspicuity of disease, but can be annoying to radiologists in three settings:

- When first becoming accustomed to the smaller film size;
- When needing to compare a smaller image to a life-sized image; and
- When needing to measure objects on the film.

Although each of these can be overcome with experience and patience, they remain an inconvenience.

Image Acquisition

Several different digital radiography technologies are under development. The only technology commercially available in the United States at this time is based on storage phosphor technology. In storage phosphor technology, the initial image capture is on a flat panel of phosphor material (called an imaging plate or IP) that replaces the conventional screen and film. Although automated cassette-less plate changers are available, most often the IP is placed into a cassette.

When exposed to an x-ray beam, this phosphor material records the pattern of x-ray exposure and stores it as energy for several hours. Because the stored energy slowly decays, the IP should be processed within several hours. The cassette containing the IP is then placed into a plate reader that exposes the IP to a focused laser beam. This laser light beam raises the energy level in the IP atoms, which then releases their stored energy, emitting light. This emitted light is captured using a light guide that is linked to a photomultiplier receptor that converts the light into electrons. These electrons are then processed electronically to produce the image. In this process, the image is divided up into small picture elements (pixels), each of which represents a very small portion of the image. In a typical system, a chest radiograph that is originally 14 x 17 inches will be divided into 2000 pixels across the 14-inch width and 2500 pixels along the 17 inch length, or a total of five million pixels. Image processing is performed on individual pixels or groups of pixels.

The imaging plate and plate reader currently accommodate various IP sizes and two different resolutions. Selected examinations (such as hands, wrists, elbows, toes, and breast images) are best performed with the higher resolution system. In others, the lower resolution system is sufficient. Higher resolution requires a three to four times higher patient exposure. It results in slower machine throughput and increases the cost of data storage. It should be used only when clinically appropriate.

Image Processing

Image processing consists of several sequential events: data clipping, spatial frequency processing, and look-up table adjustments. In some cases, histogram equalization is also performed. In some cases a special algorithm is used to identify the edge of the collimated beam. These are usually set to be performed automatically.

Data Clipping

The IP accepts and stores a wider range of exposures than does conventional radiographic film. Processing the raw data directly into an image would produce a very low contrast image, as shown in Figure 8.1. To produce an image of adequate contrast, at least two of the three commercial systems clip the total image data to remove values of very low and very high exposure. The computer algorithm that does this is complex, in that it is looking for the pattern of exposure values seen in radiographs of the body part being radiographed. In effect, the algorithm is identifying the regions of clinically relevant exposure. Because the algorithm is looking for a pattern of exposure appropriate to a body part, if the incorrect body part is entered into the identification terminal of the unit, the image that results may be substandard.

This function is illustrated in Figure 8.1, which demonstrates contrast in a chest radiograph. Compared to an abdominal radiograph, for example, a

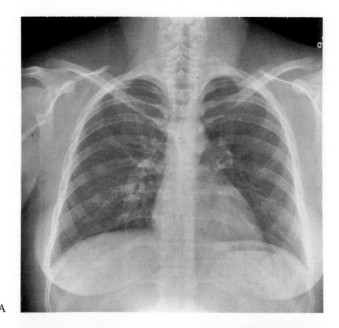

A

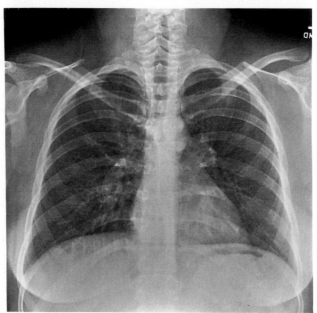

B

FIGURE 8.1. Chest radiograph processed at low and high contrasts to simulate the effect of improper clipping of data. (A) Low contrast image of the chest. (B) Standard contrast image of the chest.

conventional chest radiograph shows a wider range of optical densities in the chest image. Radiologists have long chosen to use a screen film system with different contrast scales for these two body parts. In digital radiography, the exposure range of an image plate of specific resolution is the same for all body parts. The data clipping, in part, simulates the use of different screen film combinations for different body parts.

Sensitivity: The S Number

Once the system has defined the boundaries of clinically useful exposure, it has to correct for differences of overall under-or overexposure. It does this so that the final displayed image is neither too dark nor too light. The algorithm defines a factor called the S number that reflects the average exposure within the clinically useful range. This S number is then used to adjust the values of each pixel so that the final image display will be at an appropriate optical density.

The S number is indirectly related to the exposure reaching the imaging plate. In general, an average of the S numbers of multiple properly exposed images would be expected to fall between 100 and 500 on standard resolution imaging plates and 50 to 150 on high resolution IPs. Because of the complexity of the algorithm and variations in patient size and the size of organs within the patient (e.g., large heart) the S number on an individual film has less importance.

Spatial Frequency Processing

Spatial frequency processing is used for two purposes: edge enhancement and noise suppression. In the AGFA system it also provides a method for histogram equalization.

Edge Enhancement

Slight degrees of edge enhancement produce a pleasing appearance in digital radiographs that some radiologists prefer, but which has not been shown to affect clinical diagnosis (Rosenthal, Good, Costa-Greco et al., 1990). As shown in Figure 8.2, moderate degrees of edge enhancement produce images with an overprocessed look that radiologists do not like initially. However, it can improve the visibility of specific types of structures and specific findings of anatomy or disease. It is of use in seeing large structures in low exposure regions of an image and can improve the visualization of tubes in the mediastinum or the lower cervical spine in the lateral view, as shown in Figure 8.3. Although it improves the visibility of some structures, it obscures others and should not be used as the only image viewed.

The Fuji and AGFA systems provide methods of enhancing specific ranges of spatial frequencies. High spatial frequencies are seen in sharp edged objects;

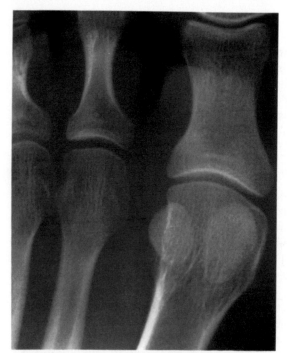

A

FIGURE 8.2. Digital radiograph of great toe. (A) No edge enhancement is used. The trabecular pattern appears slightly blurred compared to (B). (B) Mild edge enhancement has been used. The image appears of higher contrast and the trabeculae are easier to see. They appear sharper, but not distorted.

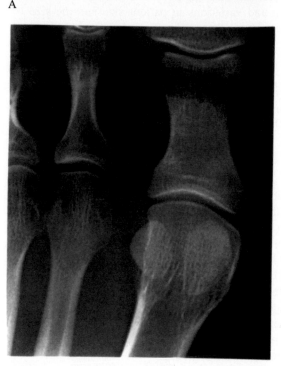

B

FIGURE 8.3. Digital radiograph of lower portion cervical spine (lateral view) to demonstrate effect of increased edge enhancement in demonstrating more of the cervical spine. (A) Standard processing with mild edge enhancement. The seventh cervical vertebra is seen, but the first thoracic vertebra is poorly seen, particularly its posterior elements. (B) Moderate edge enhancement performed to emphasize larger structures. The first thoracic vertebra and its posterior elements are better seen.

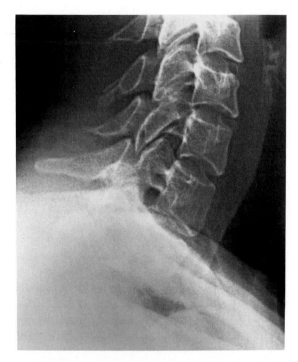

A

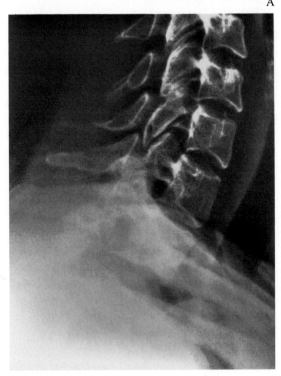

B

lower spatial frequencies are seen with less sharp objects. Adding emphasis to high spatial frequencies enhances small sharply defined objects, such as lung markings and fine bony trabeculae; adding emphasis to lower spatial frequencies enhances larger, less sharp objects, such as lung masses, the edges of bowel and kidneys, and larger bony structures.

Image Blurring

Spatial frequency processing is also used to blur objects in images. This is most often used to blur the visibility of noise so that the image becomes more pleasing to radiologists. This blurring can, however, obscure objects that would remain visible within the background noise, as shown in Figure 8.4.

Look-Up Table Adjustments

The look-up table converts the pixel values to luminance values on a monitor or optical density on a film print. These changes can be used to affect overall optical density and/or the contrast scale of the image, as shown in Figure 8.5. As an analogy to screen film imaging, look-up table adjustments are equivalent to changes in the film characteristic or "H and D" curve.

Histogram Equalization

Histogram equalization is a method of image processing in which the range of optical densities in an image are changed in such a way that a smaller range of optical densities will be present in the final image. There are several mathematical methods of histogram equalization that can be used. So far, the main clinical use has been to enhance the optical density and thereby improve the conspicuity of structures projected behind the heart and within the mediastinum on chest radiographs, as seen in Figure 8.6. Although it has not yet been proven whether this is clinically useful, there is evidence that radiologists prefer this type of image processing.

Collimator Edge Identification

Algorithms to allow the computer to identify the edge of the collimated field exist in both the AGFA and Fuji systems. This helps the image processing system identify the portion of the image dataset that contains clinically useful information. It also allows the region outside of the edge of collimated beam to be displayed as a gray background, thereby decreasing the glare around the radiographed body part. This is useful in the display of collimated images of the extremities and neonatal chest, as illustrated in Figure 8.7.

Image Storage

In a conventional radiology department, image storage is accomplished by storing the original film. Once the data is in digital form, the data can be

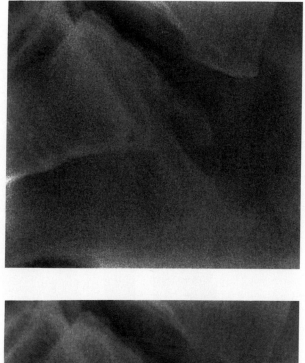

A

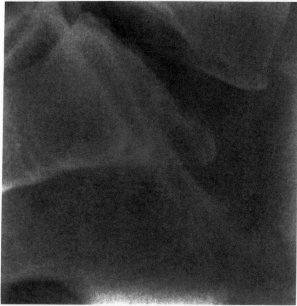

B

FIGURE 8.4. Digital radiograph of the lumbosacral junction (lateral view) to demonstrate image blurring in decreasing the visibility of noise. (A) Enhanced radiograph. The small punctate regions of noise are more easily seen. The visualized noise is mainly from quantum mottle. (B) Blurred or smoothed image. The noise is still visible, but the regions of variation in density are larger.

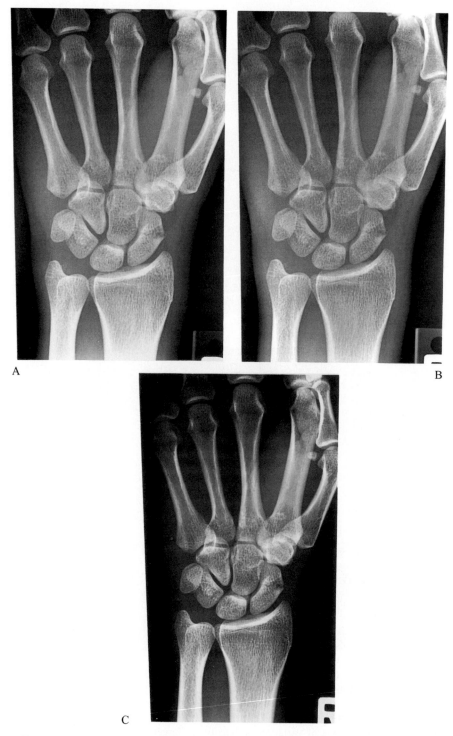

A

B

C

Figure 8.5. Digital radiograph of an undisplaced, difficult to see scaphoid fracture. (A) Standard processing. (B) Processed so that it is slightly darker. (C) Processed with a higher contrast scale. The fracture is easiest to see on the high contrast image.

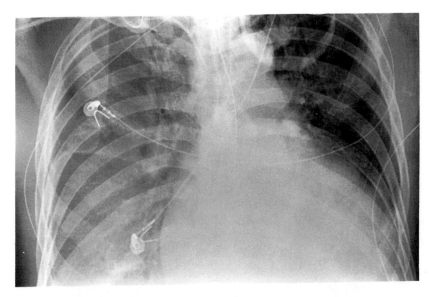

A

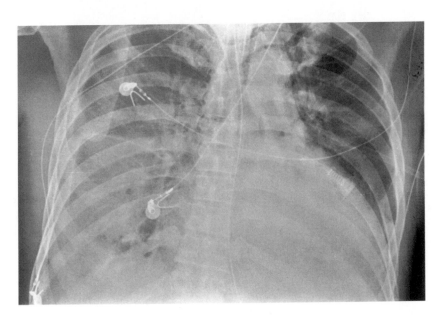

B

FIGURE 8.6. Chest radiograph in a patient with congestive heart failure showing dilated cardiomyopathy, bilateral pleural effusions, and minimal interstitial edema. (A) Standard processed image. The endotracheal tube and nasogastric tube are poorly seen. (B) With dynamic range control processing, the retrocardiac region is better seen. The endotracheal tube, nasogastric tube, and spine are more clearly seen, while the lungs show only minimal change in visualization.

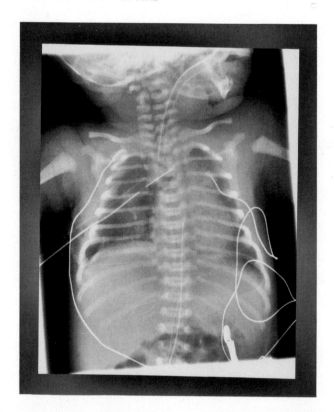

FIGURE 8.7. Digital radiograph of newborn with right pneumothorax and chest tube. The collimator edge detection algorithm creates a dark gray border around the collimated field. This would decrease the glare when viewed on a viewbox or monitor.

stored electronically. Electronic storage allows the image to be retrieved from several sites at the same time and to be transmitted to wherever the image data is needed. If the integrity of the digital storage system is maintained, the data storage is permanent. With conventional film based images, films can be borrowed or lost and therefore not be available when needed.

Image Display

Hard Copy and Soft Copy Display

Digital radiographs can be displayed as soft copy images on monitors and workstations or as hard copy produced by laser film printers. Image processing for soft copy and hard copy display needs to be individually optimized to the display device and display method. The best display size for digital radiographs is unknown. Displays can be preset at different sizes: life size, reduced in size, or enlarged. Each size offers potential advantages. Previous reports suggest that life size to two-thirds life-sized images generally do not appear to interfere with radiologists' ability to detect disease (Kehler, Albrechtsson, Andersson et al., 1989; Kehler, Albrechtsson, Andresdottier et al., 1991; MacMahon, Sanada, Doi et al., 1991). Micronodular disease is, however, harder to detect in two-thirds life-sized images, but larger nodules are easier to detect on the two-thirds life-sized images (Schaefer, Prokop, Oestmann et al., 1992). Half life-sized images have been shown to be most likely inadequate (Fisher and Brauer, 1989; Schaefer, Prokop, Oestmann et al., 1992). The interpretation of less than life-sized images and of soft copy images requires a brief period of adjustment. This seems to take several weeks of routine use. Smaller images must be viewed from a closer working distance than life-sized images.

Image Display Size and Templates of Prostheses and Catheters

When images are displayed at other than life size, radiologists and others find it more difficult to accurately measure and compare life-sized and reduced-sized images. For orthopedic and urologic applications, in which templates are commonly used, creation of templates of the correct reduced size can be made in the following way. First, expose an imaging plate of the appropriate size for the body part into which the prosthesis or catheter will be placed. (The authors use an exposure of 50 KVP, 1.6 mAs.) Place the life size template on a photocopy machine with this IP placed above the template, receptor side down. Make a single photocopy. Rapidly place the IP into a cassette avoiding too much exposure to room light. Process the IP. A small amount of edge enhancement applied at the workstation may be necessary to sharpen and adjust the optical density and contrast of the resulting template. The resulting image will be a close representation of the template reduced proportionately in size.

Clinical Digital Radiography

This section discusses digital radiography of different portions of the body, such as chest, skeletal, abdominal, renal, and gastrointestinal tract, with attention to the advantages and disadvantages of digital radiography for each region. The section also discusses the use of digital radiography in pediatric radiology and gives specific cautions, as appropriate.

Chest Radiography

Bedside Examinations

Digital radiography for bedside examinations offers several clear advantages to conventional screen film radiography. Its wider exposure latitude corrects for the under- and overexposure that can occur with bedside technique. Bedside radiography is a complicated task for radiological technologists. Mobile radiographic machines have limited KVP and mAs output. The distance between the x-ray tube and the film varies from exposure to exposure. Because views are often supine, it may be difficult to assure that the image is taken in full inspiration. With the semi-upright position, abdominal soft tissues are often bunched up over the lower chest. Phototiming is not commonly used.

Digital radiography helps to surmount the exposure-related problems of bedside radiography. Imaging plates record data from a wider range of exposures, and the automatic image processing has been designed to correct for misexposure (Freedman, Lo, Nelson et al., 1992; Schaefer, Greene, Oestmann et al., 1989). Linked to an image distribution system, digital radiography allows images to be distributed to intensive care units. Distributed image plate processors can increase productivity, because the technologists no longer need to return to the central film processing facility. Concurrent access to images can permit the radiologist to discuss findings with the intensivist in the intensive care unit while they both view the image.

Potential problems in bedside digital radiography have been studied by several groups. Current digital radiography systems provide lower resolution than the best screen film systems. Because of this, published analyses have focused on the potential diagnostic detriment that could result. These include the visibility of tubes and lines (Schaefer, Greene, Oestmann et al., 1989), the visibility of pneumothoraces (Fajardo, Hillman, Pond et al., 1989; MacMahon, Sanada, Doi et al., 1991; Marglin, Rowberg, Godwin, 1990), and the visibility of interstitial lung disease (Schaefer, Greene, Hall et al., 1991). Almost all these studies have reported either that there are no differences between screen film and digital images or that the digital images provide more complete information in viewing mediastinal structures (Freedman, Lo, Nelson et al, 1992; Kehler, Albrechtsson, Andersson et al., 1989; MacMahon, Sanada, Doi et al., 1991; Marglin, Rowberg, Godwin, 1990).

There are four potential perceptual problem areas for bedside digital radiography: (1) the visibility of noise (quantum mottle and electronic noise in the mediastinum), (2) the visibility of tubes in the mediastinum and abdomen, (3) the visibility of pneumothoraces, and (4) the assessment of interstitial lung disease. These are discussed below.

Visibility of Noise

Digital radiography images can be produced so that the noise is more visible than on screen film images. Underexposure results in visible noise, but an image is still produced. Thick regions of the body, such as the retrocardiac region of the chest can show visible noise. Whereas a conventional radiograph is clear or almost clear and captures little or no information (regions are commonly described as being white), noise can be seen on the digital image (Fig. 8.8A), providing information about the mediastinal findings. In bedside images of patients with mediastinal tubes, this information is valuable. Noise is more visible if spatial frequency enhancement (such as can be applied to improve the visibility of tubes in the mediastinum) is used.

The image processing system available with the Fuji digital radiographic system includes a blurring algorithm to decrease the visibility of noise. Using it can, however, result in decreased image information when compared to the noisy image. As an example, details of tubes and lines that can be seen through the visible noise in the mediastinum when smoothing is not used (Fig. 8.8A) become less visible when blurring is used (Fig. 8.8B).

Visible noise decreases the conspicuity of objects of low contrast. In regions where noise is visible, what is seen can be appropriately described as being present. Failure to see an object (such as a tube) in a region of visible noise does not indicate that it is not present. With experience, radiologists learn how much can or cannot be seen in a noisy image.

Visibility of Tubes and Lines in the Mediastinum and Abdomen

As illustrated in Figures 8.9A-D, image blurring can result in tubes and lines being less visible; conversely, enhancing the spatial frequency emphasis can improve the visibility of tubes. This method can be used before repeating a chest radiograph in which the position of mediastinal and abdominal tubes cannot be determined. Medium frequency enhancement may reveal the required finding and help avoid repeat chest or abdominal images.

Three image processing methods are useful for demonstrating tubes in the mediastinum: spatial frequency enhancement, black white inversion, and histogram equalization. These three methods are illustrated in Figure 8.9.

Visibility of Pneumothoraces

Small pneumothoraces can be difficult to detect on both conventional and digital radiographs of the chest. When first adapting to the smaller image format often used with digital radiography, radiologists may find it difficult to see pneumothoraces on these reduced-sized images and thus should pay special attention to the pleural margin (Fig. 8.10). Several recent controlled studies have shown no differences in pneumothorax detection (Freedman, Lo, Nelson et al., 1992; Kehler, Albrechtsson, Andresdottier et al., 1990; MacMahon, Sanada, Doi et al., 1991; Marglin, Rowberg, Godwin, 1990;). Some earlier studies did reveal difficulties in the detection of pneumothoraces (Fajardo, Hillman, Pond et al., 1989), but the reason for these differences is uncertain.

Because small pneumothoraces may not be visible on 1K monitors, we consider it necessary to zoom into the image to look at a true 2K dataset before deciding that no pneumothorax is present.

Assessment of Interstitial Lung Disease

Digital radiography, when processed with minimal edge enhancement, increases the conspicuity of normal lung structures. Pulmonary vessels can be seen further into the lung periphery, and bronchial walls are commonly visible as ring shadows in the perihilar regions. This improved visibility can result in radiologists' ascribing these normal findings as indicative of disease (Kehler,

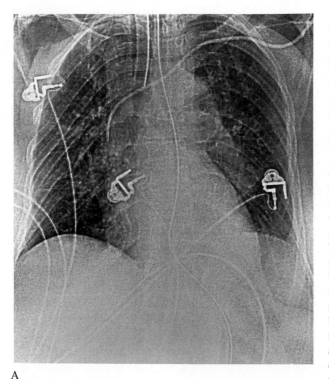

A

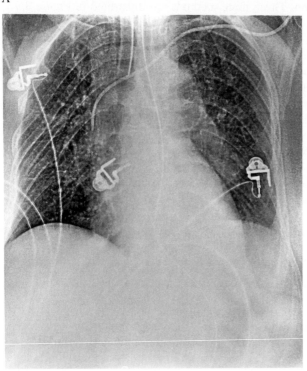

B

FIGURE 8.8. Bedside chest with endotracheal tube and nasogastric tubes superimposed on the mediastinum. (A) In this frequency enhanced image, the local contrast resulting from the edge enhancement allows the mediastinal tubes to be better seen. (B) This is the same image with the mediastinal noise purposely blurred out. The noise is less visible, but the nasogastric tube is less well seen; noise is less distinct both in the mediastinum and in the upper abdomen. This demonstrates that visible noise can contain important information and that, while blurring makes the image look more like a conventional screen film radiograph, information can be obscured.

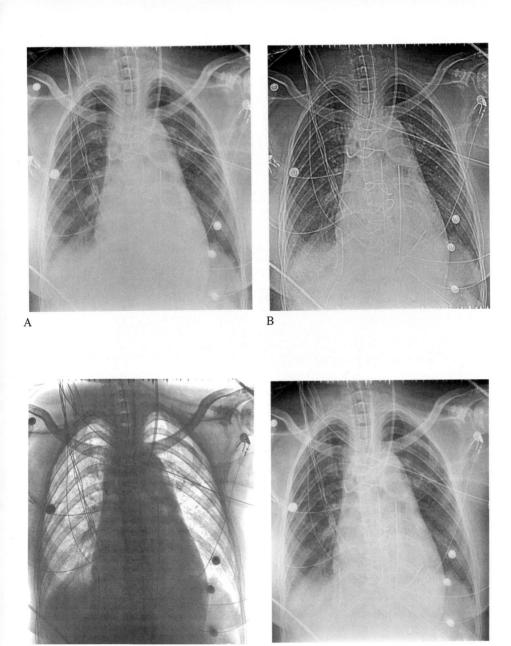

FIGURE 8.9. Digital radiograph of the chest of a patient obtained shortly following cardiac surgery. (A) Standard processing. (B) Edge enhancement to emphasize tubes. (C) Black-white inversion to emphasize tubes. (D) Histogram equalization to emphasize tubes. (B), (C), and (D) each improve the visibility of the tubes in the mediastinum and abdomen. Only in (D) does the appearance of the lungs remain almost unchanged.

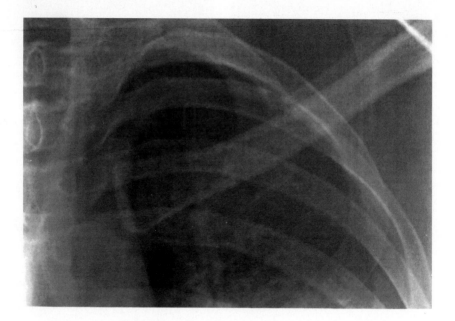

FIGURE 8.10. Digital radiograph of the chest. A small pneumothorax is present following thorocentesis for malignant pleural effusion.

Albrechtsson, Andresdottier et al., 1991). With experience, radiologists learn to look for specific findings of interstitial disease, such as Kerley lines, and learn to differentiate conspicuous blood vessels from interstitial lung disease. Most reported studies demonstrate no difference in the accuracy of interstitial lung disease detection between conventional and digital images (Kehler, Albrechtsson, Andresdottier et al., 1991; Schaefer, Green, Oestmann et al., 1990).

Schaefer (Schaefer, Greene, Llewellyn et al., 1991) reported that screen film and digital images had equal conspicuity only when a moderate degree of high spatial frequency edge enhancement was used, but not when images were unenhanced. Screen film and digital images were equivalent when the interstitial disease was minimal, but screen film images were better when the disease was moderate or marked.

Standard In-Department Chest Radiographs

Digital radiography is routinely used for in-department chest radiographs at several large sites. This has two beneficial effects. First, image processing can enhance the visibility of disease. Second, the digital form of the data allows for teleradiology and for easy entry into a picture archiving system. Its disadvantages include a smaller display size (for some such systems) and more visible noise than standard radiographs. Exposure correction features are not important because in-department chest radiographs are usually obtained with exposure automatically controlled.

Image processing of digital radiographs does increase the conspicuity of structures within the mediastinum and projected behind the heart and diaphragm, as shown above in Figure 8.9. This is most often of benefit in the detection of small pneumonias, but can also improve the visibility of small masses compared to screen film radiography (Schaefer, Greene, Hall et al., 1991; Schaefer, Greene, Oestmann et al., 1990). The effect is especially noticeable in patients with large body mass or large hearts. Studies of the use of digital chest radiography have demonstrated that it is equivalent to or slightly better than conventional chest radiography for most purposes (Kehler, Albrechtsson, Andersson et al., 1989; Schaefer, Greene, Hall et al., 1991; Schaefer, Greene, Oestmann et al., 1990).

Because digital radiography improves the visibility of the normal lung structures, it can result in the overdiagnosis of interstitial fibrosis. Radiologists must be careful to distinguish prominent blood vessels from interstitial disease. It is also likely that digital radiography demonstrates true interstitial lung disease that is present, but not visible, on conventional radiographs, as shown in Figure 8.11. With histogram equalization or edge enhancement, air bronchograms and other findings of air space disease can become more conspicuous, as is the case in Figures 8.12A and 8.12B. Although edge en-

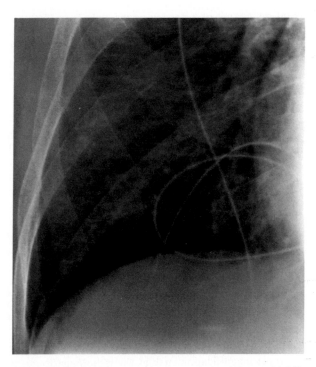

FIGURE 8.11. Digital radiograph demonstrating Kerley b interstitial lines in a patient with congestive heart failure.

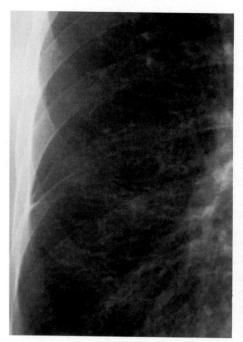 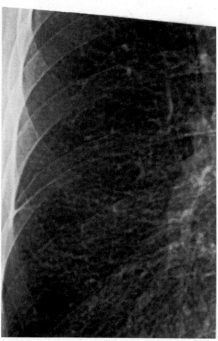

A   B

FIGURE 8.12. Digital radiograph of a portion of the right lung in a smoker with interstitial fibrosis presumable secondary to chronic bronchitis. (A) Unenhanced image. (B) Edge enhanced image. Both images show the very small holes in the lung pattern indicative of centrolobular emphysema and show changes of bronchial wall thickening. These changes are easier to recognize on the edge enhanced image.

hancement accentuates interstitial disease, small masses may become harder to detect, as illustrated by a comparison of Figures 8.13A and 8.13B.

Musculoskeletal Radiology

Extremities

Compared to conventional screen film radiography, digital radiography provides enhanced visualization of the extremities. Selection of the correct imaging plate resolution is key. In general, hands, wrists, elbows, and feet are best examined on a high resolution system. Shoulders, hips, and knees are suitable for the lower resolution, lower radiation dose system. As illustrated by Figures 8.14 and 8.15, ankles can be imaged with either resolution, although the authors prefer the high resolution system.

Digital radiography improves the visualization of the soft tissues of the extremities, and electronic magnification enables the radiologist to electronically enlarge suspect areas for more detailed evaluation. Histogram equalization effects provide a more complete view than conventional imaging can.

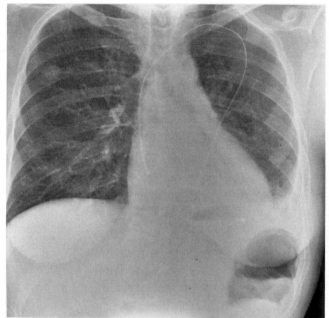

A

B

FIGURE 8.13. Digital radiograph of the chest in a woman with metastatic cancer. There is a 12 mm right upper lung mass, left lower lobe atelectasis with air bronchograms, a left pleural effusion, and a central venous line. (A) Standard processing. (B) Edge enhancement processing. The edge enhancement increases the visibility of the air bronchograms in the left lower lobe, the visibility of the central venous catheter, lung vessels, and other lung markings. It makes the lung mass harder to see.

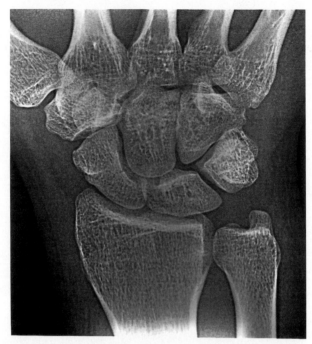

FIGURE 8.14. Digital radiograph of wrist processed with edge enhancement. A subtle undisplaced fracture of the scaphoid is demonstrated.

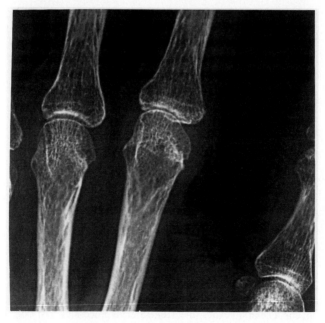

FIGURE 8.15. Digital radiograph of the second and third metacarpal phalangeal joints in a woman with rheumatoid arthritis demonstrating a small erosion.

Edge enhancement can create problems in skeletal radiographs. If lower spatial frequency structures are emphasized, the smaller trabeculae can become hidden, simulating osteoporosis, as shown in Figure 8.16. The edges of metal objects, like orthopedic screws and pins, can be overemphasized, simulating peri-metal resorption indicative of possible infection or loosening, as seen in Figures 8.17 and 8.18. In general, such images do not cause clinical confusion. However, if there is uncertainty, repeating the image without edge enhancement will remove the peri-metal radiolucency if it is the result of edge enhancement, but leave it intact if it is the result of disease. The radiologist should suspect disease if the radiolucency is eccentric or uneven in thickness or affects only one of several screws. If all metal regions show similar peri-metal radiolucency, then the radiolucency is most likely because of edge enhancement artifact.

Visualization of Soft Tissues

Soft tissue swelling is an important clue to subtle traumatic lesions of the skeleton and to infection. Visualization of such swelling, seen in Figure 8.19, is helpful in confirming findings of uncertain fractures. Visualization of soft tissue calcification, evident in Figure 8.20, is enhanced with appropriate processing of digital radiographs. Visibility of foreign bodies, soft tissue calcifications, and soft tissue masses is also enhanced (Buckwalter and Braunstein, 1992; Milos, Aberle, Baraff et al., 1989; Murphey, Quale, Martin et al., 1992; Reiner, Siegel, McLaurin et al., 1996).

Visualization of Subtle Fractures with Electronic Magnification

Electronic magnification is an optional function for the display of digital radiographs. With this system, the digital data is electronically interpolated to a larger display size. In some cases, no additional data is added; in others, additional portions of the original data are added to the image. Enlargement of the image and the ability to study it without the use of a magnifying glass can assist the radiologist in being more certain of the radiographic findings, as is the case with Figure 8.21.

Histogram Equalization

To reduce the range of image optical densities that must be displayed, histogram equalization uses image processing. Used properly, it can shift regions that on a conventional image are too dark or too light for optimal viewing into a range of optical densities that make the regions easier to evaluate, as shown in Figure 8.22.

Spine Images

In general, spine images are quite acceptable on digital radiographs. Digital radiography provides an advantage in the lateral thoracic spine view in that the use of image processing with or without histogram equalization allows more of the upper thoracic spine to be seen (Murphey, Quale, Martin et al.,

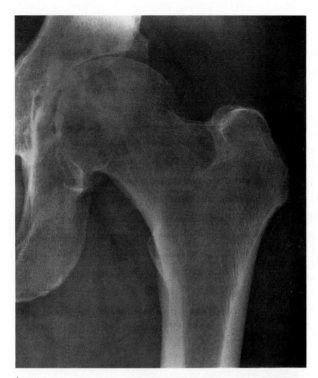

A

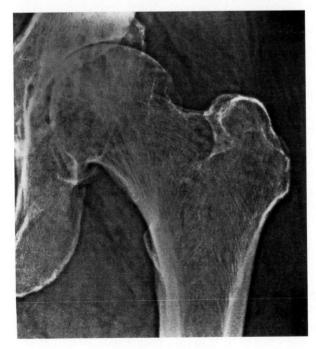

B

FIGURE 8.16. Digital radiograph of the left hip in a patient with moderate degenerative arthritis processed with marked edge enhancement. (A) Processed to emphasize small trabecular structures. (B) Processed to emphasize larger structures. The smaller trabeculae are better seen in (A). The larger trabeculae and the degenerative cysts are better seen in (B).

FIGURE 8.17. Digital radiograph of screws that transfix an intramedullary rod in the tibia. (A) Top screws show minimal lucency surrounding them caused by the edge enhancement. (B) Distal screw shows greater lucency around it because of resorption associated with loosening. The two images are processed with the same moderate degree of edge enhancement.

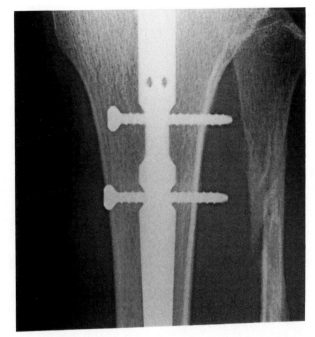

A

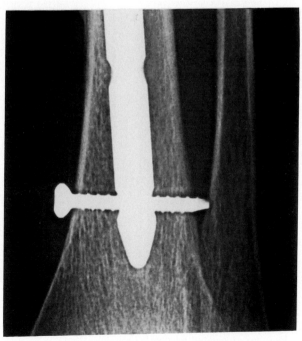

B

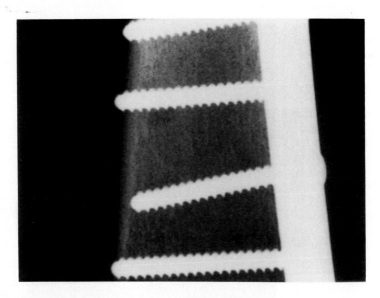

FIGURE 8.18. Digital radiograph of distal femur. Focal radiolucency near the tip of the second screw from the top is the result of resorption associated with focal infection.

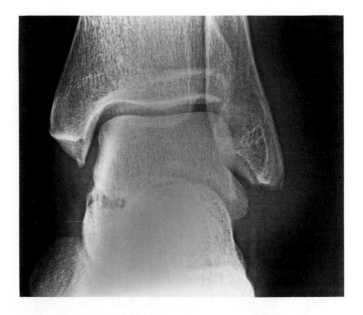

FIGURE 8.19. Digital radiograph of ankle. Subtle chip fractures of medial and lateral maleoli are associated with soft tissue swelling.

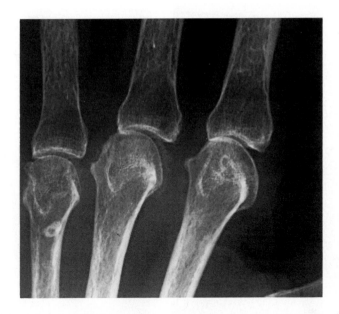

FIGURE 8.20. Digital radiograph of the metacarpal phalangeal joints in a woman with calcium pyrophosphate deposition disease. The joint calcifications and marginal osteophytes are well seen on the digital radiograph.

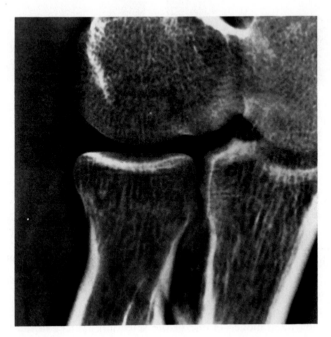

FIGURE 8.21. Digital magnification radiograph of the elbow. A subtle fracture of the radial neck is demonstrated.

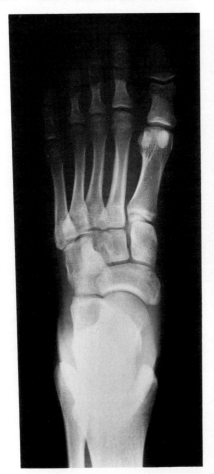
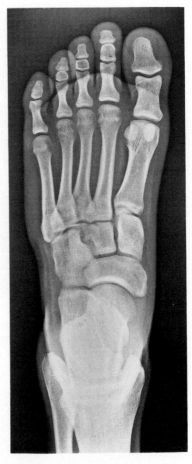

A   B

FIGURE 8.22. Digital radiograph of a normal foot. (A) Standard processing. (B) Histogram equalization. The equalized image gives a view from the toes to the hindfoot on a single image. Bone and soft tissue structures are easier to see.

1992), as in Figure 8.23. On lateral c-spine images, as in Figure 8.24, proper processing can result in the visualization of lower levels of the spine than with conventional lateral c-spine images (Murphey, Quale, Martin et al., 1992). Improvements in the visibility of the spinous processes and neck soft tissues also occurs (Wilson, Mann, West et al., 1994).

There are a few people with unusual body shapes in whom it can be quite difficult to obtain lateral lumbar spine views if one is using the automatic mode. In a few people it is necessary to use the "fixed mode" to obtain good images. The "fixed mode" is one of the selection choices in the identification terminal available to the technologist at the time the imaging plate is to

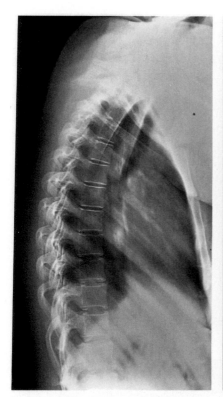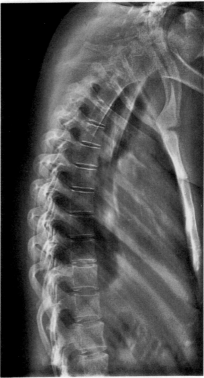

A   B

FIGURE 8.23. Lateral thoracic spine with and without histogram equalization. The equalized image (B) provides a better view of the upper and lower portions of the thoracic spine. In effect, the view extends through the shoulders and the abdominal tissues, allowing all portions of the thoracic spine to be of approximately equal optical density despite the actual difference in absorption in the body. Visualization of the sternum is improved.

be processed. In the fixed mode, the technologist indicates to the machine the exposure amount used by indicating the film-screen speed equivalent for the exposure. Thus a fixed 400 setting is equivalent to the exposure the technologist would select with a 400 speed screen film system.

Abdominal Radiography

Abdominal radiographs, as in Figure 8.25, are routinely obtained as digital radiographs. There have been no reports of special problems or advantages in the use of digital radiography in this body region.

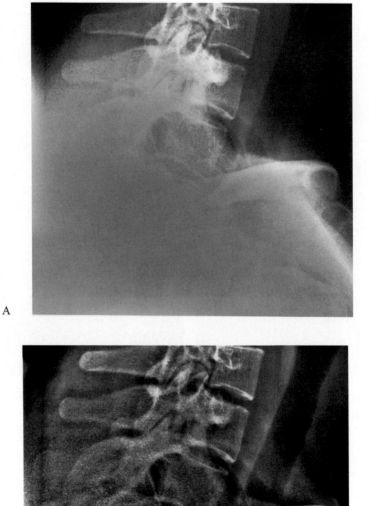

A

B

FIGURE 8.24. Digital radiograph of the lateral cervical spine. (A) Standard processing. (B) Same image with histogram equalization. The equalized image has improved visibility of the seventh cervical vertebra and first thoracic vertebra. A different technique was used in Figure 8.3 to improve the visibility of the lower cervical vertebra.

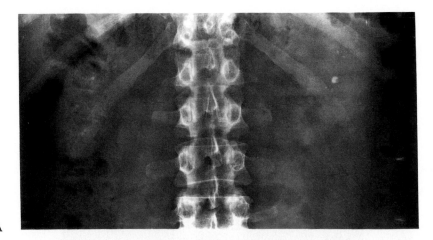

A

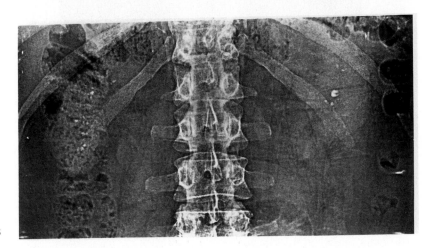

B

FIGURE 8.25. Digital radiograph of the abdomen. The region of the kidneys is selected for photography. (A) Standard processing. (B) Edge enhancement. The many renal calculi are easier to see on the enhanced images.

Intravenous Urography

When used as a replacement for conventional screen film radiography, the digital system, as shown in Figure 8.26 appears to be equivalent to the conventional. Experimental work suggests that the edges of the kidneys may be enhanced in some cases, as in Figure 8.27, by the use of special image processing designed for tomographic images of the lungs. Histogram equalization may also be of use in patients who have abundant air in their colon or stomach that overlies the kidney.

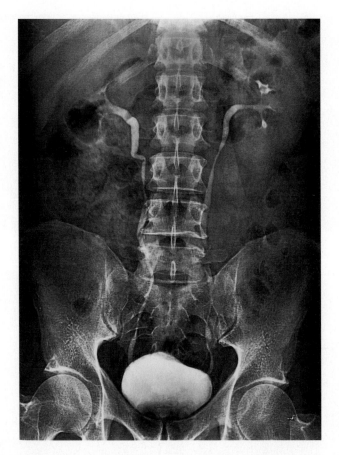

FIGURE 8.26. Digital radiograph obtained during intravenous urography 10 minutes into the urogram.

Gastrointestinal Radiography

Digital radiographs obtained as parts of upper gastrointestinal series Figure 8.28 and barium enemas are equivalent to or, in some cases, better than conventional radiographs. Advantages are seen in air-barium double contrast colon examinations. In these examinations, the digital system appears to be better in displaying the wide range of densities present on the decubitus views.

Pediatric Radiology

In children over the age of one year, digital radiography is used and generally considered acceptable (de Silva, in press; Dietrich, Boechat, Huang, 1989; Kogutt, Jones, Perkins, 1988; Stringer, Cairns, Poskitt et al., 1994).

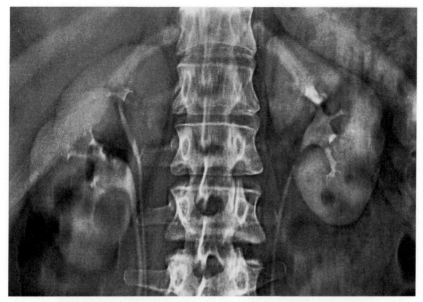

A

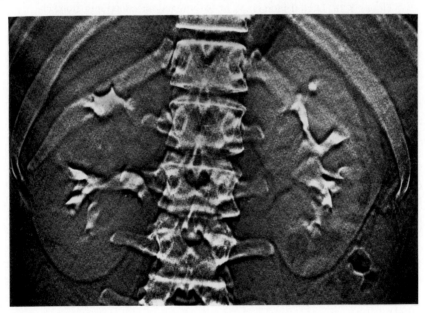

B

FIGURE 8.27. Two examples of edge enhancement of renal tomograms. In intravenous urography, one of the goals is to see the margins of the kidneys. (A) Tomographic processing type 1, normal kidneys. (B) Tomographic processing type 2,
normal kidneys.

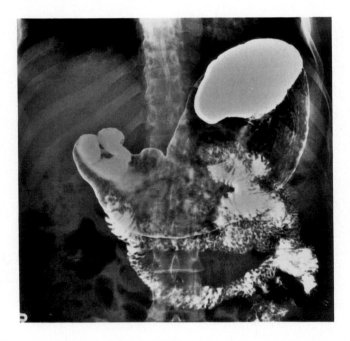

FIGURE 8.28. Digital radiograph of barium and air containing stomach.

The system provides high quality radiographs of the chest and extremities and is used exclusively in several centers (de Silva, in press).

In newborns and premature infants, there are differing reports as to its suitability (Arthur and Pease, 1992; Cohen, Katz, Kalasinski et al., 1991; de Silva, in press; Dietrich, Boechat, Huang, 1989; Merlo, Bighi, Cervi et al., 1991; Pearce, Bonner, Freedman et al., 1994). Particularly in premature infants, the small size of the images and the visibility of noise may interfere in the diagnosis of pulmonary interstitial emphysema and necrotizing enterocolitis (de Silva, personal communication, 1996). Concern is based on both the radiation dose resolution tradeoff and certain technical problems that can occur in radiographing small objects (Arthur and Pease, 1992; Pearce, Bonner, Freedman et al., 1994). Although one can obtain high quality images using the high resolution imaging plates, this system uses three to four times the radiation exposure used for conventional systems. With the lower resolution system that works at lower exposures, some observers consider the resolution marginal (de Silva, in press; Pearce, Bonner, Freeman et al., 1994).

An advantage of the digital system is its ability to correct for errors of under- and overexposure. With small field sizes, this correction can be less accurate (Arthur and Pease, 1992). We find that even with highly skilled technologists, the improvement in exposure control does not occur (Arthur and Pease, 1992; Pearce, Bonner, Freedman et al., 1994). With underexposure, there is concern that the visibility of noise could simulate either pulmonary interstitial emphysema or necrotizing enterocolitis. There are high-quality clinical sites that use digital radiography routinely for all ages (though some privately express concern of its use in neonates) and others that do not use the system in neonates. If one is willing to use the high resolution system with its increased radiation dose, the system is probably appropriate. With the low resolution system, it is considered, by us, to be marginally acceptable. When one has excellent technologists taking the neonatal examinations, there is no gain in image quality with digital radiography, and the quality may be less than screen film systems if the image is underexposed. As an entry point into a picture archive and communication system (PACS), the use of the system is acceptable.

Some papers have discussed dose reduction from the use of digital radiography in children. The papers by Kogutt (1988) and Merlo (1991) indicate that dose reduction is possible; the papers by Arthur (1992), Cohen (1991), and Pearce (1994) either found dose reduction was not possible or was detrimental to image quality. Stringer (1994) indicated there was a potential for dose reduction in scoliosis studies.

Summary

Digital radiography is in most cases equivalent to and in a few cases superior to conventional screen film radiography. The wide range of acceptable exposure and the use of image processing result in a system that, we consider, provides better image appearance than conventional screen film radiography. In most cases, it has not been possible to translate this improved appearance into statistical proof of improved diagnostic quality. In bedside examinations, the ability of the system to correct for moderate degrees of under- or overexposure is a major advantage. Digital transmission and storage of data and the ability to simultaneously view the images at several sites are additional advantages. In the future, we believe that the automatic use of computer aided diagnosis will provide even greater advantages to sites using digital radiography.

References

Arthur RJ, Pease JN. Problems associated with digital luminescence radiography in the neonate and young infant. Pediatr Radio 1992, 22, 5–7.

Buckwalter KA, Braunstein EM. Digital skeletal radiography. AJR, 1992, 158, 1071–1080.

Cohen MD, Katz BP, Kalasinski LA et al. Digital imaging with a photostimulable phosphor in the chest of newborns. Radiology, 1991, 181, 829–832.

de Silva M. Computed radiography in pediatric radiology. Sem Roentgen, 1996, 32, 57–63.

Dietrich RB, Boechat MI, Huang HK. Experience with phosphor imaging plates—

clinical experience in pediatric radiology. SPIE Medical Imaging III: Image Capture and Display, 1989, 1091, 242–244.

Fajardo LL, Hillman BJ, Pond GD et al. Detection of pneumothorax: comparison of digital and conventional chest imaging. AJR 1989, 152, 475–480.

Fisher PD, Brauer GW. Impact of image size on effectiveness of digital imaging systems. J Digital Imaging, 1989, 2, 39–41.

Freedman M, Lo SCB, Nelson MC et al. Comparative tests of two storage phosphor plate imaging systems: the AGFA ADC and the Fuji AC-1+. In Brody W and Johnston G, eds, Computer Applications to Assist Radiology: SCAR 92, Symposia Foundation, 1992a.

Freedman M, Lo SCB, Nelson MC et al. Tests of radiologist performance in interpreting bedside chest examinations on a workstation. SPIE Image Capture, Formatting and Display, 1992b, 1653, 142–158.

Kehler M, Albrechtsson U, Andersson B et al. Assessment of digital chest radiography using stimulable phosphor. Acta Radiologica, 1989, 30, 581–586.

Kehler M, Albrechtsson U, Andresdottier A et al. Accuracy of digital radiography using stimulable phosphor for diagnosis of pneumothorax. Acta Radiologica 1990, 31, 47–52.

Kehler M, Albrechtsson U, Andresdottier A et al. Digital luminescence radiography in interstitial lung disease. Acta Radiologica 1991, 32, 18–23.

Kogutt MS, Jones JP, Perkins DD. Low-dose digital computed radiography in pediatric chest imaging. AJR 1988, 151, 775–779.

MacMahon H, Sanada S, Doi K et al. Direct comparison of conventional and computed radiography with a dual-image recording technique. Radiographics 1991, 11, 259–268.

Marglin SI, Rowberg AH, Godwin JD. Preliminary experience with portable digital imaging for intensive care radiography. J Thoracic Imaging, 1990, 5, 49–54.

Merlo L, Bighi S, Cervi PM et al. Computed radiography in neonatal intensive care. Pediatr Radio 1991, 21, 94–96.

Milos NJ, Aberle DR, Baraff LJ et al. Initial clinical experience with computed radiography imaging in an emergency department. Appl Radiol 1989, 18, 32–37.

Murphey MD, Quale JL, Martin NL et al. Computed radiography in musculoskeletal imaging: state of the art. AJR 1992, 158, 19–27.

Pearce D, Bonner C, Freedman M et al. Comparison of storage phosphor and screen-film images in the neonatal intensive care unit: a multiple observer preference study. SPIE Medical Imaging: Image Perception 1994, 2166, 111–118.

Reiner B, Siegel E, McLaurin T et al. Evaluation of soft-tissue foreign bodies: comparing conventional plain film radiography, computed radiography printed on film, and computed radiography displayed on a computer workstation. AJR 1996, 167, 141–144.

Rosenthal MS, Good WF, Costa-Greco MA et al. The effect of image processing on chest radiograph interpretations in a PACS environment. Invest Radiol 1990, 25, 897–901.

Schaefer CM, Greene R, Hall DA et al. Mediastinal abnormalities: detection with storage phosphor digital radiography. Radiology 1991, 178, 169–173.

Schaefer CM, Greene R, Llewellyn HJ et al. Interstitial lung disease: impact of postprocessing in digital storage phosphor imaging. Radiology 1991, 178, 733–738.

Schaefer CM, Greene RE, Oestmann JW et al. Improved control of image optical density with low-dose digital and conventional radiography in bedside imaging. Radiology 1989, 173, 713–716.

Schaefer CM, Greene RE, Oestmann JW et al. Digital storage phosphor imaging versus conventional film radiography in CT-documented chest disease. Radiology 1990, 174, 207–210.

Schaefer CM, Prokop M, Oestmann JW et al. Impact of hard-copy size on observer performance in digital chest radiography. Radiology 1992, 184, 77–81.

Stringer DA, Cairns RA, Poskitt KJ et al. Comparison of stimulable phosphor technology and conventional screen-film technology in pediatric scoliosis. Pediatric Radiology 1994, 24, 1–5.

Wilson AJ, Mann FA, West OC et al. Evaluation of the injured cervical spine: comparison of conventional and storage phosphor radiography with a hybrid cassette. Radiology 1994, 193, 419–422.

9
Digital Mammography

MATTHEW T. FREEDMAN, DOROTHY STELLER ARTZ, JAQUELYN HOGGE, REBECCA A. ZUURBIER, AND SEONG KI MUN

Digital mammography is the outgrowth of the convergence of two different paths represented by conventional screen film mammography and digital projection radiography. Each path has been characterized by progressive improvements. Conventional mammography has been marked by improvements in contrast and thereby the conspicuity of normal and abnormal tissues within the breast. Digital mammography represents an extension of trends already evident in conventional mammography toward higher contrast images and higher lesion conspicuity. Radiologic diagnosis done on digital mammograms uses the same signs for the detection of breast cancer as conventional mammography, but appears to show the findings with greater conspicuity and perhaps at a slightly smaller size.

Like all digital imaging, digital mammography requires additional clinical training to understand the value and limitations of computer processing, the artifacts that can be produced, and the ways in which computer processing can hide disease. In a fundamental sense, this is no different from learning about conventional screen film mammography—its values and limitations, its artifacts, and the ways in which a badly exposed, handled, or processed film can obscure disease. Digital mammography requires additional quality control procedures to assure that image quality is preserved and artifacts are limited. These must be machine specific.

At Georgetown University Medical Center, for example, procedures have been specifically designed for the machine in use. With that equipment and very high standards of quality assurance, digital mammography appears to provide a small but measurable improvement in the conspicuity of the signs of breast cancer. The improvement is so slight, however, that the system is not likely improve the accuracy of mammographic detection or classification of possible breast cancer lesions as interpreted by radiologists highly skilled in the mammographic detection of breast cancer. Nonetheless, digital mammography performed with this system is as accurate as conventional mammography, and improvements in lesion conspicuity may increase the accuracy of less skilled radiologists or nonphysicians screening mammography images prior to review by a radiologist.

In a recent study of digital mammography at Georgetown, six radiologists evaluated 24 cancer cases, 25 benign biopsy cases, and 48 clinically normal mammograms. Of the 24 cancer cases, 15 were 1 cm or less in size. The areas under the ROC curve averaged 0.7197 for the digital system and 0.7192 for the screen film system. This study showed that the accuracy of the digital and screen film mammograms were essentially identical (Freedman, Artz, Hogge et al., 1998). Systems now being developed may provide a slight additional increment in image quality compared to screen film mammography and may provide diagnostic advantages.

Trends

Conventional Screen Film Mammography

Conventional screen film mammography has changed dramatically over the past 25 years, with improved understanding of how to achieve in a single image the greatest visibility of the signs of small cancers. The trend has been toward the production of high contrast images, with adequate spatial resolution obtained at a radiation dose as low as reasonably achievable (ALARA). The exacting demands of conventional mammography have led to progressively higher contrast screen film combinations, improved methods for film processing, and better x-ray mammography machines. Mammography machine development led to dedicated mammography machines with small focal spot sizes, low KVP output, special targets and filters, improvements in breast compression, improvements in scatter rejection (by use of a grid), and the use of phototimers to assure adequate exposure. Although the name mammogram has not changed over these 25 years, the method of producing a mammogram and the appearance of the mammographic image are now vastly different. Digital mammography represents the next stage in this development. In a few years, the descriptor digital will be dropped, as digital mammography becomes the new standard for mammography.

Digital Projection Radiography

Digital projection radiography using storage phosphor plates was clinically introduced approximately 15 years ago for applications in bedside chest radiography. It has since evolved toward machines that can perform all projection examinations (e.g., chest radiographs, abdominal radiographs, musculoskeletal radiographs, mammography) previously obtained with conventional screen film projection radiography. Digital projection radiography has been accepted by many radiologists throughout the world because it provides excellent control of the optical density of the final image, thereby resulting in a more consistent appearance of the resulting radiograph. It provides a robustness to the imaging process, so that variations in exposure, KVP, and patient size produce very little change in final image appearance.

It provides this consistency by

- Providing an image receptor that can accept a much larger range of exposures than screen film receptors, and
- Using computer based image processing to correct for some of the changes resulting from misexposure.

Digital projection mammography is reported to be in clinical use in Japan, England, Switzerland, and Denmark (Bidstrup, 1992; Brettle, Ward, Parkin et al., 1994; Voegeli, 1992). Newer methods of digital mammography will incorporate many of the principles of digital projection radiography using phosphor plates.

Image Processing

Most of the computer based image processing methods used by digital projection radiography are computer implementations of the analog processes used to affect screen film image appearance. The first digital projection radiography machines were developed by the research laboratory of a major x-ray film company. The developers designed the machines to make the computer based performance of these systems mimic—through computer algorithms—the best features of the screen film system. The analogies between these two systems are as follow:

- Use of an appropriate film characteristic curve to affect contrast ~ computer based changes in the look-up table to affect contrast.
- Use of extended film processing to increase contrast ~ use of an appropriate look-up table.
- Choice of screen film combination to reduce visible noise ~ computer based noise filtering.
- Selection of a lower or higher resolution screen film combination ~ selection of a detector of appropriate inherent resolution.
- Use of a bright light to see darker regions of an image ~ (a) use of different window levels to bring the optical density of an image into a range that would not require the use of a bright light combined with the printing of two different images or (b) the use of histogram equalization to balance the optical densities within an image so that a bright light is not needed.
- The use of a hand held magnifier ~ electronic zoom to enlarge an image.
- Edge emphasis of Xeromammography[R] ~ electronic unsharp masking.

Image Quality Improvement

Digital radiography and conventional screen film radiography differ in how they handle the three functions of image formation: acquisition of the image data, image processing, and image display. With its chemical processing, film incorporates all three functions. Radiologists can change the character of each component of this image formation through the implementation of changes in film, screens, developer chemistry, processing temperature, and processing time. However, these changes must be made prospectively, prior to the mammographic exposure and prior to having knowledge of the tissue composition of an individual woman's breast. With digital mammography, on the other hand, these changes can be made after the image data has been acquired, allowing the radiologist to adjust image appearance to be patient specific (Freedman, Artz, and Mun, 1996). The best image appearance for a fatty breast is different from that for a heterogeneous or dense breast, as shown in Figures 9.1 and 9.2. The electronic adjustment in image appear-

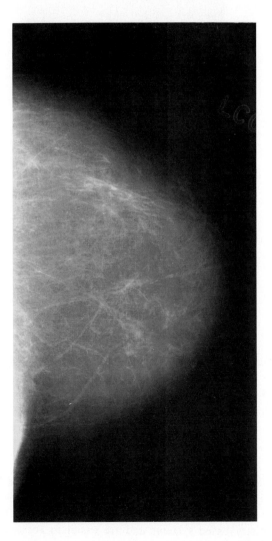

FIGURE 9.1. Digital mammogram of fatty breast. The range of optical densities is not great. One can see from the skin line to the interior of the breast in a single view.

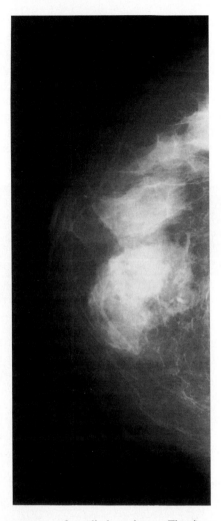

FIGURE 9.2. Digital mammogram of a radiodense breast. The tissue density range varies from light gray to dark gray. The digital mammogram corrects automatically for the different ranges of tissue density.

ance can be done automatically by the computer or manually by the technologist or radiologist (Freedman, Pe, Zuurbier et al, 1994). In addition, certain of the desired changes in image processing are difficult to accomplish in chemistry based systems and are easier to accomplish with computer algorithms.

New Hardware in Digital Radiography

Image Acquisition

The initial implementation of digital projection radiography was done using imaging plates that were sensitive to x-radiation and could store the information for later retrieval; they used storage phosphor methodology. The imaging plate stores the information in analog form, but it is extracted and converted into digital form. Other methods of recording x-ray data in digital form or converting it from analog to digital form include film digitization, charge coupled devices (CCD), and other direct x-ray detectors not based on phosphors. Because CCDs are not themselves good detectors of x-radiation, they use a phosphor or cesium iodide layer to convert the x-ray photons into light, which is then, in turn, transferred to the CCD chip directly or through a fiber optic or lens linkage. Most systems depend on the use of a phosphor, either identical or quite similar to the phosphors used in radiographic screens. Cesium iodide is commonly used in the image intensifier tubes of fluoroscopes. Still newer systems are based on the use of selenium receptors, amorphous silicon, and thin film transistors. Some of these devices directly record the x-ray exposure without the production of light as an intermediary. Others use a light producing phosphor or cesium iodide to produce light that is then recorded by the receptor.

While each of these methods is separate in its engineering methodology and requires different quality control methodologies for manufacture and clinical use, the final images should look quite similar and be of similar clinical value. The methods of machine operation, types of artifacts, and image appearance may differ slightly between systems; thus, machine specific training is desirable. Proper exposure factors for these different devices may differ and should be individually evaluated.

Pixel Size

These devices have different pixel sizes for acquisition of image data. Currently planned or existing digital mammography systems have pixel sizes 25 to 100 µm in size. The choice of pixel size affects five parameters of image quality: size of smallest detectable object, separability of adjacent objects, contrast of smallest detectable object, required exposure, and image noise (or signal to noise ratio). These concepts are discussed later in this chapter.

Image Display

Image display is usually done by printing the digital data on laser cameras, the same equipment used for printing CT and MR images. Because of the exacting quality demands of mammography, only the best laser printers can be used. Although soft copy displays for digital mammography interpretation are under development, the authors are unaware of any study showing soft copy displays to be adequate for primary diagnosis. The display of mammography requires a system that can show a wide range of display luminence or optical density. This is necessary so that the display can project the wide range of exposures that occur in mammography. In general, soft copy display devices do not provide an adequate range of display luminence for this purpose.

Clinical Utility

In conventional mammography, the radiographic signs of potential breast cancer are

- Clusters of five or more microcalcifications of appropriate size and shape.
- A mass, which may or may not have a spiculated edge.
- Architectural distortion.
- Certain types of increased tissue since a prior exam.

The digital mammographic signs of breast cancer are identical. Digital mammography research, to date, has not discovered any new signs that are useful in the detection of breast cancer. The conventional signs are used, but because image processing can provide a higher contrast image, it may increase the conspicuousness of a lesion and make it easier for the radiologist to see it. To date, however, there is no study that shows that digital mammography is better than conventional mammography. Studies by Freedman (Freedman, Artz, Hogge et al., 1997), Brettle (Brettle, Ward, Parkin et al., 1994), and Jarlman (Jarlman, Samuelsson, and Brew, 1991) support the conclusion that digital and conventional mammography are equal in diagnostic accuracy.

Evaluative Studies

The evaluation of new radiologic devices that are evolving from existing devices usually involves comparing images of geometric test objects from the old and new systems, followed by studies comparing clinical images produced by both systems. When the signs of disease are well known and the changes made in the new image reflect past trends in image improvement, full-scale outcome studies are rarely done and would probably represent a waste of resources. In conventional mammography, there is a general consensus as to what images should look like and how to differentiate a good from a bad image. The signs of breast cancer on mammograms are well understood, but radiologists would like to be able to see these signs of breast cancer more easily and with better definition.

If digital mammography could improve the conspicuity of the accepted mammographic signs of breast cancer and, especially, if it could better dem-

TABLE 9.1. Table of smallest object seen: screen film versus direct digital 50 and 100 µm systems.

Test object	screen film	100-µm phosphor	50-µm CCD
CDMAN	130. 100 at 5× mag	100 at 1 micron thick	100 at 0.8 microns thick
CIRS Detail	240	160	160
RMI 156	240 (3/6)	240 (3/6)	240 (3/6)
CIRS Half Round	160	160	160

CDMAM test object from Nuclear Associates, Carle Place, New York; CIRS, Norfolk, Virginia. Fuji (Tokyo) Kyokko UM Fine Screen with Fuji UM-MA-HC film. The 100-µm device is a whole breast storage phosphor machine [Fuji (Tokyo) FCR 9000]. The 50-µm CCD is a digital spot device purchased by Georgetown University Medical Center in 1995 (Fischer Imaging, Denver, CO).

onstrate the signs that distinguish benign from malignant, it would and should replace conventional mammography. Digital mammography is not yet at this level of quality, but it is close. There is evidence in geometric test objects that digital mammography can equal or slightly exceed conventional screen film mammography in the conspicuity of the details in geometric test objects. Table 9.1 represents data from several geometric test objects (Freedman, Steller, Jafroudi et al., 1995).

There are slight improvements in the visibility of smaller object details in some of the test objects with the digital methods. Recent work by Roehrig confirms the slight advantage of a 50-µm CCD system over screen film mammography in tests using the CDMAM test object (Krupinski, Roehrig, and Yu, 1995; Roehrig, Krupinski, and Yu, 1995). A look at the images of these test objects makes it quite clear that, while the conventional and digital systems performed similarly in the detectability of small objects, the contrast of the details is visibly higher in the digital images. Together Georgetown and Roehrig have tested three different digital systems with essentially the same findings. Image processing can enhance the visibility of micro-calcifications. Figure 9.3 demonstrates the enhancement of calcifications that can occur from a change in image optical density and a slight degree of added edge enhancement.

Desired Improvements

Practicing clinical radiologists prefer digital mammographic systems to current mammography and consider them likely to improve detection or classification if the breast images provided contained the following changes:

- Improved conspicuity of microcalcifications and small masses.
- Improved definition of the shape of microcalcifications.
- Improved definition of the appearance of the edge of small masses.
- Improved conspicuity of architectural distortion.
- The ability to interpret accurately more mammograms per day.
- Direct magnification or zooming to eliminate the need to use a magnifying glass.

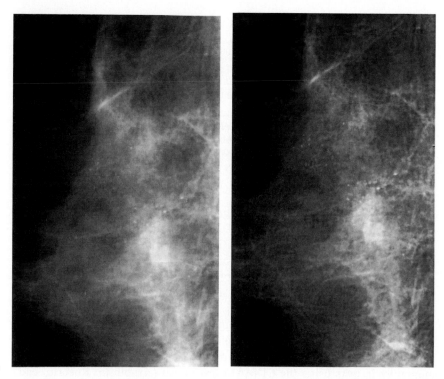

A   B

FIGURE 9.3. Benign breast calcifications. (A) Standard image, mild edge enhancement. (B) Image enhanced for better demonstration of microcalcifications

There is the potential for digital mammography to do each of these if the trends in digital mammography already demonstrated continue.

Optimum Image

The goal of mammography is to produce an image that is the optimum for each woman's breast (Freedman, Artz, and Mun, 1996). Breasts vary in composition. In broad categories, they can be predominately fatty, predominately dense, or heterogeneous. With conventional mammography, the composition of the breast cannot be accurately predicted prior to imaging (although physical examination of the breast can provide significant clues). Thus, each mammogram represents a compromise in image technique so that all breasts can be imaged moderately well. Some newer conventional mammography machines measure the composition of the breast prior to imaging it by a brief, low energy exposure, and then adjust the KVP, mAs, target, and filter to be breast composition specific. Digital mammography systems can accomplish the same goal through automatic image processing. The digital images in a recently reported study (Freedman, Artz, and Mun, 1996) used automatic contrast correction for breast composition. The goal is an image that achieves maximum contrast for the breast.

Quality Control Issues

Digital systems and conventional systems can both produce artifacts that mimic or, conversely, obscure the signs of cancer. Both systems can create calcium-like and mass-like artifacts or obscure true findings. Quality control procedures for digital systems overlap procedures needed for screen film systems and also impose additional quality control requirements. Differences between digital systems make it difficult to describe the quality control requirements for all systems as a group. Each of the following types of artifacts can be produced in digital mammograms by incorrect image processing or improper exposure. It is important that these problems are covered in procedure manuals for digital mammography systems and that radiologists receive training in addressing them.

- If the digital system can produce artifacts that can be misinterpreted as microcalcifications, training should be provided in how to decrease or avoid such artifacts and how to recognize them when they occur.
- If the digital system can produce artifacts that can be misinterpreted as small masses, training should be provided in how to decrease or avoid such artifacts and how to recognize them when they occur.
- If the image processing can be adjusted to obscure small masses or microcalcifications, training should be provided in how to decrease or avoid such artifacts and how to recognize them when they occur.
- If under- or overexposure of the breast can occur and be obscured by the image processing of the system, it would be preferable to redesign the machine to avoid such possibility. Should that not be possible, training should be provided in how to decrease or avoid such under- or overexposure and how to recognize it should it occur.

Technical Considerations

Pixel Size

Pixel size affects resolution, the detection of small objects, the evaluation of the shape of small objects, the exposure required for digital mammography, and the machine and data handling costs of the machines. The larger the pixel, the less the data handling costs; (in general) the less the required radiation, the lower the visibility of shape and edges, and the lower the visibility of noise in the image.

Pixel Size and Smallest Detectable Object

Given the importance that pixel size has on image quality, there are surprisingly few scientific studies of this question. Articles in the late 1980s by HP Chan (Chan, Vyborny, MacMahon et al., 1987) suggested that 100-μm digitized film was not adequate for the detection of the smallest micro-calcifications seen on screen film mammography, and work by Oestmann (Joerg, Oestmann, Kopans et al., 1988) suggested that with storage phosphor technology 100-μm pixels could, in a test object, detect all the calcification clusters seen on screen film mammography systems, but not each individual microcalcification.

The authors have presented data that show that the use of a 50-μm versus. a 100-μm pixel potentially would result in slight improvements in the contrast of detected objects and a small improvement in the definition of the shape of objects. No decrease occurred in the minimal size of objects seen, probably because this effect is slight and the available test objects did not have small enough decrements in size to allow this effect to be detected. A slight decrease in detectable object size would be expected, however. In geometric test objects, images made with a 100-μm pixel show objects equal to or slightly smaller than screen film images, depending on the test object, as shown in Table 9.1.

Pixel Size and Object Shape

Shape determination is related to pixel size. The more pixels contained within the shadow of the object, the more accurately its shape will be depicted (see Fig. 9.4). At the moment, the Georgetown data, which need independent confirmation, suggest that the improvement that results from the use of a 50-μm pixel is real, but small when compared to screen film and 100-μm pixel mammography. Because the improvement in shape definition is slight, it is unclear what effect this will have on the detection of breast cancer by a

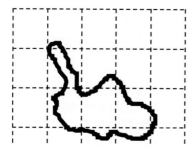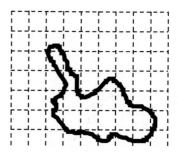

FIGURE 9.4. The greater the number of pixels, the more accurately a shape will be depicted.

human observer. There are data that show that detection accuracy in computer aided diagnosis algorithms is improved by the use of digitized film with pixel sizes of 25, 35, and 50 μm, compared to a pixel size of approximately 100 μm (Chan, 1995; Fujita, Endo, Matsubara et al., 1995). In a recently reported study, the use of a 100-μm detector compared to a conventional screen film system did not decrease the ability of radiologists to distinguish between benign and malignant lesions, but it is unknown whether a 50-μm detector is better (Freedman, Artz, Hogge et al., 1997).

Resolution versus Detection

Pixel size is related to resolution— the ability to separate two adjacent objects. Detection is related to object contrast, the amount of noise in the background, and the variability of the background. Object contrast is related to pixel size. If an object is of high enough contrast, it can be detected even if it is smaller than a single pixel. This is analogous to the partial volume effect seen in other digital imaging systems. It is anticipated that decreased resolution would result in a decreased capability to separate or count microcalcifications, but would not affect their group detectability. A study of this issue (Freedman, Artz, Jafroudi et al., 1996) found that more of the readers preferred the digital system for detecting microcalcifications, but preferred the screen film system for counting the microcalcifications.

Exposure

Decreased Exposure

Early reports on digital mammography suggested that the exposure to patients might be reduced by the use of digital mammography methods. This is a complex issue. The 100-μm digital system used at Georgetown does perform better than screen film systems at lower exposures; however, it is not functioning with its maximal quality at these lower exposures. The machine does provide conspicuity equal to screen film mammography at the usual screen film dose and appears to perform slightly better than conventional mammography at a still higher dose. Because the tested 100-μm system performs better than screen film mammography at low exposures as shown in geometric test objects, it seems likely that digital systems would provide better detection of small objects in areas of increased breast radiodensity if the comparison screen film mammogram was underexposed in the same region. No advantage would be expected if the region in question were properly exposed, as shown in Figure 9.5 (Freedman, Steller, Jafroudi et al., 1995).

Because information is recorded in the digital data at lower exposures equivalent to regions of increased breast radiodensity, it becomes possible to use image processing to display this information. Figure 9.6 shows the effect of this reprocessing in enhancing the visibility of microcalcification. Digital radiography also allows the use of special image processing to "remove"

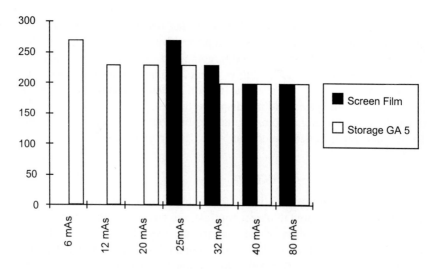

FIGURE 9.5. This chart demonstrates that at mAs less than 25, the storage phosphor system could demonstrate objects, but the screen film failed to demonstrate any of the objects. At 25 and 32 mAs, the storage phosphor demonstrated smaller objects than screen film. At 40, and 80 mAs, the two systems performed equivalently. In this experiment, 40 mAs corresponds to a screen film optical density of 0.42. Under these test conditions, the storage phosphor system provided more information at low exposures than did the screen film system. [Fuji (Tokyo) Kyokko UM Fine Screen with Fuji UM-MA-HC film.] The 100-μm device is a whole breast storage phosphor machine. (Storage = Storage Phosphor Radiography. GA = gradient angle of the look-up table.)

much of the white material present in the breast leaving an image in which the microcalcifications and breast fibers become more visible. This is demonstrated in Figure 9.7 (Freedman, Artz, Jafroudi et al., 1996).

Increased Exposure

For the digital system in use at Georgetown, the standard mammographic exposure is below the optimum level (Jennings, Jafroudi, Gagne et al., 1996). Higher exposures will allow the detection of smaller objects. This could result in the improved detection of small breast cancers, but much research still needs to be done to justify this increase in dose. As a general rule, smaller pixels will require increased patient exposure. There are several methods of avoiding this problem, but it is important that if an increase in patient exposure is required that it be justified by improved diagnostic accuracy.

Treatment Implications

Current screening mammography is an excellent clinical tool. It has a relatively high sensitivity, but is less than ideal because of its relatively low

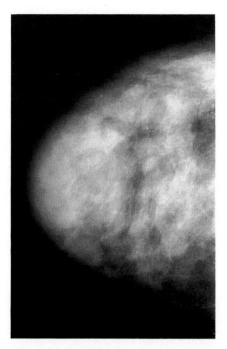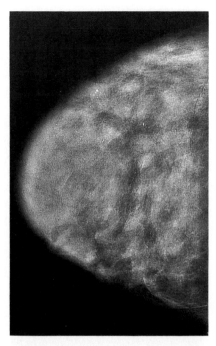

A   B

FIGURE 9.6. A radiodense breast with benign microcalcifications. (A) Standard processing. (B) Enhanced processing. The standard processing shows the calcifications in the
less radiodense regions of the breast without difficulty, but in the anterior portion of the
breast, the radiodensity is sufficient to obscure the calcifications. The enhanced image
better demonstrates these many benign calcifications.

specificity and relatively high cost, particularly if the costs of biopsies resulting from its low specificity are included. Detection of breast cancer when
a lesion is small improves patient outcome (Bedwani, Vana, Rosner et al.,
1981). Improvements in mammography that allow the detection of smaller
cancers will improve survival and should decrease health care costs. It is
also known that breast cancer has smaller microcalcifications than those
currently detectable by any imaging method in vivo (Egan, McSweeney, and
Sewell, 1980; Millis, Davis, and Stacey, 1976; Powell, McSweeney, and
Wilson, 1983;). If digital systems could allow the detection of smaller calcifications, more and smaller cancers may be detected.

Detecting Smaller Lesions

Finding smaller microcalcifications or smaller masses might shift the proportion of such lesions that represent cancer, altering the cost of finding cancer
through screening. If the proportion of cancers was decreased, this would increase both the psychological and physical trauma of unnecessary breast biop-

sies. Currently, clinicians at Georgetown do approximately three biopsies of masses or calcifications for each cancer detected. In other centers, it can be one in five. In one series, only 17 percent of biopsies done for microcalcifications showed cancer (Powell, McSweeney, and Wilson, 1983). Finding smaller microcalcifications and smaller masses could increase or decrease the frequency of biopsies demonstrating cancer. The authors are aware of no data on this potential problem.

As shown in Figure 9.8, there are several potential outcomes if technology allowed the detection of smaller lesions. In this drawing, let (A) represent the current detection of microcalcifications and small masses. If we increase the detection rate as shown by the larger circle in (B) (representing an increase in sensitivity with no change in specificity), then the percentage of cancers remains the same and we have not altered the expected cost of detecting cancer. Ideally, as shown in (C), better definition of detail would allow us to improve the proportion of cancers detected (an increase in sensi-

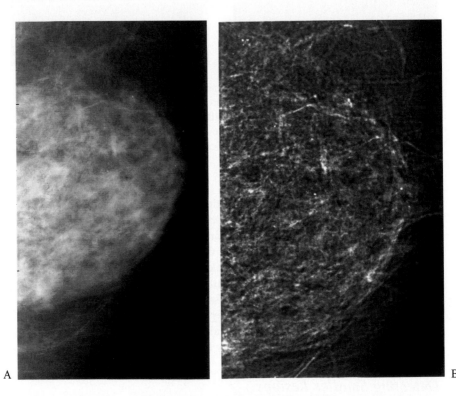

A   B

FIGURE 9.7. Digital mammogram of a radiodense breast containing groups of benign calcifications. (A) Standard digital image. (B) Special image processing with histogram equalization. On the equalized image, the microcalcifications are easier to see. The dense breast tissue is "removed" from the image.

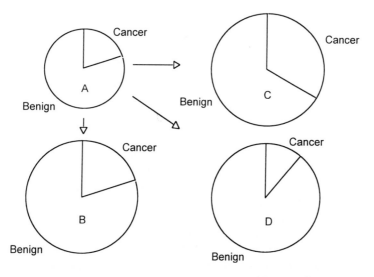

FIGURE 9.8. Delection of small lesions: possible scenarios.

tivity and specificity or just an increase in specificity). But, as shown in (D), the proportion of cancers might decrease resulting in an increased number of breast biopsies with little or no improvement in the detection of breast cancer (no change in sensitivity, decrease in specificity). Which of these scenarios will occur is unknown.

Improving Diagnostic Accuracy

Sensitivity

Although there is currently no supporting evidence, it is believed that digital mammography will improve the sensitivity of mammography for the detection of breast cancer. Reasons to believe so relate to the improved conspicuity of lesions whose mammographic appearances currently are used as indicators of the possible presence of breast cancer. Improving the conspicuousness of such findings makes them less likely to be missed.

Specificity

To improve the specificity of mammography, classification of detected lesions into benign and malignant categories must be done with greater precision than now possible. Current findings used to improve this categorization are related to the shape of microcalcifications, their number, the shape of the edges of identified masses, and the presence or absence of change from the prior mammogram. Digital mammography at 50 μm, as supported by preliminary data and not yet independently confirmed, appears to provide slightly greater information about shape to the human observer than conventional mammography. In a recently reported study, the classification of lesions as malignant was more accurate with the digital system, albeit not at a statistically significant level (Freedman, Artz, Hogge et al., 1997).

Computer Aided Diagnosis

The use of computer analysis to assist the radiologist in the detection of breast cancer and in the categorization of breast lesions into benign and malignant categories is currently in clinical trial at several sites. Preliminary data suggest that computer aided diagnosis will become an important aid to the radiologist, who will use it to provide a second opinion or second reading of the mammogram and predictive statistics as to whether a lesion is benign or malignant. Acquiring the mammogram in a direct digital form will make it substantially easier to implement computer aided diagnosis methods into clinical practice. Improved classification of identified lesions into benign and malignant categories should help prevent some unnecessary biopsies (Chan, Wei, Lam et al., 1995; Lo, Grisson, Floyd et al., 1995; Tsujii, Wu, Freeman et al., 1996; Wu, Lo, Zuurbier et al., 1994). This computer based improved classification should result in improved specificity of mammographic findings.

Cost Related Factors

Lead Time Bias

When improvements in digital mammography allow the detection of smaller cancers, the clinical outcome may not really change because of lead time bias. Although extensive future testing and confirmation would be necessary, this lead time effect may allow the interval between screening mammograms to be safely increased without affecting long-term outcome. If detecting breast cancer at a smaller size can be done with high sensitivity but does not affect its long-term prognosis, lengthening the interval between screening would have no effect on outcome, but would decrease the cost of breast cancer screening programs proportionately.

Cost Impact

At this time it is not possible to evaluate the long-term effect of the introduction of digital mammography on the cost of health care. The initial effect would be increased cost because of the need to acquire new equipment. In the longer view, this initial equipment cost may be offset by the following potential, but, as yet, experimentally unproved benefits:

- Improved specificity based on better information about shape, decreasing the number of biopsies for benign disease.
- Detection of cancer at an earlier stage.

- Use of lead time bias to increase the spacing between screening mammograms.
- Detection of cancer at an earlier stage in women with dense breasts, especially younger women.

Based on preliminary work with computer aided classification of mammographically identified lesions, improved specificity seems likely. Smaller cancers, it is expected, would proportionately be shifted toward those in a lower stage. Recent work on exposure effect differences between conventional screen film and digital mammography (Freedman, Steller, Jafroudi et al., 1995) suggests that digital mammography might offer advantages in the dense breast. The contrast enhancement that allows smaller and lower contrast objects to be detected digitally (Freedman, Pe, Zuurbier et al., 1994) could benefit the earlier detection of breast cancer in dense breasts. Clearly further research is needed to explore the full potential of digital mammography.

Summary

Digital mammography is the outgrowth of the convergence of two different paths represented by the progressive improvement of conventional screen film mammography and the progressive improvement of digital projection radiography. The improvements in conventional mammography have been directed towards improvements in contrast and thereby improvements in the conspicuity of normal and abnormal tissues within the breast. Digital mammography represents an extension of trends already evident in conventional mammography toward higher contrast images and higher lesion conspicuity. Radiologic diagnosis done on digital mammograms uses the same signs for the detection of breast cancer as conventional mammography, but appears to show the findings with greater conspicuity and perhaps at a slightly smaller size.

Digital mammography, as with all digital imaging, does require additional clinical training to understand both the value and limitations of computer processing, the artifacts that can be produced, and the ways in which computer processing can hide disease. In a fundamental sense, this is no different than learning about conventional screen film mammography—its values and limitations, its artifacts, and the ways in which a badly exposed, handled, or processed film can obscure disease. Because digital projection imaging is not extensively explored in most radiology residencies, courses would be needed to properly train radiologists in the proper use of digital mammography machines.

Digital mammography does require additional quality control procedures to assure that image quality is preserved and artifacts are limited. We believe that these must be machine specific, and we have devised them for the machine we use. Physicists, radiologic technologists, and service engineers will need training in the specific requirements of the digital mammography machine they will be using.

Experience at the Georgetown University Medical Center suggests that, with high level quality assurance, digital mammography can provide a small but measurable improvement in the conspicuity of the signs of breast cancer. The difference is so slight, however, that it probably will not improve the accuracy of mammographic detection or classification of lesions that might be due to breast cancer, especially when the interpreting radiologists are highly skilled in the mammographic detection of breast cancer. However, the quality of digital mammography performed with the Georgetown system is equivalent in accuracy to conventional mammography. Improvements in lesion conspicuity may improve the accuracy of less skilled radiologists or nonphysicians providing initial screening of mammography images prior to their review by a radiologist.

On the near horizon, systems are being developed that may provide a slight additional increment in image quality. The physician's creed is to do no harm to patients, but harm can occur both by delaying the introduction of an appropriate new technology and by proceeding with the inappropriate introduction of technology to replace a proven test. Digital mammography systems are complex. Improperly designed or used, they can either hide the findings of breast cancer or produce the appearance of lesions that can be misinterpreted as signs of breast cancer. Radiologists interested in digital mammography should be prepared to:

- Accommodate the progressive quality improvement that will occur as these machines improve over the next few years.
- Recognize the need for tests in geometric test objects, but realize that different test objects provide different information and that no test object truly reflects the complex composition of breast tissue or the mammographic signs of breast cancer. In the final analysis, clinical trials will be needed.
- Remain vigilant that radiation exposure is controlled to the minimum amount necessary.
- Evaluate clinical trials to be certain that these trials:
  - include a reasonable sample of breast cancers less than 1 cm in size.
  - include breasts of different parenchymal patterns.
- Be certain that the manufacturer supplies manuals for machine specific specialty training and machine specific quality control procedures.

References

Bedwani R, Vana J, Rosner D et al. Management and survival of female patients with "minimal" breast cancer. Cancer 1981, 47, 2769–2778.

Bidstrup P. Clinical Experience. In: Busch HP, Georgi M, eds. Digital Radiography Workshop. Schnetztor-Verlag GmbH, Konstanz, 1992, pp. 16–17.

Brettle DS, Ward SC, Parkin GJS et al. A clinical comparison between conventional and digital mammography utilizing computed radiography. Br J Radio 1994, 464–468.

Chan HP. Personal communication regarding effect of pixel size of film digitization on accuracy of computer aided diagnosis, Feb. 25, 1995.

Chan HP, Vyborny CJ, MacMahon H et al. Digital mammography: ROC studies of the effects of pixel size and unsharp mask filtering on the detection of subtle microcalcifications. Invest Radiol 1987, 22, 581–589.

Chan HP, Wei D, Lam K et al. Computerized detection and classification of microcalcifications on mammograms. Proc SPIE Medical Imaging: Image Processing, 1995, 2434, 612–620.

Egan RL, McSweeney MB, Sewell CW. Intramammary calcifications without an associated mass in benign and malignant diseases. Radiology 1980, 137, 1–7.

Freedman M, Artz DS, Hogge J et al. Storage phosphor digital mammography: a receiver operating characteristic (ROC) study (submitted) 1998.

Freedman M, Artz D, Jafroudi H et al. Digital mammography: an evaluation of the shape of microcalcifications. Proc SPIE Medical Imaging: Physics of Medical Imaging, 1996a, 2708, 626–632.

Freedman M, Artz D, Jafroudi H et al. Digital mammography in the radio-dense and complex pattern breast. Proc SPIE Medical Imaging: Image Processing, 1996b, 2701, 783–793.

Freedman M, Artz DS, Mun SK. Image processing in digital mammography: the optimum image for each woman's breasts. In: IEEE Colloquium on Digital Mammography. The Institution of Electrical Engineers: London, Jan. 1–3, 1996.

Freedman M, Pe E, Zuurbier R et al. Image processing in digital mammography. Proc SPIE Medical Imaging: Image Capture, Formatting, and Display, 1994, 2164, 537–554.

Freedman M, Steller D, Jafroudi H et al. Digital mammography: the effects of decreased exposure. Proc SPIE Medical Imaging: Physics of Medical Imaging, 1995a, 2432, 488–500.

Freedman M, Steller D, Jafroudi H et al. Digital mammography: tradeoffs between 50- and 100-micron pixel size. Proc SPIE Medical Imaging: Physics of Medical Imaging, 1995b, 2432, 114–125.

Fujita H, Endo T, Matsubara T et al. Automated detection of masses and clustered microcalcifications on mammograms. Proc SPIE Medical Imaging: Image Processing, 1995, 2434, 682–692.

Jarlman O, Samuelsson, Braw M. Digital luminescence mammography: early clinical experience. Acta Radiologica, 1991, 32, 110–113.

Jennings RJ, Jafroudi H, Gagne R et al. Storage phosphor-based digital mammography using a low-dose x-ray system optimized for screen-film mammography. Proc SPIE Medical Imaging: Physics of Medical Imaging, 1996, 2708, 220–232.

Joerg W, Oestmann JW, Kopans D et al. A comparison of digitized storage phosphors and conventional mammography in the detection of malignant microcalcifications. Invest Radiol 1988, 23, 725–728.

Krupinski EA, Roehrig H, Yu T. 1995. Observer performance comparison of digital radiograph systems for stereotactic breast needle biopsy. Acad Radiol 1995, 2, 116–122.

Lo JY, Grisson AT, Floyd CE et al. Computer-aided diagnosis of mammograms using an artificial neural network: merging of standardized input features from the ACR lexicon. SPIE Medical Imaging: Image Processing, 1995, 2434, 571–578.

Millis RM, Davis R, Stacey AJ. The detection and significance of calcifications in the breast: a radiological and pathological study. Br J f Radio 1976, 49, 12–26.

Powell RW, McSweeney MB, Wilson CE. X-ray calcifications as the only basis for breast biopsy. Ann Surg 1983, 197, 555–559.

Roehrig H, Krupinski EA, Yu T. Physical and psychophysical evaluation of digital systems for mammography. Proc SPIE Medical Imaging: Image Perception, 1995, 2436, 124–134.

Tsujii O, Wu YC, Freedman M et al. Classification of microcalcifications in digital mammograms for the diagnosis of breast cancer. Proc SPIE Medical Imaging: Image Processing, 1996, 2710,794–804.

Voegeli E. In: Busch HP, Georgi M, eds. Digital Radiography Workshop. Schnetztor-Verlag GmbH, Konstanz, 1992, pp. 90–91.

Wu YC, Lo S-CB, Zuurbier RA et al. Classification of microcalcifications using a hybrid neural network. Proc SPIE: Medical Imaging: Image Processing, 1994, 2167, 630–641.

10
Quality Assurance and PACS

John C. Weiser

The advent of PACS and filmless radiology has made it necessary for us to rethink the way we provide radiology services both within and between medical facilities. In the same manner, this new technology has caused us to step back and take a fresh look at the concepts of quality assurance and quality control. In 1988, the National Council on Radiation Protection and Measurements (NCRP) published its recommendations on quality assurance for diagnostic imaging and defined the term *Quality Assurance* as follows (NCRP, 1988):

> Quality Assurance is a comprehensive concept that comprises all of the management practices instituted by the imaging physician to ensure that: (1) every imaging procedure is necessary and appropriate to the problem at hand; (2) the images generated contain information critical to the solution of that problem; (3) the recorded information is correctly interpreted and made available in a timely fashion to the patient's physician; and (4) the examination results in the lowest possible radiation exposure, cost, and inconvenience to the patient consistent with objective (2).

A large part of quality assurance involves dealing with human performance issues, such as training, efficiency, or policies and procedures. Those specific areas of quality assurance that can be addressed by monitoring the performance of equipment are collectively referred to as Quality Control.

Equipment Performance and Quality Control

Because equipment performance has a major effect on the information content of the image and on the radiation exposure to the patient, we can see that part (2) and part (4) of the definition are related to quality control. In a film-based radiology department, part (3) of the definition, which deals with the interpretation of the image and the distribution of the image and the report, is beyond the scope of quality control, because it has little dependence on equipment. The alternator or lightbox on which the film is hung for interpretation is the last point in the workflow, where our traditional view of equipment quality control applies.

In contrast, a filmless radiology department continues to depend on equipment performance throughout the interpretation phase and for the delivery of both the images and the report to the patient's physician. The ability to provide the radiologist with appropriate previous examinations to aid in the interpretation is dependent on the performance of the PACS archive and the accuracy of the PACS database. The ability to make the interpretation and the images available to the patient's physician in a timely fashion is dependent on the speed and reliability of the hospital-wide network. In a filmless department, there is a continuous flow of digital information through a chain of networked devices that starts with the acquisition of the image and ends with the display of the image and the report on the desktop of the physician who ordered the examination.

The definition of quality control in the filmless department must be expanded to include all of these equipment components. Their performance must be monitored, both as a system and as individual parts. We must be able to evaluate not only how each individual component performs, but also how the components collectively perform to meet the criteria of the definition of quality assurance.

The Department of Defense (DoD) published a PACS specification for the Medical Diagnostic Imaging Support (MDIS) project, which can serve as a guide for developing a quality control program in a filmless radiology department (DoD, 1991). The MDIS specification breaks the PACS down into four subsystems:

- Image Acquisition Subsystem,
- Image Output and Display Subsystem,
- Image Database and Storage Subsystem, and
- Communications Network Subsystem.

This categorization provides a convenient way of focusing on the performance of groups of equipment items that have a similar function within the PACS, while still retaining the concept that they are all interrelated parts of an integrated system. The acceptance testing protocol for the MDIS contract made use of this dual focus on both component and system aspects of performance by having one set of measurements called the Component Performance Test and another set called the System Integration Test (Romlein, Weiser, Sheehy et al., 1994). The ability to integrate the various components into an overall system capable of supporting the complex flow of information that delivers an interpreted radiology examination to a requesting physician is the major challenge of PACS. The success or failure of a filmless hospital system depends, to a large degree, on the success or failure of this system integration.

The Image Acquisition Subsystem

Many of the imaging modalities in a modern radiology department are inherently digital, and thus require a minimal change in quality control management at the component level when the department transitions to filmless operations. Some modalities, such as computed tomography (CT) and magnetic resonance (MR), are often sold configured as a mini-PACS, with a dedicated image review workstation, database, and archive within a vendor proprietary network. Computed radiography (CR), a recent addition to many departments, is usually installed with a quality control workstation. Thus, we are already accustomed to performing certain quality control tests in soft copy form on a workstation, and many vendors have incorporated image analysis functions into their workstation software for this purpose. Recently, these mini-PACS configurations have also been offered for ultrasound and nuclear medicine systems. Other digital modalities, such as digital fluoroscopy or digital subtraction angiography, are not usually configured as a mini-PACS, but instead are set up for direct output to a laser film printer. In either case, in the filmless radiology department, there needs to be an interface from the vendor's equipment into the main PACS network, which can distribute the images to the appropriate locations throughout the hospital. To integrate equipment from various manufacturers into a functional system, a DICOM compliant interface should be specified (NEMA, 1993).

This interface can assume various forms, depending on how closely the modality vendor embraces the DICOM standard or on the age of the equipment to be connected. Regardless of the form it takes, this network connection becomes a new image production pathway that must be incorporated into a quality control program. The most desirable form is to have a DICOM network connection that is an integral part of the vendor's operating software. It is not unreasonable to specify this type of interface on all new equipment purchases, since the DICOM standard has been in existence for several years and there has been ample time for vendors to incorporate this feature into their product lines. If a built-in DICOM connection is not available, the next approach is to install a gateway that translates the vendor's proprietary network protocol to the DICOM standard. These gateways are sometimes offered by the modality vendor or they can be purchased from third party vendors who specialize in network integration. For situations in which images cannot be obtained in a format that can be converted to the specific DICOM modality standard, DICOM has a more general category called secondary capture. Secondary capture images are usually obtained by intercepting the modality's printer output, either by digitizing a video signal (a video frame grabber) or by connecting to a digital camera interface. When setting up a quality control schedule for network modality interfaces, the following points should be considered:

- Check for any configurable parameters in the modality and interface software that can affect the transmitted image, such as display look-up tables and default window/level settings. Record these settings and check them after any reload or upgrade of software. Put in place procedures to ensure that the quality control supervisor is notified whenever software is modified. If the vendor providing service has access to a remote dial-up modem on the network, take special care to control software changes that can be made by this method.

- Measure the transfer rate of the interface at a time of the day when the network is not busy and measure it again after any software changes. Realize that slight changes in communication protocol timing can have a significant effect on interface performance.
- Make a digital test image, such as a SMPTE Pattern (Gary, Lisk, Haddick et al., 1985), available on the modality side of the interface to send through to a PACS display workstation. Transmit this image at least weekly to verify proper operation of the interface.

The Image Output and Display Subsystem

The main components of the Image Output and Display Subsystem are the various configurations of display workstations that are connected to the PACS network. These workstations are generally subdivided into two general categories: diagnostic workstations and clinical review workstations. The distinction is not based as much on the quality of the workstation as on its intended function. The diagnostic workstation is designed to support the workflow required to perform primary diagnosis and render a report. These workstations normally have two or four monitors; they may have 2K or 1K resolution, depending on the type of images to be reviewed. In a filmless hospital, the CRT monitors of the PACS workstation replace the functions of the film processor and the lightbox; thus the tests that are performed on these two pieces of equipment in a film-based department must be transformed to an equivalent series of tests on the workstation. When we perform film sensitometry and densitometry, we are producing a series of calibrated gray levels that, in conjunction with the intensity of the film illuminator, determine the overall gray scale performance of the film-based display system. When we display a SMPTE pattern, or other type of gray scale test image, on a PACS workstation, we are performing the same function. With the film-based system, we separate the quality control measurements into two parts. One measurement determines the brightness of the unobstructed lightbox; the other determines the log of the relative transmission of light through the different gray scale blocks that the sensitometer placed on the film. Of course, we do not refer to this second measurement as "log of relative transmission"; we simply call it optical density. With a CRT monitor, the test image and the illumination source are not separable, so these two measurements are combined into one. The measurement of the brightness of the test pattern is made with a luminance meter, and the brightness is reported in units of foot-Lamberts (fL) or candela per square meter (cd/M^2).

The initial step in checking the performance of a CRT monitor is to adjust the minimum black level and the maximum white level, using the contrast and brightness controls. This is equivalent to checking the maximum optical density and the base plus fog level of the sensitometric strip on a film. Because we are accustomed to thinking in terms of optical density, it is useful to express the luminance range of the monitor in equivalent terms. We can define an equivalent optical density range of the monitor as

$$OD_{eq} = \log (L_{max} / L_{min})$$

where L_{max} and L_{min} are the luminance measurements of the maximum white level and minimum black levels, respectively. For example, the manufacturer's specifications for a typical monitor call for the black level to be set at 0.05 fL and the white level to be at 70 fL. The equivalent optical density range for this monitor is determined to be

$$OD_{eq} = \log (L_{max} / L_{min}) = \log (70/0.05) = 3.15$$

In other words, the dynamic range of the monitor is equivalent to that of a film whose maximum optical density is 3.15 above base plus fog. Because an SMPTE test pattern displays ten equally spaced steps of gray scale value, the luminance measurements at each of these steps can be used to construct a characteristic curve for the monitor response in the same manner that we use the optical density measurements of the sensitometer steps to construct an H&D curve for film. The equivalent optical density at any of the SMPTE steps is found by taking the log of the ratio of L_{max} to the luminance of the step. These values can then be plotted to construct an equivalent monitor response curve. In general, this response curve has a toe, but no shoulder. The normal response of a CRT monitor reduces contrast in bright parts of the image and enhances contrast in the darker parts of the image. For this reason most workstations have an inverted gray scale or black bone display option that allows the lighter parts of the image, such as bone, to be observed in the darker gray scale range. When the workstation contains two or more monitors, then the luminance response of each of the monitors should be in agreement to an acceptable tolerance. The MDIS specification required that the luminance of the monitors be matched to within 5 percent. Brightness uniformity is the final quality control check to be performed with the luminance meter. This criterion measures the difference in luminance between the center and the edges of the display. The maximum allowable difference for brightness uniformity in the MDIS specification was 15 percent.

The Image Database and Storage Subsystem

The image database and storage subsystem is the digital equivalent of the film file room, the clerks who are responsible for filing the film with the report and associated records, and the system that is used to track the status of these records within the department and throughout the hospital. This subsystem is the heart of the PACS, or perhaps, more appropriately, the central nervous system. The storage part of the subsystem usually has two parts:

short-term storage and long-term storage. Short-term storage is most often an array of magnetic disk devices that provide rapid access to active exams. Active exams include those for which an approved report has not yet been rendered, related older exams to be referred to when rendering a report on a new exam, inpatient exams for the entire patient length of stay, and exams to be used in conjunction with scheduled clinic appointments. This amount of data can require anywhere from 20 to several hundred gigabytes of storage, depending on the workload of the department and the extent of the outpatient clinics. Long-term storage is usually a library, sometimes called a jukebox, of tape cartridges or optical disks that are accessed by robotic retrieval mechanisms for reading and writing. Long-term storage contains all of the exam records that must be maintained by the hospital for a specified length of time. The MDIS specification required that the long-term storage system be able to maintain the current year plus the previous four years of examination information for most patients, and maintain certain records even longer. The memory requirement for long-term storage is usually measured in terabytes. A terabyte is equal to 1024-gigabytes. On some long-term storage systems, the disks or cartridges that contain the oldest data are removed and stored externally when the capacity of the jukebox has been reached. The location of the information on these disks or cartridges is still known to the database, and when needed, they must be fed back into the jukebox for retrieval. The terms online, near line, and off line are sometimes used to designate short-term storage, long-term storage in the jukebox, and long-term storage out of the jukebox, respectively.

Keeping track of such a large amount of information gathered from various sources, including imaging systems, radiology information systems, and hospital information systems, is no small task. As a quality assurance check in a film-based department, one might randomly pick a number of patients and see if the film jacket can be located, related older exams can be found, and the reports are filed with the films. One might also check for backlogs in filing or delivery of film folders. These same types of checks must be performed in a filmless department, but the focus is on the integrity of the database, rather than on the operation of a film file room. To manage effectively the operation of a PACS, it is essential to have the capability to produce various reports of the transactions occurring in the database. These reports should be designed to highlight undesired conditions in the database that need to be corrected.

For example, there may be images in the PACS that can not be associated with a particular scheduled exam, or there may be exams that should have been completed but have no images. These situations, known as orphaned exams, are the equivalent of misfiled information in a film-based hospital. This situation often occurs when an entry error is made by the technologist at the operator's console of one of the imaging devices, such as misspelling a name or interchanging two digits of a patient ID number. When these images are sent to the PACS, the information typed in by the technologist is used to match the images with examination data that was most likely obtained through an interface to the hospital or radiology information system. If the PACS database cannot get a good match of the data fields it uses to link these information elements, an orphaned exam is created. Such a condition then requires manual intervention by a person who is authorized to determine the source of the error, correct the data elements, and properly link the images with the examination information.

Orphaned exams can be avoided if the imaging system has the capability to interface to the information system used to schedule the exams. With such an interface, the technologist operating the imaging system does not type in the patient's name or any other patient demographics. Instead, an acquisition work list is provided at the operator's console based on data received from the scheduled examination data on the information system. An interface such as this avoids the possibility of typographic error and assures that the data associated with the images matches the data associated with the examination. These HIS/RIS interfaces are now available for some computed radiography systems, but manufacturers of other imaging modalities have been slow to incorporate this capability into their products. Other, more generalized reports can also be constructed that can indicate symptoms of problems with the archive and database. Statistics on the volume of information being retrieved from long-term storage or on the average age of the information in short-term storage can point to systemic problems if outside of an acceptable range of values. A properly integrated PACS/HIS/RIS can be a valuable tool for providing insight into the operation of the filmless radiology department.

The Communications Network Subsystem

The final subsystem that connects all of the parts is the communications network subsystem. This system deals with the physical and logical connections among all of the input devices, the display devices, and the database and archive. It is the digital equivalent of the "sneaker net" that is used in a film-based department to carry films and records from one place to another. Before a PACS is installed in any medical institution, a large amount of data about the volume and rate of image generation and image usage is obtained. This data is then used to model the bandwidth requirements and network design for the PACS. In the MDIS specification, clinical scenarios were developed for each of the three original installation sites, and generic scenarios were developed for typical small, medium, and large medical treatment facilities within the U.S. Army and Air Force. These scenarios described the image production rates of the facilities in terms of images per day and images per year for each modality, and also estimated the peak throughput in images per hour at the busiest time of the day. Estimates of the rate at which studies would be reviewed at workstations within the department of radiology and the hospital emergency and critical care units were also provided. Based on the PACS vendor's model of how their system operates, they will then design the network so that it can support the existing workload and have sufficient excess capacity to allow for future expansion or configuration changes. As a quality control measure, it is necessary to have means in place to monitor network activity and identify potential problems before they can affect clinical operations.

There are various commercial software products available which provide this type of network management information, and most PACS vendors have incorporated one of these products into their PACS software package. In addition, it is useful to have a standard set of images that can be used to test the overall end-to-end system performance on a scheduled basis at various times of the day. The MDIS specification defined a standard chest study and a standard CT study for purposes of bench marking system performance. The chest study consisted of two newly acquired images and four images in previous exams that had to be retrieved from long-term storage. The CT study consisted of a new exam and an old exam in long-term storage, each consisting of 50 images. The bench mark requirement was that no more than five minutes could elapse between the time of initiation of the transfer of the new study from the acquisition device until both the new study and the relevant old study were available for review at the diagnostic workstation. The test was to be performed under loaded network conditions. The real problem with objectively performing such a test is in the definition of loaded network conditions. However, if this test is performed repeatedly as a quality control check at various times on an operating system, some sense of the normal range of performance can be obtained.

Conclusion

This chapter has provided an overview of the concepts of quality assurance in a filmless radiology department. It can be seen that the same methodology and philosophy that is presently used in the quality assurance program of a film-based department has logical equivalents in the filmless system. In many ways, quality assurance is much more straightforward in the filmless environment because the physical design of the PACS requires us to think of radiology as an integrated process. A well-designed and well-maintained PACS database can provide radiology department managers with reports and statistics that point out potential problems before they become a serious issue. Radiology is a service activity. The product is the interpretation of a radiologic examination, and the customer is the referring physician. A well-designed quality assurance program promotes the delivery of this service in the most efficient and timely manner.

References

Department of Defense (DoD). Medical Diagnostic Imaging Support (MDIS) system. Contract No. DACA87-91-D-0047, U.S. Army Corps of Engineers, Huntsville, AL, 1991.

Gary JF, Lisk KG, Haddick DH et al. Test pattern for video displays and hard copy cameras. Radiology, 1985, 154, 519–527.

National Council on Radiation Protection and Measurement (NCRP). Quality assurance for diagnostic imaging, NCRP report no. 99. Bethesda, MD: NCRP, 1988.

National Electrical Manufacturers Association (NEMA). Digital Imaging and Communications in Medicine (DICOM), NEMA standards publication PS 3.x. Washington, DC: NEMA, 1993.

Romlein J, Weiser JC, Sheehy M et al. Acceptance testing design execution and results for large-scale PACS installations. Proc SPIE, Medical Imaging, 1994, 2165, 569–581.

Section 4

11
PACS and the End User: A Study in Two Demanding Environments

STEPHEN M. POMERANTZ, ZENON PROTOPAPAS, AND ELIOT L. SIEGEL

Diagnostic imaging has historically been hostage to the limitations of film. The digital medium used by picture archiving and communication systems (PACS) promises to free radiologists and clinicians from many of the constraints of the hardcopy image. As PACS allow clinicians easy and direct access to images, the utility and acceptance of PACS will depend on how well these end users' specific requirements are satisfied. In addition to the need for adaptability to the varied end users (e.g., different physician specialists, nurses, technicians, physical therapists), the PACS must function equally well in different hospital environments whether it be the medical ward, intensive care unit, emergency department, operating room, or outpatient clinic.

Relying on the film paradigm to design large-scale PACS may result in poor utilization of the capabilities of digital image management and display. Potentially this could result in a system that does not meet the requirements of all its diverse users. Most traditional film-based imaging is oriented toward the radiologist and the radiology department in which the majority of imaging related activity occurs. A PAC system will disperse a greater proportion of this activity throughout the hospital and associated facilities and the system's design should reflect this. Although experience with film-based radiology should be a design influence, the opinions of the specific end users and the experiences of users in existing PACS-based hospitals should also heavily influence design. For a PAC system implementation to be successful, it must provide an overall functionality that meets or exceeds that of film in all of the hospital areas in which it operates.

This chapter draws on the experiences of end users, both radiologist and nonradiologist, with implementation of a hospital-wide PACS at the Baltimore Veterans Affairs Medical Center (BVAMC). Special attention is paid to two of the more challenging areas of deployment.

The Baltimore Experience

A 300-bed teaching hospital performing 60,000 imaging studies per year, the Baltimore Veterans Affairs Medical Center has operated a hospital-wide PACS installed by General Electric (Milwaukee, WI) since 1993. Its 42 workstations utilize MacIntosh IIFX or Quadra 950 computers (Apple Computer, Cupertino, CA). These are distributed throughout the BAMC, including the diagnostic imaging department, patient care wards, conference rooms, surgical and medical outpatient clinics, the emergency department (ED), intensive care unit (ICU), and the operating room (OR).

The workstations display both images and report text and are bidirectionally linked to the hospital information system/radiology information system (HIS/RIS). Workstations are linked by fiberoptic cable to a central server using a proprietary network protocol that enables rapid image retrieval and display. Images are initially stored online for approximately two to three months after acquisition on a central high-performance image file server. Studies are then automatically archived to an optical jukebox from which retrieval times are somewhat longer (1.2 minutes versus 1.5 seconds for a CR image). A separate HIS/RIS PACS utilizing separate workstations is available throughout the hospital. It displays and stores patient information as well as clinical images such as digitized photographs, endoscopy, bronchoscopy, and laparoscopic images. Radiology images are stored (at lower resolution than the radiology PACS) on this second PACS serving as a backup in case of failure of the radiology PACS.

Our experience in two of the more challenging hospital environments, the operating room and the emergency department, will be detailed in an attempt to provide insight into the benefits and challenges of a large-scale PACS for the radiologist and nonradiologist end user. The challenges facing successful filmless operation will be explored with attention to those measures that can be taken to better tailor a large-scale PACS to all of the varied hospital environments. Measures implemented or proposed to address problems encountered will be described as a model to illustrate how to best match a PAC system's capabilities to its end users.

Operating Room (OR)

The OR is a particularly demanding environment for PACS. The system must satisfy diverse personnel in an often tense atmosphere. Any interruption or malfunction in system operation would at best waste expensive OR time and complicate the OR schedule. Potentially, a system problem could have adverse effects on a patient's well-being. Surgeons and staff may have difficulty operating the workstation simultaneously with the surgical tasks they are performing, especially given sterility considerations. Ergonomic issues, such as component location, may affect the utility and acceptance of the system.

PACS offer considerable advantages for the OR. Perhaps most important is the capability to display all of a patient's images and reports on demand, thereby dispensing with the common OR problem of inability to locate the pertinent films. Workstation tools have the ability to significantly improve the quality of intraoperative images, which are classically of poor quality.

The BVAMC contains six general-purpose operating rooms each containing a two-monitor 1152 x 1078 pixel workstation. Two urology ORs share an additional workstation. Although most surgeons at the BVAMC agree that the PAC system has been successful in the OR, satisfaction levels have varied among different surgical specialties and differing types of OR support staff when these personnel have been surveyed.

Tailoring a PACS to any specific type of user requires knowledge of their patterns of image review. In the OR, these patterns vary by specialty and procedure. Image review often occurs outside of the OR, perhaps in the surgical clinic, patient care ward, or near the surgeon's office where the site, scope, and approach of the surgical procedure are determined. Preoperative images are often rereviewed in the OR just prior to surgery. Use of images during surgery varies considerably. The PAC system is used intraoperatively either to display images as a "roadmap" to guide the procedure or to display intraoperative imaging studies such as cholangiography, cystography, prosthesis/hardware positioning, or stereotactic brain biopsies. Overall, the BVAMC general surgeons tend to utilize the PACS during surgery infrequently (<15 percent), whereas the orthopedic, vascular, and neurosurgeons use PACS during surgery in more than 90 percent of cases. Interestingly, many preoperative images that would be displayed on the OR lightbox during surgery in a film-based hospital are not displayed in the PACS OR. Surgeons admit that in the film-based hospital these images are often hung as "window dressing, more for ambiance than utility." They do, however, consider their ready availability for potential use essential.

Image Quality

The PACS workstations in the BVAMC's ORs utilize relatively lower resolution monitors (1152 × 1078 pixel) when compared to the "diagnostic" monitors used in the radiology department (1536 × 2048 pixel). Despite this difference, there is general satisfaction with the quality of the images. This may be explained by the advantages that result from being able to extract additional information from images with workstation tools, such window/level controls and magnification. This is especially true in the case of portable intraoperative studies that are typically of limited quality on film because of deficiencies in exposure, contrast, and overlying artifact. The number of repeat interoperative images required has been reduced with the PACS when compared to film. There have been occasional complaints by orthopedic surgeons that the monitors cannot resolve fine structures in bone that need to be visualized during surgery. Higher resolution monitors in the orthopedic operating rooms would address this problem.

Image quality only partially depends on the workstation itself. It also relies on the technologists' attention to quality and their understanding of the capabilities of the workstation. Attention to proper imaging technique has declined somewhat at the BVAMC since PACS implementation because of some technologists' notion that workstation tools, such as window/leveling, can correct any deficiency. Although some deficiencies in technique can in fact be corrected to some degree (e.g., exposure), other elements of technique, such as proper positioning, cannot. Because the technologist in a film-based hospital must bring films back to the OR once they are processed, surgeons there have an opportunity to complain when images are suboptimal; this has a quality assurance (QA) advantage. In a PACS based hospital, the technologist would not have to return to the OR after placing the imaging plate in the reader unless needed for additional x-ray examinations. Educating technologists in advance of the true capabilities and limitations of the PAC system with regard to image quality is essential. Additionally, requiring them to return to the OR to display images on the workstation may address the accountability issue.

Workstations

Operation

The degree to which the surgeon operates the workstation personally or delegates this task to OR staff varies widely. Often the surgeon will display and arrange images just prior to surgery and have a nurse use the workstation during the surgery, usually to page through already arranged and formatted images. Frequently one of the assistant surgeons will "break scrub" to operate the workstation. Alternatively, the primary surgeon will often don a second pair of gloves to operate the workstation. Magnification, window/level, and measurement are the image manipulation tools used most frequently. Angle measurement capabilities are often used by orthopedic surgeons.

Component Location

The level of satisfaction with the location of the workstation keyboard, pointing device, and monitors tends to vary based on personal preferences of surgeons and staff as well as on the layout and workstation location within a given OR. Most BVAMC surgeons and staff believe workstation components could be arranged in a more ergonomic fashion than was originally implemented. Issues raised have included the distance of the monitors from the OR table, inappropriate monitor height, and inconvenient placement of keyboard and pointing devices with respect to the operating table. Nurses and OR technicians in particular have complained that the workstations sometimes obstruct OR traffic flow. Installing the monitors on ceiling-mounted articulated arms would allow variable positioning, including the ability to bring the monitors to eye-level close to the OR table. Use of a wireless keyboard/pointing device (with a sterile covering) located at the OR table and/or a foot pedal have been requested by many surgeons and staff.

Tools

Surgical staff at the BVAMC have found workstation operation complicated and have had difficulty using many of the workstation tools. Although many feel that this could be improved through training, there is a desire for less complex, more automated controls. The most common complaint is that inability to properly operate nonintuitive window/level controls results in poor image contrast. Radiologists have often observed surgeons and staff who were unaware that they were viewing markedly suboptimal images as a result of poor window/level settings. Automated image display or window/level setting presets (already available on workstations within the radiology department) could reduce this problem.

Lighting

Lighting conditions in the BVAMC OR have been less than optimal for viewing the PACS monitors. Image conspicuity is degraded by glare from ambient light. Improved nonglare monitors and/or the ability to dim the lights with a foot pedal could address this problem.

Manipulation of Multiple Studies/Sequences

Comparing images from multipart studies or between different studies has confounded surgeons and staff. For example, there have been difficulties observed comparing CT or MRI scans from different dates. Viewing and comparing different sequences on MRI examinations has been particularly cumbersome. More sophisticated image navigation software would to assist with this problem. Although some surgeons have suggested more monitors per workstation, most surgeons believe that this would only contribute to increased OR clutter.

Inactivity Settings

To prolong monitor life, all hospital workstation monitors were originally designed to go blank after five minutes of nonuse. Many of the surgeons and staff interpreted the screen blanking as a workstation malfunction. This resulted in frantic calls from the OR to the radiology department. Resetting the default workstation inactivity timer to eight hours easily solved this unanticipated problem.

Component Damage

Frequently, containers of fluid, such as blood, specimens, and pathology chemicals (e.g., formaldehyde), are placed near PACS components, where a spill could cause considerable damage. Keyboard and pointing devices are vulnerable to wet hands/gloves. Currently, mice rather than trackballs are used because of difficulty manipulating a trackball with gloves on.

Component Cleaning and Maintenance

Workstations are considered dust collectors by many surgical staff members, because regular OR and clinic custodial staff tend to avoid cleaning the PACS components for fear of damaging the equipment. Cleaning and proper maintenance is essential in this critical area and may need to be provided almost entirely by radiology department personnel.

Intraoperative Examinations

Logistical Issues

Most intraoperative image acquisition at the BVAMC utilizes conventional portable x-ray machines using computed radiography (CR) plates. As with other x-ray examinations in the hospital, the imaging plate must be delivered to a CR image reader where it is read into the PACS. This requires that the technologist carry the plates from the fifth floor ORs to image readers located on other floors (one is near the ICU one floor below and two others are in the radiology department on the first floor). Surgeons and staff perceive that there is a longer period between OR image acquisition and availability for review when compared to a film-based OR. Several explanations have been offered for this difference:

- Lack of a film reader adjacent to the operating rooms. In a large film-based hospital, a film processor is usually located in or near the OR. Because of the equipment expense, the PACS hospital may be limited in the number and location of CR readers. Significant delay may result from time spent carrying image plates to a remote image reader.
- Loss of technologist accountability. As discussed, in a typical film-based system, the technologist obtains the intraoperative x-rays, takes them to be processed, and returns with them to the OR. The idea of impatient surgeons waiting for the films represents a strong incentive for the technologist to process and return with the films expeditiously. In the PACS setting at the BVAMC, the technologist's responsibility originally ended at the film reader. Not having to face the surgeons again resulted in a decrease in technologist speed (and as discussed, image quality).
- Inability to easily determine when images are ready for review. Because the technologist does not return with the images as they would in a film-based system, the surgeons and staff do not know when the images are ready for review without repeatedly checking the on-screen exam lists for the image status. Additionally, images may be ready but

the surgical staff delayed in reviewing them because of difficulty locating them within the system.

Solutions

Given the above experience, the plate reader has been relocated to an area adjacent to the OR suite. This move was difficult to accomplish due to the constraints of a busy OR environment. This is one of the better examples of how additional attention to efficient design of PACS prior to implementation could have avoided considerable expense and inefficiency.

As for technologist accountability, a solution would be to require technologists to return to the OR after processing the image plates in the reader. At this point they could bring up the images on the workstation, thereby obviating the problem of surgeons not knowing when images are ready and where they are located in the system. It would also free the OR personnel from the inconvenience of having to interrupt their activities to operate the workstation. In the absence of this, software and/or hardware could be configured to give an audible or visible indicator that images are ready. Finally, having intraoperative images come up on the workstation monitors automatically is a solution offered by BVAMC surgeons that appears to have validity.

A C-arm fluoroscope is used for a small subset of portable OR studies. A direct interface with the PACS is not available at the BVAMC and these images are therefore not archived. Interestingly, when surveyed, this was not a capability that the BVAMC surgeons considered necessary or desirable.

Other OR Issues

Orthopedics

Orthopedic surgeons have registered the most dissatisfaction using the PACS. This is in part because specific functions of film are not duplicated by workstations. Proper size selection of prostheses and other hardware involves placing a clear plastic template over a film image. They are unable to use these templates at the BVAMC because laying the template over the image on the monitor has been unreliable. This would require the image to be formatted with a 1:1 aspect ratio. They have requested that the software be modified to allow this. Orthopedic surgeons often superimpose pre- and postprocedure films to assess adequacy of intervention. For example, in the case of a fracture, a prereduction film is often superimposed over the postreduction image to assess for change. Currently the workstation software does not support this superimposition of images.

Review of Previous Examinations

At the BVAMC, images acquired or reviewed within a two-month period can be accessed from the rapid image server and brought up on the PACS workstation within seconds. This accounts for the vast majority of images needed in the OR. Occasionally, images not recently acquired or reviewed are needed and must be fetched from the long-term optical disk jukebox archive. This usually occurs in less than a minute. However, in practice, longer waits are possible because of other requests for images from all over the hospital. Surgeons have approached this problem by assigning a member of their staff to "prefetch" any studies that they might possibly need prior to surgery so they will be available from the rapid image server if needed. The current BVAMC system gives retrieval priority to radiologists over other users. Surgeons have requested that OR users have a similar priority, as well as an emergency fetch that would allow them to gain immediate access to archived images before other users. Automated prefetch protocols could be devised that would automatically trigger examination retrieval from the long-term archive whenever a preset event occurs. Such events could include hospital admission or OR procedure posting. Faster hardware and software should also improve retrieval speed.

Fear of System Malfunction

There is a natural tendency among the computer literate and noncomputer literate alike to fear total dependence on a computer system to provide images for an area as critical as the OR. Although there is no record in BVAMC OR logs of a procedure postponement or cancellation because of PACS malfunction, the potential for system failure is of considerable concern to surgeons and staff. Availability of a PAC system engineer is essential 24 hours a day, especially given the critical activities that take place in areas such as the OR. The BVAMC provides in-house PACS repair and troubleshooting staff members during regular working hours and on call technical support during off-hours. On-call staff members have remote access to the PACS via modem and are available to come to the hospital in person when necessary. Other safeguards at the BVAMC include the proprietary HIS/RIS PACS available in all of the ORs, which contains all diagnostic images (at lower resolution) and therefore provides necessary system redundancy. The hospital maintains emergency generators to provide backup electrical power to all critical hospital systems including the PACS. Given the potential for a system failure with loss of ability to retrieve and display images, surgeons and staff consider the ability to print film as a backup critical.

Potential for Three-Dimensional Imaging

Surgeons, to a much greater extent than radiologists, are accustomed to a three-dimensional perspective. The PACS workstations can provide them with this perspective via rapid sequential image display (cine mode). Three-dimensionally reconstructed images from CT and MRI studies can be displayed on the workstation in the form of rotating images. Although only a small percentage of studies are reconstructed and displayed in this manner, the feedback from surgeons has been very favorable. An additional advantage of the cine mode is the ability to display angiograms, ultrasound studies, nuclear cinecardiographs, and magnetic resonance angiograms in motion to facilitate interpretation. Making these capabilities more available would be an asset.

PACS Training for Surgeons and OR Staff

Tailoring PACS training to the specific needs and requirements of those in the surgical setting is essential. Formal PACS training is offered at the BVAMC on a one-to-one basis by appointment during working hours. Initially offered to physicians and physician assistants only, only a small number of the surgeons took taken advantage of the formal training, stating that OR-related time limitations and scheduling conflicts prevented training session attendance. PACS workstation operation is consequently learned from colleagues or is "self-taught." Interestingly, all physician assistants surveyed took the training and reported that it was valuable. The initial lack of nursing staff training was felt to be particularly detrimental in the OR because surgeons frequently call on the circulating nurses to operate the workstation. Training of nurses was implemented after the need was recognized, and the majority of nurses have completed the tutorial. Despite the training, most nurses consider their PACS skills less than optimal. A common frustration is situation where a nurse struggles with operation of a workstation with an impatient surgeon looking over his or her shoulder.

Solutions for addressing the poor utilization of training resources by surgeons center on making training sessions more convenient and accessible. Although computer based training modules have been introduced to assist in this regard, the surgeons and staff have not significantly taken advantage of them. Reasons for this include poor communication of the modules' availability and an inconvenient placement on the computers in the radiology department. Surgical staff have suggested that these modules be accessible on any PACS workstation within the hospital. There is consensus among OR and radiology staff that training should be site-specific with more in-depth teaching of functions typically used in the OR. Training personnel could visit the OR on a regular basis to provide guidance on-site and answer questions as they come up. Certain OR personnel could be more highly trained and act as a resource for other staff. Making operation of the workstation less complex would in turn make training easier.

Security

System security is essential to prevent tampering with the PACS software and data and to protect patient medical record confidentiality. Although all appropriate OR staff are required to have unique passwords for PACS access, OR staff often use a common password. This could be addressed by having the system periodically force the user to change passwords or by having the system deny access when the sign-on codes are already in use. Surgeons report difficulty keeping track of the many passwords a staff member has for the different computer systems at the BVAMC and the adjacent University of Maryland Hospital. A unified password for all systems including PACS would be advantageous.

Emergency Department (ED)

As is the case with the OR, the ED presents many unique challenges for a PACS system. Speedy triage, evaluation, and treatment require dependable, ready access to images and imaging reports. When compared to traditional film-based imaging, PACS has many definite advantages in accomplishing these goals. However, given the critical nature of ED activity, not meeting these standards can have significant consequence.

The Baltimore VAMC Emergency Department provides a full range of emergency services, serving approximately 35,000 patients and ordering 10,000 imaging examinations per year. Emergency Medicine attendings, residents, and medical students staff the ED. Additionally, there are nurses, physician assistants, technicians, clerks and orderlies.

The BVAMC ED contains two imaging workstations, each with two medium resolution (1024 × 1280 pixel) monitors. The following paragraphs reflect experience gleaned over the past three years in this fast-paced high pressure hospital environment.

Image Quality

A typical x-ray image contains areas of widely varying density. The static nature of film requires a compromise in technical factors that will allow an acceptable but not optimal level of contrast for all parts of the film. With a digital image on a PACS workstation, the user can evaluate each part of the image with contrast settings optimal for that area. This ability to window and level over any area of an examination is especially helpful with extremity examinations for trauma that are very common in the ED setting. For example, a fracture on a foot x-ray might be overlooked on film because of poor contrast in the affected area. With PACS, all areas can be examined with multiple window level combinations for better visualization. In a survey of BVAMC ED physicians, 54 percent were more confident interpreting an image on PACS rather than film, 24 percent preferred film, and the rest had no preference or had no response.

ED examinations often are predisposed to poor image quality as a result of the nature of the typical ED patient. Because of a patient's condition, examinations often must be taken portably and or with less than optimal patient positioning. Uncooperative patients are common. Frequently, images must be acquired through clothing, neck stabilization collars, or backboards.

PACS offer the ability to adjust contrast to the point that diagnostic images are attainable where images on film would have been unacceptable. This is reflected in the decrease in the BVAMC radiograph retake rate from 5 percent prior to PACS to 0.8 percent after PACS implementation. Although this has not been quantified for the ED alone, ED physicians estimate their retake rates were significantly higher than the 5 percent with film but match the less than 1 percent rate currently.

Image Loss

The ED in a film-based hospital typically is one of the areas most affected by film loss. Given the acute nature of the ED activity, films are often removed from the radiology department without being signed out. The films often are taken farther afield by ward clinicians when patients are admitted to their service. Examination loss prevents a report from being generated, resulting in potential financial and medicolegal repercussions. PACS virtually eliminates this problem by making the images available to all who need them at the same time without the prospect of film loss. The undictated examination rate at the BVAMC has decreased from 8 percent in 1993 before PACS to 1.5 percent in 1994 after PACS went into operation and subsequently has dropped to less than 0.3 percent.

Image Review Time

As is the case with the OR, delays in patient care because of imaging related problems are poorly tolerated. The vast majority of ED physicians are of the opinion that reviewing images with a PACS workstation is faster than when reviewing film. This is in large part the result of time saved by not having to retrieve the films. The film library, a constant source of complaints and delay in a typical film-based hospital, is taken completely out of the loop. The stacks of film jackets that an ED physician typically has to search through to find a stat exam do not exist in the filmless environment. Often, previous films are unavailable for comparison in the ED. However, with PACS, they can be retrieved from the archive. In similar fashion to the OR, protocols for prioritization of retrieval, emergency fetch capability, automated prefetching, and improved hardware and software would be helpful.

Comparison to Film

ED staff have had some difficulty when comparison is necessary between images on the workstation and film. This becomes necessary in two instances: when previous BVAMC examinations were acquired before PACS implementation and when patients bring examinations from other institutions. While the former instance has been almost completely eliminated by the passage of time, the ED is unique in the large number of films from outside facilities that are brought in with the patient. Film viewboxes are positioned on the wall near the workstations, but the proximity is not optimal. Soft copy images and outside films are not immediately adjacent as would be the case in an all-film or all-PACS environment. ED staff complain that the difference in lighting between the viewbox and the monitor also make comparison difficult. Radiologists have suggested that the problem be alleviated by digitizing the outside films. This would allow direct comparison on the monitors and would assure that the images are archived. Currently at the BVAMC, the ED film must be taken to the radiology department where the film digitizers reside and locate personnel trained to properly digitize and attach appropriate demographic information. The time involved in this process makes this impractical for the busy ED staff often attending to very sick patients. A solution would be to place a digitizer in the ED and have the radiology technologist trained to operate it.

Reporting Time

PACS provides the potential for radiologists to report ED examinations as soon as they are available. True real-time reporting has been realized during working hours, in which radiologists interpret studies as soon as they appear on the exam list. Keeping an empty or near empty queue has become a source of pride for BVAMC radiologists. Immediate interpretation allows ED physicians to be contacted more quickly with a positive finding. Electronic annotation on the image including text, arrows, and circles calling attention to positive findings has been very helpful to the ED clinicians. Although the official report generation time has decreased significantly because of the efficiencies of the PAC system, it still is not rapid enough for ED personnel to have a dictated report at the time of patient care. Currently, BVAMC reports are reported on a digital dictation system and transcribed directly into the HIS/RIS. Clinicians can access the radiologists dictation immediately using the telephone. Reports are then available on the HIS/RIS system and on the PACS linked to the appropriate images, typically within two hours. Near real-time dictation capability will be necessary to provide a final dictated report at the time of patient care. Automated voice recognition systems would accomplish this goal and could be integrated with a PAC system. Because clinicians are less likely to visit the radiology department in the PACS environment, they are also less likely to directly consult the radiologist for an opinion. The consultative role of the radiologist might therefore be diminished. Near real-time dictation would allow the report to be available to the clinician at the time of image interpretation. They are more likely to then read the report than if it comes several days after the image has been reviewed.

Coverage

There is ongoing controversy regarding the responsibility for immediate radiology consultation. In many areas, radiologists are not compensated if they do not provide reporting at the time of patient care. Although coverage is not an issue at the BVAMC, where an in-house radiologist provides night and weekend coverage, teleradiology capabilities of PACS address the need for immediate radiologist consultation in other settings. Currently, two other VA facilities are linked with the BVAMC; telemedicine is important for ED physicians in assessing potential patient transfers for emergency treatment.

Time Savings

Of those ED physicians surveyed, 84 percent believe that they save time using a PAC system when compared to a film-based system. More time savings could result from having more workstations available, more intuitive and automated workstation controls, faster retrieval of old examinations, and more integration of radiology images with other medical information. The PAC system containing medical records and clinical images is separate from the radiology PAC system. Combining the two systems would be more efficient.

PACS and Change

PAC systems have the advantage of allowing images to be immediately available wherever a workstation is sited without the inconvenience of retrieving film or fear of lost films. This has profound consequences for how clinicians and radiologists interface with imaging studies. The potential is for better patient care because of better access to and analysis of diagnostic images. But as clinicians and radiologists benefit from these advantages, they will also have to adjust to the constraints and peculiarities of PACS. Clinicians and radiologists must become facile with workstation operation. This may be more difficult for those that are more technophobic. Workstation availability may be more limited than desired. Radiologists may lose a measure of control they have enjoyed until now; no longer is control of the image (formerly the film), predominantly within their domain.

Clearly the implementation of PACS at the BVAMC has resulted in significant changes in the relationship of radiologists and clinicians to each other and to imaging in general. As illustrated in two critical areas of the hospital, the OR and ED, there are substantial benefits to having a PAC system and many potential problems. To best serve the patient, the radiologist, and the clinician, the problems must be minimized. There must be fast, convenient, user-friendly workstations that are suited to the environment in which they are sited. It is anticipated that most desktop PCs will be able to function as workstations (nondiagnostic), improving availability significantly. Retrieval of archived images must be rapid, and there must be technical support available at all times. As might be expected, given the lack of large numbers of already established large-scale PACS, the BVAMC PAC system could not anticipate all of the varied needs of different end users. As experience mounts, the minor and major modifications to the system that might tailor it to its many users are becoming evident. Many of these modifications (e.g., location of monitors in the OR) would be of negligible expense if anticipated before system installation. A one-size-fits-all system will serve none optimally.

A successful PACS implementation can be accomplished by carefully examining those systems already installed with attention to the requirements of different hospital environments and users. Clinicians must be involved in the design and planning of a hospital-wide PAC system from the start so that it better reflects their needs. In addition, they will be more invested in the success of the system. With a greater understanding of the PACS, they are less likely to resist changes in their practice patterns that will result from the introduction of a PACS. Once a system is installed it should be continuously monitored so that ongoing improvements can be made. Continued technological advances and careful attention to serving the needs of the radiologist, clinician, and patient will all contribute to the success of PAC systems as they become the norm.

Bibliography

Gay SB, Sobel AH, Young LQ, Dwyer SJ III. Processes involved in reading imaging studies: workflow analysis and implications for workstation development. J Dig Imag 1997, 10(1), 40–45.

Gur D, Fuhrman CR, Thaete FL. Requirements for PACS: users' perspective. Radiographics 1993, 13, 457–460.

Honeyman J, Staab EV. Operational concerns with PACS implementations. Appl Radiol 1997, 26(8), 13–16.

Honeyman JC, Frost MM, Huda W et al. Picture archiving and communication systems (PACS). Curr Probl Diagn Radiol 1994, 23, 101–158.

Horii SC. Electronic imaging workstations: ergonomic issues and the user interface Radiographics 1992, 12, 773–787.

Huang HK, Andricole K, Bazzill T, Lou SL, Wong AW, Arenson RL. Design and implementation of a picture archiving and communication system: the second time. J Dig Imag 1996, 9(2), 47–59.

Kuroda C, Yoshioka H, Kadota T, et al. Small PACS for digital medical images: reliability and security in a clinical setting. Comput Methods Programs Biomed 1994, 43, 101–106.

Pomerantz SM, Siegel El, Protopapas Z, Reiner BI, Pickar ER. Experience and design recommendations for picture archiving and communication systems (PACS) in the surgical setting. J Dig Imag 1996, 9(3), 123–130.

Protopapas Z, Siegel EL, Pomerantz SM, Reiner BI, Pickar E, Doherty RJ. PACS in the emergency room: experience at the Baltimore VA Medical Center and design considerations for the future. Proc S/CAR 412–414.

Protopapas Z, Siegel EL, Reiner BI, Pomerantz SM, Pickar ER. Picture archiving and communication system training for physicians: lessons learned at the Baltimore VA Medical Center. J Dig Imag 1996, 9(3), 131–136.

Ramaswamy MR. Wong AW. Lee JK, Huang HK. Accessing picture archiving and communication system text and image information through personal computers. AJR 1994, 163(5), 1239–1243.

Reiner BI, Siegel EL, Hooper F. Pomerantz SM, Protopapas Z, Pickar E. Killewich L. Picture archiving and communication systems and vascular surgery: clinical impressions and suggestions for improvement. J Dig Imag 1996, 9(4), 167–171.

Siegel EL. Plunging into PACS. Diagn Imaging 1993, 15, 69–71.

Siegel EL, Diaconis JD, Pomerantz SM et al. Making filmless radiology work. J Digit Imaging 1995, 8, 151–155.

Yamamoto I, Kaneda K. The practical use and evaluation of picture archiving and communication system in the department of orthopaedic surgery. J Dig Imag 1991, 4, 25–2.

12
PACS and Training

ZENON PROTOPAPAS, STEPHEN M. POMERANTZ, AND MICHAEL WILSON

When healthcare providers begin employment at a film-based medical center, they typically receive an informal orientation on radiology procedures from their colleagues. They learn how to order radiology examinations, find reports, and locate the films in various film libraries. Radiology technologists register studies, once completed, at the appropriate film library. Film library personnel present studies to the radiologist for reporting and locate films for healthcare providers who order them.

Filmless medical centers are different. Healthcare providers new to filmless imaging have much to learn. To begin with, there are no film libraries. Images are not managed by file room personnel. Radiology technologists enter the images into the PACS database for retrieval and subsequent review by the interpreting radiologist and the requesting physician. Transcriptionists enter reports into the PACS directly or through the interface with the hospital information system (HIS) or the radiology information system (RIS). Healthcare providers have to know how to retrieve images and reports from the database.

In this new setting, PACS training is required for a wide range of hospital personnel:

- Those inputting examinations into the PACS, including all imaging technologists and anyone operating a digitizer.
- Those requiring access to radiological examinations and their accompanying reports, including radiologists, other physicians and caregivers, and ancillary personnel, such as operating room technologists who may have to retrieve images during procedures when the surgeon is scrubbed.

An imaging department strives not only to produce high-quality imaging studies, but also to make these studies and their accompanying reports readily available to healthcare providers. In a filmless imaging department, these are stored in the PACS. To view them, healthcare providers need to be able to navigate the patient database, identify the patient, and then display images and report.

Training providers to become proficient with the PACS has a number of benefits. From the patient care standpoint, it ensures that clinicians are able to access images and reports as they are needed for optimal care. If the

PACS has been recently installed, user acceptance is critical. Experience shows that familiarity with any system generally improves acceptance. If the system is being newly installed, training healthcare personnel to use the PACS makes the transition from the film-based environment to a filmless environment easier. This is especially important during the introduction of the system, when there are no "experienced users" (except trainers) available to help other users having difficulties with the system.

It is typically the imaging department that gives healthcare providers logon and password identification for PACS, thereby granting the privilege to use the system. In effect, the department is acknowledging the proficiency of a given individual to use the system. For this reason, PACS training is the responsibility of the department and the hospital, although it is often delegated to the PACS vendor.

Training at the Baltimore VA Medical Center

This chapter provides an overview of PACS training at the Baltimore Veterans Administration Medical Center (BVAMC), one of the first facilities to adopt hospital-wide filmless radiology. The 300 bed tertiary-care facility provides medical services to veterans in Maryland. The outpatient volume is 260,000. There are approximately 7000 admissions annually resulting in approximately 60,000 radiological examinations. The hospital is situated on the campus of the University of Maryland Medical School with which it is fully integrated. Staff physicians, as well as resident staff from the University of Maryland rotate through the various clinical services at the Baltimore VAMC.

The Baltimore VAMC center utilizes a large-scale, radiology, nuclear medicine, and cardiology PACS, which was installed in June 1993. This system has resulted in near "filmless" operation with the exception of mammograms and a portion of magnetic resonance imaging (MRI) examinations. Imaging workstations are located throughout the BVAMC including the radiology and nuclear medicine departments, the operating rooms, the emergency room, all medical and surgical wards, outpatient clinics, the auditorium, medical media, and the radiology conference room at the University of Maryland. The PACS is bidirectionally interfaced to the hospital and radiology information systems (Protopapas, Siegel, Reiner et al., 1996; Siegel, Diaconis, Pomerantz, Allman, 1995).

Installation of the new PACS was accompanied by extensive training efforts, as the department worked to take full advantage of the new technology. The center also conducted studies to measure the economic impact of PACS and to document the changes in the practice of medicine. Not surprisingly, preliminary studies indicated that healthcare providers who undergo formal training are more proficient in the use of the PACS than those do not. Untrained individuals scored lower on a standardized test and were slower performing basic functions on the system. These latter findings suggest that PACS training may result in increased productivity of healthcare providers. Details of the training program at the Baltimore VAMC follow, along with information on training principles and implementation.

Training Objectives

All PACS users need to be able to navigate within the system to locate specific imaging examinations and to display images and reports. Clearly the imaging needs of various healthcare providers vary according to specialty and duties. The PACS skills needed by the radiologist differ greatly from those required by the operating room personnel accessing images for surgeons during a procedure or those needed by clerical personnel entering patient data or printing a report. Training objectives for any PACS should take into account the type of healthcare personnel being trained and focus on two critical areas: database skills and workstation skills.

Database skills include examination/image entry into the PACS, database query, and retrieval of radiological examinations and reports. These skills are basic for radiology personnel responsible for scheduling exams, image acquisition, examination entry, and examination quality assurance. Database query and retrieval skills are required by any PACS user who wishes to find a current or historic radiological examination with its accompanying report. For radiologists, query, retrieval, and display of unreported examinations on a workstation must precede reporting. Once a report has been completed, the exam should be marked "dictated" and the report should be entered into the PACS directly or through a HIS/RIS interface.

Workstation skills needed by PACS users vary greatly depending on several factors. First is the type of images that are to be displayed. Computed radiography (CR), computed tomography (CT), and magnetic resonance imaging (MRI) all have different requirements. The imaging requirements of the medical specialty practiced by the user are also important. Whereas orthopedic surgeons need to be able to measure angles and to master the tools that allow them to do so, most internists do not. A third critical factor is whether the user is the primary reader of the images, as are radiologists. As primary readers, they must be proficient in the use of all available workstation tools that can be used to enhance image display. In addition, they should be adept in using automated image display protocols and other shortcuts that can increase their productivity.

Except for unusual cases, in which skills unique to a medical specialty are required, clinicians and nurses who are not radiologists or radiology personnel need master only a subset of basic workstation skills in order to utilize PACS effectively. These include the ability to:

- Logon to the PACS.
- Locate the patient's folder in the database.

- Locate a current examination and any historic images.
- Display associated radiological reports.
- Display images of current and historic radiological examinations from the short term memory.
- Fetch historic examinations not currently available in short-term memory.
- Use workstation tools for window and level change, magnification, image flip and rotate, image format.

Radiology technologists require more extensive training, including additional skills in:

- Examination entry into the PACS using various interfaces between the PACS and the radiology equipment.
- Image quality assurance.
- · Verification of exam and demographics after quality assurance.
- Printing of images for outside consultation or transfer of patients to outside institutions.

To maintain productivity and accuracy of image interpretation, radiologists need in-depth training in the structure and use of the PACS, including:

- System overview.
- Database structure: various worklists containing examinations to be interpreted, changing examination status to "dictated" and thus removing examinations from unread examination worklists.
- Use of academic and conference folders.
- System administration tools including "fetch" and printing status of various examinations or lists.
- Use of all workstation tools for optimal image interpretation.
- Image annotation to mark subtle findings on the image for other healthcare providers (e.g., a small pneumothorax or a small nodule on a chest radiograph).
- Macro or speed commands to facilitate rapid interpretation of images.

In addition, the American College of Radiology (ACR) Standard for teleradiology suggests that radiologists should "understand the basic technology, its strengths and weaknesses (as well as limitations) and should be trained in the use of teleradiology" (ACR, 1995, pp. 57–62).

Methods

PACS training can be offered in three ways: computer-based training, online training, and traditional training. To date, the Baltimore VAMC has experimented with the first two and utilized the third most extensively.

Computer-based training (CBT) has been used by a relatively small number of physicians with encouraging results. Its main advantage is its availability to clinicians around the clock, thus avoiding scheduling difficulties. This method also has the potential of being tailored to a particular physician's specialty. The main drawback at our institution currently is that this training is offered only on a small number of workstations and is not convenient to most clinicians.

Although online training method may intuitively seem ideal for PACS training in a hospital environment, it is currently available in only very limited form at the Baltimore VAMC. Clinicians are taking advantage of the ability to invoke online help menus and "balloons" or "wizards" as they use PACS. One significant benefit of online training is its availability. With workstations located in convenient areas, users can access online training 24 hours a day, 7 days a week.

With the traditional method, a dedicated trainer works with small groups or, ideally, one-on-one, adapting the training to the trainee(s). Sessions are tailored according to the level of computer expertise of the user and the specific needs for each specialty. To adapt the training effectively, the trainer should ideally have a background in teaching as well as radiology. To better understand user needs that may be site or specialty specific, the trainer should spend time prior to the formal sessions observing physicians and other healthcare providers who will be using PACS in the clinics, inpatient wards, and other care settings, such as the intensive care unit or the operating room. After the formal training sessions, the trainer should make follow up visits to these same sites, both to reinforce the training and to understand further the PACS needs of each user group. This is helpful in tailoring future training sessions. Formal training has several drawbacks. It is administered at set times, limiting access for physicians who are caring for patients. Scheduling can be difficult during periods of high staff turnover, such as the beginning of the academic year in teaching hospitals. In addition, a trainer knowledgeable in education and radiology and PACS can be expensive and hard to find.

Results

At the Baltimore VAMC, the PACS vendor supplied a full-time trainer, a registered radiographer and sonographer with extensive experience in training in a radiology department as an MRI applications specialist. The trainer was responsible for operating the training program, including individual tutorials and group sessions with clinicians, radiologists, technologists, and other authorized healthcare workers. Training was mandatory for all PACS users before obtaining a sign-on identification and password; sessions were conducted using a PACS workstation.

Nonradiologists were trained in groups of one to four; training was limited to an hour, including a 30- to 45-minute demonstration of the workstation and its features followed by a 15- to 30-minute period during which the trainee was given the opportunity to use the workstation. Review of the log sheets revealed that, for nonradiologists, an average of two physicians were trained per session.

All of the radiologists (residents, fellows, and attending staff) were trained individually. Training for radiologists was accomplished in two sessions, each lasting approximately one hour and covering the use of the database structure in detail. For example, radiologists were taught to use conference folders, create teaching files, and use the annotation tool to "draw" on the image like drawing on film with a wax pencil. The main focus of the sessions was to equip the radiologists with the necessary expertise to use workstation tools for optimal image interpretation. They were also taught to use macros to perform certain repetitive tasks and the use of default display protocols ("intelligent" display of current and previous images on a multiple monitor workstation) to increase throughput.

In addition to the formal training sessions, the training staff made themselves available to answer questions and provide further guidance to physicians during outpatient clinic hours. This provided supplemental training for the physicians and simultaneously gave the trainers the opportunity to observe the clinicians using the PACS and to determine specific needs for different groups of physicians.

Review of training log sheets indicated that all of the radiologists and technologists received formal training. However, less than 25 percent of the physicians throughout the medical center had been through the formal PACS training course. Physicians had the lowest training rate and the highest turnover rate due at least in part to the constant turnover of residents shared by the University of Maryland Hospital and the Baltimore VAMC.

This poor compliance may be the result of a number of factors. Experienced PACS users are available around the clock to provide "peer" training, and user friendly workstations enable PACS users to perform basic functions without any formal training. Scheduling training sessions during regular working hours remains problematic, especially for physicians. Also, widespread use of generic logon codes and sharing of logon codes allows PACS users to bypass the mandatory training.

A questionnaire was distributed to all medical house staff with responses from 58 of 95 (61 percent) persons surveyed (Protopapas, Siegel, Reiner et al., 1996; Siegel, Protopapas, Pomerantz et al., 1995). As shown in Figure 12.1, 22 percent of the respondents indicated they had attended the formal training course, 32 percent identified themselves as having been "peer trained," and 41 percent described themselves as "self taught." There was a 5 percent no response rate.

Despite the relatively low number of residents trained, a significant majority of those who availed themselves of training found it useful in their daily clinical duties. According to the survey, 92 percent of the trained residents judged the formal training useful; the remaining 8 percent did not indicate their assessment.

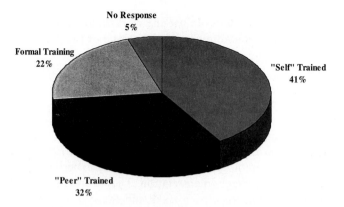

FIGURE 12.1. Housestaff survey. Results of question "Did you attend formal training?"

The low compliance with the mandatory PACS training prompted a study comparing PACS proficiency in trained and untrained physicians. Twenty-nine subjects with no prior PACS experience were recruited for the study from rotating housestaff. Of these, 10 were given standard PACS training of 1 hour within 3 days of starting their rotation at the BVAMC. All subjects were tested at the end of weeks one and four of their clinical rotation. Testing included database and workstation skills. Database skills tested included the ability to locate a patient and a particular study, display images and reports, and determine the availability of images in short term memory. Workstations skills tested were the ability to determine when tools are required and to use them properly, including window level, zoom, flip and rotate, and format.

Prior to data collection, agreement was reached on an arbitrary scoring system. Six database tasks had to be performed in less than 2 minutes each for a total of six possible points. Five workstation tool tasks had to be performed in less than 2 minutes each for a total of 10 possible points. Pass-score was arbitrarily set at a total of 11 of 16 points. At least 5 of the 11 points were dependent upon database skills.

PACS Skills at 1 Week

As would be expected, there were differences in PACS skills between trained and untrained subjects at 1 week. Statistically significant differences between trained and untrained subjects were observed in the global scores (Fig. 12.2). Statistically significant differences between the two groups were observed at one week when the data was further analyzed according to database (Fig. 12.3) and workstation skills (Fig. 12.4), as well as speed to perform certain basic database tasks at the workstation (Fig. 12.5).

PACS Skills at 4 Weeks

Global score differences between trained and untrained subjects at 4 weeks remained statistically significant (Fig. 12.2). This was both reflected in work-

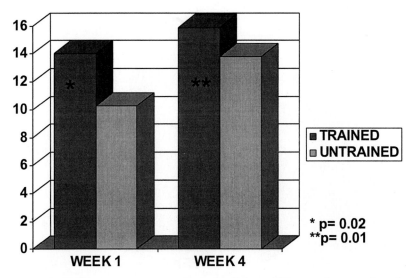

FIGURE 12.2. Global scores versus experience. Proficiency differences between the trained and untrained subjects persist at four weeks. Score includes both database tasks and workstation skills.

station skills as well as speed using the workstation (Figs. 12.3–12.5). There was significant improvement in all measured parameters over time irrespective of their training status suggesting a learning effect over the observed

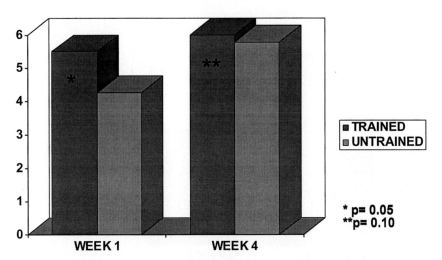

FIGURE 12.3. Database scores versus experience. Score derived from the database skills at week 1 is lower for the untrained group ($p = 0.05$). At four weeks there is no significant between the trained and untrained subjects. (Database skills tested included the ability to locate a patient and a particular study, display images and reports, and determine the availability of images in short term memory.)

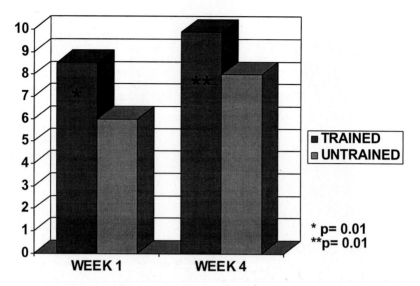

FIGURE 12.4. Workstation-tool scores versus experience. Statistically significant differences in workstation tool score were observed between trained and untrained subject at one and four weeks. (Workstations skills tested were the ability to determine when tools are required and to use them properly, including window level, zoom, flip and rotate, and format.)

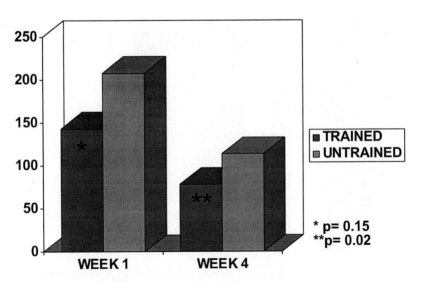

FIGURE 12.5. Time required to perform database tasks versus experience. At one week there was no statistically significant difference between trained and untrained subjects. At four weeks the trained subject performed the required database tasks faster ($p = 0.02$).

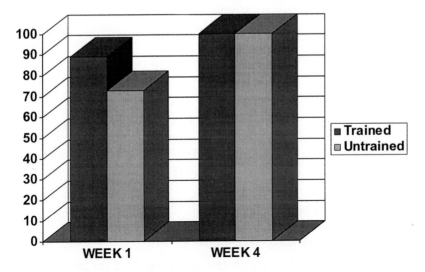

FIGURE 12.6. Pass rate versus experience. Pass rate after the first week showed statistically significant differences between the trained and untrained groups. Note that at four weeks all the subjects passed the test irrespective of their training status.

period either by "peer" or "self" training. All subjects passed the PACS proficiency test at 4 weeks.

The present study is limited because of small number of subjects tested, an arbitrary scoring system, and the inherent learning experience during testing of the same skills. However, the data suggest the following:

- Speed and proficiency benefits of training persisted at 4 weeks. Because of these differences at 4 weeks between trained and untrained physicians, we continue to offer a mandatory training course for all physicians.
- Speed and proficiency improvements were observed over 4 weeks in both trained and untrained individuals irrespective of training status. This suggests a learning curve of at least 4 weeks for nonradiologist physician PACS users.
- In spite of the significant differences in scores, all subjects passed the PACS proficiency test at 4 weeks. This suggests that adequate PACS skills could be achieved without the use of "formal training." After 1 week, there was a significant difference in pass rate (Fig. 12.6).

Subjects in this study were primarily recent medical school graduates with advanced personal computer skills. Such basic computer skills are surely helpful in becoming a proficient PACS user. Such computer skills may have allowed untrained subject to benefit more from "self" and "peer" training and may have therefore lessened the effect of training on PACS proficiency.

The presence of more senior residents on the wards and clinics in an academic setting allows for more opportunities for "peer" training as well than would be expected in a smaller hospital with no housestaff. This would also make training more important.

Conclusions

Based on its experiences implementing the PACS, the Baltimore VAMC faculty believes that training should be mandatory for all users before they are given identification and password for logging on to the system. Such training is required to:

- Assure PACS user proficiency.
- Fulfill possible medicolegal obligations.
- Enhance clinician acceptance of PACS.

PACS training should be customized to the needs of the particular user group and the specific hospital site. User training should be further tailored to the computer skills of the individual trainee. The BVAMC trains radiologists one on one and other PACS users in small groups of two to four. This type of training is very labor intensive and can be offered only when the PACS applications specialist is available.

The trainer makes frequent visits to the various clinics and wards. This practice increases the trainer's understanding of the needs of PACS user groups and hospital sites. In addition, the trainer has the opportunity during these visits to answer questions from PACS users and reinforce training objectives as necessary.

The availability of technical assistance for users is important for general acceptance of PACS, especially at the introduction of the system or after major system upgrades, when experienced users are not available throughout the hospital to offer "peer" training to their less experienced colleagues.

The BVAMC is considering expanded use of computer based training (CBT) and online training. Experience with both methods, although limited, has been favorable. CBT can be made available around the clock and to certain degree be customized to the needs of particular PACS user group. Computer-based testing at the end of training sessions can also measure the proficiency of potential users before they are given a PACS logon identification and password.

Training at the BVAMC continues to be mandatory because of proficiency differences between trained and untrained individuals at 4 weeks. These differences could potentially be greater in a nonteaching hospital setting where physicians may spend a much smaller part their working day in the hospital using the PACS and may not be as familiar with computers in general, as our subjects were. Moreover, in a nonteaching hospital, a physician not familiar with the PACS may not have the same opportunity for "peer" training as in a teaching hospital.

For these reasons we would recommend PACS training for all users, particularly in a setting where experienced users may not be readily available at all times.

References

ACR Standard for Teleradiology in American College of Radiology Standards. 1995, 57–62

Protopapas Z, Siegel EL, Reiner BI et al. PACS training for physicians: lessons learned at the Baltimore VA Medical Center. J Digital Imaging 1996, 9(3), 131–136.

Siegel ES, Diaconis JD, Pomerantz SM et al. Making filmless radiology work. J Digital Imaging 1995, (8), 151–155.

Siegel EL, Protopapas Z, Pomerantz SM et al. Clinician acceptance of PACS at the Baltimore VA medical center. RSNA paper presentation, Nov, 29, 1995.

13
Clinical Aspects of Workstation Design and Operation

Steven C. Horii

The use of electronic workstations to replace the display function of film for medical imaging is steadily increasing. In part, this is because of the growth in the use of digital processes in most areas of medical imaging. Also, the ability of picture archiving and communications systems (PACS) to handle the management of images has made use of workstations more practical.

This chapter focuses on the history, roles, evaluation, and future of workstations for medical imaging. Chapter 14 on Workstation Functions and System Capabilities, describes the issues related to workstation hardware and software design, the functional requirements for workstations, and the physical environment in which workstations are used.

In 1976, Larsen (Larsen, 1976) described the application of an image processing workstation to computed tomography (CT) scans of the head, noting the potential of interactive capabilities to giver users rapid visual feedback from the processing performed. In 1979, Lemke (Lemke, Stiehl, Scharnweber et al., 1979) presented what may be the first medical picture archiving and communications system (PACS) in the literature. Designed to perform image processing on head CT images for enhancement and automated extraction of features such as ventricles, the system included workstations for image processing and evaluation, a computer network for communicating the images, and a filing system for storing them. Lemke also addressed the management of images and the integration of text and voice annotation of images into the medical record.

By the time of the first International Workshop and Conference on PACS for Medical Applications in 1982 (Duerinckx, 1982), the concept of a PACS had spread through much of the radiology research community. At that meeting, Maguire (Maguire, Zeleznik, Horii et al., 1982) described a system much like the one outlined by Lemke; the workstation prototype was constructed using a minicomputer, graphics display subsystem, and a magnetic tape drive. Dwyer and colleagues (Dwyer, Templeton, Anderson et al., 1982) outlined many of the requirements for a radiology PACS, including the data on retrieval rates for radiological examinations that formed the basis of many designs for archives.

Roles of the Workstation

Within a PACS, the workstation has one of the more difficult jobs. Certainly, all components of a PACS are needed for the system to operate, but the workstation has the unique function of serving as the human interface for the display role. As such, it has to support a user interface that is readily learned and used, yet it must be flexible enough to meet the varied needs of different healthcare professionals. The film-based environment so familiar to radiologists, shown in Figure 13.1, has evolved to the point where the user interface is well known and the roles played by support personnel are transparent unless there is a problem. In the filmless environment, workstations must be able to display faithfully the information they are sent or, if they cannot, somehow indicate to the user that there may be changes to the original data.

The speed of workstation operations has to be fast enough to avoid user frustration, but not so fast as to drive costs for the hardware to impractical levels. Above all, workstations must offer users a clear advantage over film, whether in speed, functions performed, or ability to do tasks not possible with film. If this is not the case, the impetus to switch from hardcopy to softcopy will be weak or even nonexistent.

Of the several roles a workstation fulfills, the diagnostic role may be the most demanding; it is also the role best known to radiologists. When the workstation is used for primary reading of examinations, anything that detracts from the accuracy of the radiologist is likely to become a reason for rejecting the workstation. Basically, roles for workstations parallel those filled by conventional lightboxes and films.

Traditionally there are three types of review. The first is done by the radiologist on examinations that have already been interpreted. This may be done for groups in a conference, or for individuals when consulting specialists seek a radiologist's opinion. A second type is performed by the referring physician, usually on examinations already interpreted by the radiologist. This is often done for learning or confirming treatment decisions. A third involves other healthcare professionals, including physical therapists, nurse practitioners, and respiratory therapists. All three types of review are important; they help determine what levels of performance and functions will be needed as well as help shape the user interface design.

Some workstation applications, such as those in an operating room, require special hardware configurations designed to meet special electrical safety requirements and a user interface tailored to hands-free (or sterile operable) controls.

To date, studies focus on two fundamental roles, each with variations to suit particular applications. The first is the primary interpretation role, with workstations designed to be used by the radiologist or other medical imaging specialist who interprets the imaging study at the request of the referring

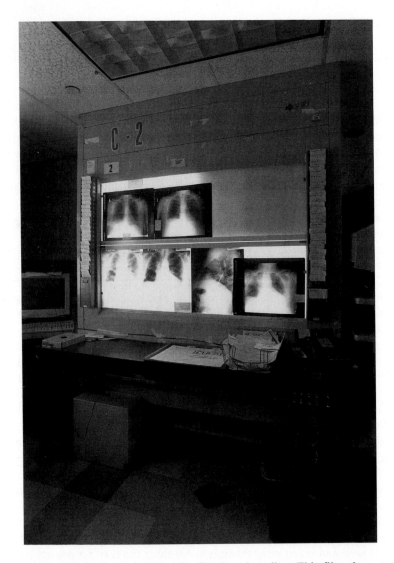

FIGURE 13.1. This is the workstation for film-based reading. This film alternator (or multiviewer) shows up to two panels of four 14 ´ 17 inch (35 ´ 43 cm) films at one time. Switches at the lower right of the work surface allow any combination of the eight light boxes behind the films to be turned on or off. A foot pedal (barely visible on the floor) causes the mechanism to move through the panels to display a particular set. The vertical trays to the right and left hold cards that display the name of the patient and the panel location of the films. This is analogous to the image navigation tools on workstations. The wire basket on the work surface holds the requisition forms for the examinations that have been read. The medical history and reason for the examination are summarized briefly on these paper forms. Radiologists are so used to this environment that it is hard for them to enumerate all of the tasks performed in addition to reading the films.

physician. The second is the review role, with workstations that support the features used for viewing images that have already been interpreted. The author of this chapter compared medical intensive care unit (MICU) physicians with radiologists (Horii, Feingold, Kundel et al., 1996) using a workstation for portable chest radiographs done on CR plates. In the task evaluated, the radiologists were doing primary interpretation of the images. The study showed the two groups differed in their use of workstation functions. The radiologists used the grayscale adjustment (window and level) more frequently than did the MICU physicians, while the MICU physicians used the other workstation image manipulation functions (zoom, invert, and full-resolution display) more frequently than did the radiologists.

Such studies tend to be limited to specific image categories or reading conditions and should not be used to generalize a list of workstation functions, but they may be useful in determining which functions are likely to be selected under different workstation use scenarios.

Clinical Factors in Workstation Design

The "first approximation" approach to designing workstations is to emulate what is done with film on lightboxes or alternators. Although this approach has flaws that will be discussed, it nonetheless provides a good starting point. One of the most useful tools in performing the analysis needed for this approach is a detailed time–motion study. In a landmark study, Rogers (Rogers, Johnston, Brenton et al., 1985) found that the reading process could be divided into three stages:

- Stage 1: General information gathering, including a review of the patient's history, radiological examination history, and other data, along with a rapid sort through the films of the current study.
- Stage 2: Rapid review of the image set to detect candidate pathological states.
- Stage 3: Focused attention on those candidate abnormalities with the dismissal of some as nonpathological and recognition of others as significant—what most would think of as the actual "reading" or diagnostic phase.

In a study of the information gathering stage, Levin (Levin, Horii, Mun et al., 1990) did a workflow analysis of all of the activities required to bring together the information needed to support the interpretation of nuclear medicine ventilation/perfusion lung scans. This was done as an example to determine which were steps that could be done within a PACS, which were handled by other information systems, and which were manual operations. Levin found that there are extensive interactions with multiple information sources to support examination interpretation. Haynor and Saarinen (1989) focused on the problem of finding prior examinations of the same type for the patient and any correlative (cross-modality) examinations the radiologist might want during reading. Compared to outpatients, inpatients had a higher frequency of prior (plain film) studies and their "old" studies that were "younger," an average of 15 days as opposed to 53. Analysis of cross-modality examinations indicated that for plain films, ultrasound, and neuroradiologic magnetic resonance (MR), the correlative study was a prior CT examination. For neuroradiologic computed tomography (CT), it was a prior MR or myelogram. This study suggested that relatively simple rules can be constructed for the automated retrieval of these needed cases from a PACS archive.

Both Levin and Haynor focused primarily on activities taking place in support of the reading task, and less on the actual reading process. Nonetheless, without such support processes, radiologists would be reluctant to interpret examinations. There are several possible approaches for determining the requirements of diagnostic workstations:

- Interviewing radiologists in addition to observing what they do.
- Using the actions identified in time-motion studies or building functional models of the radiologist's working tasks and combining these with human–computer interaction principles
- Building models or prototypes, having them evaluated by radiologists, refining them based on such evaluation, and repeating this cycle until requested changes reach a minimum, or the users express a high degree of satisfaction with the result.

The interview and observation approach was taken by Horii (Horii, Schimpf, Isles et al., 1984), Hohman (Hohman, Johnson, Valentino et al., 1994), and Honeyman (Honeyman, Arenson, Frost et al., 1993) among others. Horii's study, conducted when the author was at New York University (NYU), was done when there were only prototype workstations in the Department of Radiology at the NYU Medical Center; most radiologists did not use them, but they did use the independent consoles of the CT machines to view images. The work by Hohman was done using the developmental PACS in place in the Department of Radiological Sciences at the University of California, Los Angeles (UCLA). Honeyman compared the features of four workstations installed at the University of Florida's Shands Hospital and surveyed attendees of the workstation exhibits at the Radiological Society of North America InfoRAD area.

Although ten years elapsed between the Horii and Hohman papers, many of the responses were similar, most notably the finding that control of the grayscale of the display (window width and level adjustment) was the most frequently used function. For the Honeyman survey, the importance of window/level, magnification, and flip/rotate functions was thought to be high enough that users were told to assume that the workstation had these features. One major difference seen between the Horii and Hohman studies is the change in acceptance of the mouse and menu for control of the user interface. In the Horii study, the mouse ranked least desirable, exactly the opposite was true in the Hohman survey. This difference, the author believes, is readily explained by the rapid growth of personal computers with graphical user interfaces for which the mouse and menu is the predominant control mechanism. The Honeyman study also asked about "higher level" workstation functions involving organization of images or their management; the study found the most important function to be the ability to view multiple studies on the same patient simultaneously.

Meyer-Ebrecht (Meyer-Ebrecht and Wendler, 1983) used the time–motion study coupled with human–computer interaction principles. This approach to functional requirements modeling is based on more informal observation combined with ergonomic design. Meyer-Ebrecht proposed to use a well-defined set of image processing primitives to implement workstation functions. Rogers (Rogers, Johnston, Brenton et al., 1985) analyzed the time–motion analysis they did and determined a basic set of functions that workstations supported by a PACS should perform. Included were access to patient history (text and prior images), window/level presets, controllable automatic progression through series, temporary image markers to return quickly to a marked image, display of multiple images, magnification, and measurement (pixel value and dimensional). With the possible exception of patient history (other than what is provided on the radiology requisition), most of these functions have been implemented. Of interest is the "controllable automatic progression through series," now familiar as the "stack view" mode in which a user can move through a series of images very rapidly. For cross-sectional imaging, this display mode allows for very rapid review of studies and provides a three-dimensional sense of anatomic structures.

Most researchers using the model and human factors methods have arrived at a similar conclusion (Beard, Pizer, Rogers et al., 1987; Gee, DeSoto, Kim, 1989; Kasday, 1986; McNeill, Seeley, Maloney et al., 1988; Schuttenbeld and ter Haar Romeny, 1987; Steinke, Nabijee, Freeman, Prior, 1990): a user interface developed from a simple or intuitive mental model is easier to learn and use with a minimum of errors. Overall, work using this approach has suggested that the radiology reading task is a complex one, both from the point of view of the radiologist (the internal processes) and the infrastructure to support the radiologist (the external processes).

The third approach, developing a prototype user interface and refining it by having different users work with it, has also been well used (Belanger, Robertson, Coristine et al., 1989; Braudes, Mun, Schnizlein et al., 1989; Feingold, Seshadri, Arenson, 1991; Huang, Mankovitch, Taira, Kangarloo, 1986; Johnston, Rogers, Creasy et al., 1987; O'Malley, 1989; ter Haar Romeny, Raymakers, van Waes et al., 1987; van der Voorde, Arenson, Kundel et al., 1986). In effect, this same cycle happens with products installed by vendors, but with a longer cycle time. In the prototyping method, trial user interfaces are constructed and refined before they are committed to production hardware. Using this method, Belanger (1989) and van der Voorde (1986) spent a great deal of time with radiologists and nonradiologists at Ottawa Civic Hospital and the Hospital of the University of Pennsylvania, respectively. They focused on evaluating or developing the user interface, and developed workstations that would be used extensively by referring physicians. Rather than assume that functional requirements were the same as for radiologists, they sought the advice of the physician population that would be using the workstation. The result in both instances was a high degree of acceptance by nonradiologist users.

Diagnostic Accuracy

A debate is ongoing as to whether digital imaging workstations yield the same results in diagnostic accuracy as film-based interpretation. Combining studies that made certain assumptions and met certain statistical criteria, Kundel (1993) did a metaanalysis of comparison studies of film compared to digital hard copy. Because of the spatial resolution issues of digital plain radiography, this analysis did not compare film against softcopy, but it offered a useful comparison. The study could not show a statistically significant difference between conventional and digitally produced film, except for skeletal abnormalities imaged with a 512 ´ 512 pixel matrix. These were significantly poorer in observer performance than their conventional film equivalents. In the studies used by Kundel in his metaanalysis, the digital hardcopy was produced from digitization of an analog hardcopy original. All of the studies favored film to a slight degree; although this was not statistically significant, the differences in observer performance were not equally distributed around zero, suggesting a slight overall disadvantage of digital imaging.

Slasky (Slasky, Gur, Wood et al., 1990) used receiver operating characteristic (ROC) analysis to evaluate observer performance with conventional film, digitally produced film, and workstation viewing. For individual observers, no significant differences between the digitally produced film and workstation viewing could be identified. However, when observer data were combined, the workstation viewing had a poorer diagnostic accuracy (judged by the area under the ROC curve, called A_z) for pulmonary interstitial disease and pneumothoraces. Performance was not significantly different for pulmonary nodules.

Scott (Scott, Bluemke, Mysko et al., 1995) compared observer performance on film and workstation viewing of radiologists and emergency room physicians at different levels of training. This study showed that observer performance on the workstation was inferior to that from film. However, the workstation display resolution was 1200 × 1600 pixels, less than the 1536 × 2048 pixels used by Slasky. The focus of the Scott study was on the evaluation of a teleradiology workstation; it concluded that the workstation was unacceptable for primary diagnosis of the class of radiographs used for the study, which were primarily emergency department musculoskeletal, abdominal, and thoracic images.

For teleradiology applications that use workstations for primary interpretation of images, the American College of Radiology (ACR, 1994) has recommended in their standard that pixel array size and display monitor size should be such that the displayed resolution of the image is not of lower spatial resolution than the original image.

Reasons for the poorer diagnostic performance of workstations compared to conventional film are not all known. A reduction in spatial resolution is one possibility, though in studies where the monitors matched film resolution (e.g., some of those cited in Kundel, 1993), observer performance was still inferior on workstations. One likely factor is the difference in luminance. High luminance grayscale cathode ray tube monitors may have an output of 100 to 200 foot-Lamberts (ftL) (343–685 candelas per square meter), still less than the 400 to 600 ftL (1370–2056 candelas per square meter) of conventional fluorescent-tube illuminated lightboxes (Sezn, Yip, and Daly, 1987). Human visual perception is known to have a contrast-detail response, in which the contrast required to see some level of detail decreases as luminance increases (Taylor, 1973) until very high luminance levels are reached. Less luminous flux for an image also means that the signal-to-noise ratio will be inferior for that image compared to one of higher luminous flux.

Rossmann (1969) has noted that the signal-to-noise ratio of an image is likely to be a major determinant of perceived image quality and observer performance. The lower luminance of workstation monitors also makes effects of glare more dominant. Because extraneous illumination is known to degrade observer performance in detecting abnormalities on radiographic images (Alter, Kargas, Kargas et al., 1982; Baxter, Ravindra, Norman, 1982; Ravindra, Norman, Baxter, 1983; Rogers and Johnston, 1987), environmental considerations are more important for workstations than for film-based reading.

The User Interface

The most heavily discussed aspect of workstations for medical imaging is the user interface design. In part, this is because there is wide opinion about how such an interface should work. The classic idea has been to emulate the operation of a film alternator. Countering this is the concept of going beyond what can be done with film. Manufacturers have tended to use the user interface design to differentiate one product from another, as the hardware is often the same or similar across multiple manufacturers.

One difficulty with user interface design is that objective study of the resulting interface is difficult and time consuming. Users find the obvious problems with a design almost immediately. The more subtle difficulties may not have immediately evident impact, and only thorough examination reveals them. At best, they cause problems such as longer reading time or complaints of fatigue. At worst, they degrade diagnostic accuracy.

Researchers at the University of North Carolina (Beard, 1990; Beard, Hemminger, Perry et al., 1993; Beard, Pisano, Denelsbeck, Johnston, 1994; Beard, Pizer, Rogers et al., 1987) and the University of Arizona (Krupinski and Lund, 1996) have applied well-validated methods of industrial psychology to the evaluation of user interfaces for medical imaging workstations. The results are sometimes counterintuitive. For example, Beard (Beard, Pizer, Rogers et al., 1987) found that a very fast single screen workstation could be as effective for reading CT studies as multiple films on lightboxes. This is in conflict with the widely held opinion that multiple monitor workstations are needed for CT reading.

In a study of visual gaze fixation during the image reading task, Krupinski and Lund (1996) found that it took longer to fixate on an abnormality on workstation displays and that overall viewing time was longer on the workstation. They also found that for film all eye fixations were confined to the image area, while for the workstation display approximately 20 percent of the fixations were in the area of the menu that displayed the image processing functions. In other words, the radiologists set their gaze on a nonimage area for about a fifth of all fixations. If they were to spend the same amount of overall time looking at the image, those additional gaze fixations would add to the viewing time per image. A more serious problem could occur if the gaze fixations on the control menus were to decrease the number of fixations on the image, and possibly decrease detection of abnormalities. This study should give pause to workstation designers who have continued to add controls and functions to on-screen menus or buttons.

The study of how humans interact with computers is not new. The scientific study of human–computer interaction (HCI) grew out of earlier industrial psychology methods for examining human–machine interactions of other types. Applications of such studies resulted in improved safety and efficiency of industrial machinery. The keys to such studies are in quantitative examination of time and motion and in detailed task analysis. For the viewing of images, eye tracking experiments are added to time–motion studies. Such examinations can tell experimenters what it is that radiologists and others viewing images do. As different user interface elements are added or changed, repeat measurements can show whether the change is likely to have a positive or negative impact.

From such research, several key points have emerged. A basic principle of HCI is that the user interface should follow a logical and simple mental model. Because the task of reading from a workstation is likely to be different from reading from film, the mental model of the workstation interface should be simple to learn. If radiologists are confronted with an unfamiliar film alternator (or multiviewer), they are likely to make a few mistakes until they learn how to advance or back up the panels and how to turn on and off the separate illuminators. The number of errors they make until they become facile with the system is a measure of how simple the interface is to learn. An example of a common user interface control is the familiar computer mouse. On a flat desk, moving the mouse away from the user generally moves the cursor on the screen in an upward direction with mouse movement towards the user being down, and right and left corresponding to those directions. Switching these directions is very difficult for almost all users to get used to; the controls run counter to the mental model. This sort of control inversion can have disastrous consequences. Aircraft that use a joystick respond to pulling back on the joystick by climbing and to pushing forward on the joystick by diving. If the airplane becomes inverted and the pilot disoriented, the reversal of the control responses may not be realized; pulling back on the joystick will then put the airplane into a dive.

The writer of this chapter has often proposed the following test of a user interface: if a person can figure out how to use it without having to refer to a manual, it is probably based on a good mental model. In the model popularized by Apple Computer's Macintosh, developers were told to adhere to a particular set of interface guidelines. This meant that most application programs operated in a similar fashion. Whether preparing text in a word processor or numeric data in a spreadsheet, users learned that, to print the resulting document, they pulled down the "File" menu and found "Print" among the choices. If software developers adhered to these principles, it was possible for users to accomplish most basic operations in any program without having to read volumes of documentation. Unlike other operating systems of the time (e.g., DOS and Unix), the user did not have to remember commands or the syntax of many of them. Keywords in the menu were reminders of functions to be performed. If additional input was needed from the user, selecting a menu item would then bring up a dialog box in which the user would make additional choices by clicking on "buttons" or checking "check boxes." The Macintosh environment was, and is, highly graphical and, though not the first graphical user interface (GUI), it became the first widely popular one.

From the mental model of "how do I make this thing do what I want?" comes the development of logical controls to perform those tasks. It is this process, turning operations done in a conventional system into controls and their effects in the computer based system that constitutes development of a user interface. The trend in medical imaging workstations has been to adopt the GUI based user interface. As noted by Krupinski and Lund (1996), however, that may not be the best possible choice. There have been, mostly in historical workstations, significant departures from the GUI paradigm. Examples include the General Electric Medical Systems Independent Console (G.E. Medical Systems, Milwaukee, WI) for which multiple keys were traded off against a GUI, shown in Figure 13.2. The plasma panel of that console allowed for flexible "soft" buttons to be used as well, vastly increasing the number of things that could be done without making the number of function keys impossibly large. The idea used for this console, that commonly used

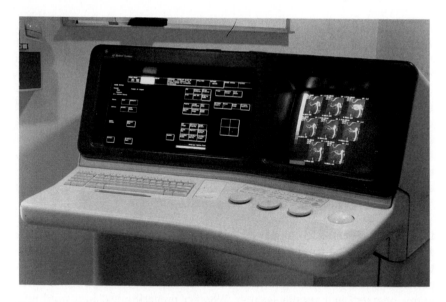

FIGURE 13.2. This is an independent viewing console that was sold as an option with General Electric CT and MR machines (General Electric Medical Systems, Milwaukee, WI). It is shown as an illustration of a display that has no menus on the image screen (the monitor on the right). Instead, all functions were moved to keys, knobs (the three knobs are for controlling image grayscale display), a trackball (for cursor movement and other functions depending on what function was selected), and a large touch-sensitive plasma panel (on the left). The plasma panel allowed for "soft" keys that displayed legends under control of the software of the console. Touching the key activates the function shown in text on the "button." The value of this system is a vast increase in the number of functions possible without having them all physically present on buttons. A human factors advantage for this sort of design is that the functions can be grouped by category (e.g., all image distance and pixel statistics measurements). This console was not intended for primary interpretation of CT and MR examinations.

functions would be represented on dedicated keys and those that were needed for specific operations would be on the plasma display, has also been translated into more modern workstation designs. Many current systems have "soft" keys displayed in a fixed portion of the menu on the monitor(s) to perform the common functions. Operation-specific functions are selectable from menu portions that change with the operation being done. The very commonly used functions, such as window width and level adjustment, are usually always available under mouse control. The work by Krupinski and Lund (1996) for display of radiographic images on workstations and that of Beard for CT images (Beard, Hemminger, Perry et al., 1993) would argue for a minimal set of controls that do not require users to look at them to operate them. Such a control set is not available from medical imaging workstation manufacturers at the time this chapter was written, though one manufacturer (Aurora Technology, Lake Forest, IL) has incorporated a foot pedal to change to the next or prior examination on the worklist.

The navigation method most commonly used is based on the model of the film jacket. In a hierarchical display, the electronic patient "jacket" is shown with the studies it contains. The user then selects the study (and sometimes the series) to be displayed, as in Figure 13.3. An additional organizational layer on top of this is the worklist. This model parallels the lists or index cards kept at film alternators to show which examination is on which panel. On most workstations, the worklist shows a list of patients and selecting a patient then displays the "jacket." The worklist is potentially a very powerful tool; with appropriate workstation software and an interface of the PACS to a radiology information system, worklists could be used to help manage workflow. That is, examinations to be read could be directed to particular workstations or shown on the worklist of a particular radiologist when he or she logs on. A worklist could also be used to show referring physicians which examinations have been read and have reports available. Information such as the time the patient has been waiting, "stat" status, the patient's appointment time with the referring physician, and so on, could be used to help the radiologist prioritize reading order. A "lockout" could prevent two radiologists inadvertently trying simultaneously to read the same examination while still allowing "viewing" access. Some of these features are currently implemented in commercial workstations, but others are still on this author's "wish list." By paying more attention to the design of the navigation process, workstations can improve on film-based methods. Beard (Beard, Walker, Bell et al., 1989) developed a rapid prototyping and evaluation method in part for examining the human–computer interactions involved in the navigation process.

A significant part of image navigation is some form of automated arrangement of the images in an examination when there are multiple images. This has come to be called the "hanging protocol" after the manner in which films are arranged on lightboxes or alternator panels for reading. For sectional imaging, such as CT, MR, and nuclear medicine PET and SPECT, the ability to sort images by series, by time of acquisition, by anatomic location, and by imaging protocol (such as pulse sequence for MR) is of great importance. In the conventional film-based operation, this sorting is often done by the technologist as the examination is filmed. Automation of such sorting will facilitate interpreting these examination types at workstations. For plain radiographic images, the "hanging protocols" are also of some importance. For the trauma patient with multiple radiographs, sorting them by examination time may be wholly inadequate and other criteria, such as anatomic area, may have to be considered. In addition, the sorting of sectional images and the arrangement of radiographic ones are governed to some extent by the individual desires of the radiologist. All these requirements dictate that such sorting and arrangement is both automated and customizable.

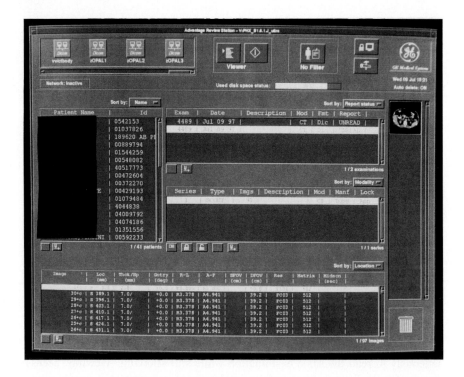

FIGURE 13.3. An example of a screen for selection of patients and their examinations. This particular screen is from a General Electric Phoenix (General Electric Medical Systems, Milwaukee, WI) workstation. Four major text windows dominate the display. The one on the far left with the vertical list of numbers is the list of all patients who have examinations on the particular system being queried (patient names have been blacked out, but would appear to the left of the associated medical record numbers). To the right of this window are two smaller ones that provide details about the examinations a particular patient has had (top of the two windows) and the series within the examination (bottom of the two windows). The wide window at the bottom of the screen shows details of the individual images within a series. To the right is a vertical window that shows representative images from different series. All of these windows have scroll bars since the lists may be longer than can be displayed within the window. The "buttons" just above the right upper corner of each window show the option selected for the display, and if "pressed" by pointing to the button and holding the mouse button down, a list of all options is shown and a different one may be selected. For example, the patient list may be sorted by patient name (as shown) or by medical record number. Across the top of the display are a window on the left showing the devices that the workstation may query, a selection tool for the "browser" (the name of this whole display) or the viewer (which displays the images when selected), a button that allows a filter to be applied to the list of patients (for example, those with examinations from "today," "last 24 hours," "last 72 hours." etc.), and buttons for locking a display and displaying the list of additional tools for image display. Displays such as this illustrate the difficulty of trying to produce a workstation navigation tool that is comprehensive yet not too "busy."

Controls and displays in general could benefit the user if they were customizable. The number of images displayed simultaneously for sectional imaging, the window width and level preset values, the initial image display parameters (very useful for MR imaging), and even the location and arrangement of on-screen controls could all be based on who logs in, so that personalized "setups" are automatically set. If this sounds extravagant, readers should recall that many such functions are done currently in film-based operation and are done in a fashion "transparent" to the radiologist by technologists, file room clerks, and radiology residents who quickly learn the preferences of the radiologist with whom they are working.

An important aspect of user interfaces is error recovery. In the best of circumstances, users may still make mistakes. How a user interface allows the correction of such errors is important; if the user deems the error correction process to be "too taxing," it may be ignored and errors may propagate. Aside from preventing erroneous conditions that are detectable, there is the matter of reversing a function or operation that was inadvertently selected. There are two levels of such reversal; the "undo what I just did" version that can be thought of as allowing a user to back up a step, and the "take me back to where I started" choice that resets starting conditions.

In the case of the "undo" function, some things, such as selecting a preset image arrangement choice can be reversed fairly simply. Others, particularly operations that manipulate pixel data, may be irreversible. Some forms of edge sharpening, for example, cannot readily be reversed. In some instances, warnings to the user prior to executing such an operation may be warranted. Erasing images is a typical example, although a well-designed user interface will provide a safety option for even this action.

The "reset" function, analogous to a "panic button," is useful when a user has gotten so far off the desired functional direction that only resetting to the starting conditions will be helpful. Such a reset, however, should ordinarily not be the equivalent of shutting down and restarting the workstation; a well-designed reset should just reestablish starting conditions and do so quickly.

A manner of quantifying the user effort required to invoke undo and reset functions is based on a model proposed in the MDIS Specification (1991). This model relies on the number of keystrokes or their equivalent (a mouse button click) used to implement workstation functions and has also been used by Beard in developing workstation designs (Beard, Walker, Bell et al., 1989). For users contemplating the purchase of PACS workstations, determining the number of "keystroke equivalents" needed to perform common functions is a good method of comparing the effort involved in using different workstations. For example, if a workstation required six keystroke equivalents to perform the window width and level functions, this would be, by almost anyone's measure, far too cumbersome. Typically, such a commonly used function would be either always available or one- to two-keystroke equivalents away at a maximum.

User interfaces are a complex subject and, many believe, a matter of personal choice. Nonetheless, principles including simplicity of the mental model behind the interface and minimum actions to perform common functions are applicable across many users and levels of experience. These are discussed at length in Chapter 14.

The Future of Workstations

One problem with the development of user interfaces and specification of workstation functions is that the model used is film-based operation. Although this is a good base upon which to build, it tends to obscure the things that can be done with digital imaging workstations that cannot be done with film. Some techniques, such as window width and level adjustment, have become a routine function used on workstations that is not possible with film without photographing the image at multiple window width and level settings (which is typically still done in film-based CT reading). For ultrasound, nuclear medicine, and cardiac angiography, the use of cine or dynamic displays can be done with film or videotape, but is much simpler on workstations. The "stack view" mode (Beard, Hemminger, Perry et al., 1993; Beard, Pizer, Rogers et al., 1987; Chang and Hoffman, 1993), in which cross-sectional images are viewed rapidly as though moving through a stack, is also readily accomplished on most workstations.

The author has experimented with a technique from the aerial reconnaissance field, sometimes called the "window shade" display (Horii, Kishore, Stevens et al., 1994). Potentially this could allow a display of two images to be compared on one monitor. A movable bar or region of interest (ROI) would show the image "underneath." Though formal studies of this technique have not been done in radiology, those radiologists who tried the prototype expressed interest in it. One advantage is that the viewer does not have to turn his or her head to view the comparison image on another monitor.

A method employing the registration and subtraction of two temporally spaced images (temporal subtraction) has been demonstrated by Kano and colleagues (Kano, Doi, MacMahon et al., 1994) from the University of Chicago. In this technique, the two images to be subtracted are first registered so that differences due to patient position are minimized. The subtraction image then shows areas of change as black. Such areas can be used to direct the viewer's attention during inspection of the image to be read.

The University of Chicago has also pioneered the use of computer aided diagnosis (CAD) (Doi, Giger, MacMahon et al., 1994; Giger and MacMahon, 1996). Software for automated detection of lung nodules and breast masses has been demonstrated. Such software is not intended to replace the radiologist, but rather to reduce the false negative rate in circumstances in which the consequences of such a false negative are severe. The programs can display what they detect as a graphic overlay on the image. The size of the graphical elements used can indicate the computed likelihood of a real lesion based on the decision criteria the program uses. The radiologist would then evaluate these areas on the image and decide whether or not the detected structure represents pathology.

Aside from functions and methods employed to enhance usability or diagnostic accuracy, workstations must also address the problem of image availability in diverse locations. Haskin noted some years ago that most hospitals have a very large number of lightboxes (Haskin, Haskin, Laffey et al., 1985); this finding implies there are a large number of locations in which images are viewed. Contemporary healthcare systems involve very large networks of facilities of varying sizes, from physician offices to large medical centers (Greenes and Bauman, 1996). Becasue the patient population will be served by combinations of these facilities, some manner of distributing images and other information is needed to support the level of service that such networks are advocating.

One choice that is receiving increasing interest is to use the Internet or a private version of it (often called an intranet). A good history of the Internet is provided by Hafner and Lyon (1996) and serves to provide some scale for this world-wide "network of networks." The advantages of an open and readily accessible network, especially the multimedia World Wide Web that operates on the Internet, are counterbalanced for medical information by a lack of security and privacy. Although technological solutions for some of the problems posed by the general issue of security "gaps" are available, moving the technology of the Internet to a private intranet helps solve the problem. Any connection between the private network and public communications carriers (necessary for wide-area service) can be carefully controlled. The advantages of Internet technology for workstations are that "browsers," or the software used to retrieve information from remote World Wide Web (WWW) servers, are available for multiple types of machines, are capable of handling images, and have a user interface well-understood by a large segment of the population. Several authors have described using personal computers with a browser to access medical information (Feingold, Grevera, Mezrich et al., 1997; Li, Valentin, So et al., 1995; Mascarini, Ratib, Trayser et al., 1995). The low cost of personal computers and the wide variety of communications choices to access the Internet or an intranet mean that the goal of wide availability of images and other medical information can be met. It is likely that the majority of future workstations used outside of radiology, or other specialties that do not do primary diagnosis from workstations, will be personal computer-based and access needed information using an Internet browser. Recently, movement of the Internet WWW search service software to intranets (DeJesus, 1997) means that the capability to search even very large databases will be available for intranets.

Workstations also permit on a desktop what used to require a mainframe computer; reconstruction of two-dimensional slice data into three-dimensional images that may be manipulated in real time. This is, in itself, a large topic deserving of much greater explanation than can be given here. This author notes that computer graphics methods add yet another dimension to abilities beyond what film can accomplish. The reference by Vannier and Marsh (1996) provides a contemporary overview of the subject.

Conclusion

Those who are impatient for workstations to replace film-based reading should recall that radiologists have a hundred-year experience with film. There are those who pessimistically note that the "paperless office" and "bookless library" have not come to pass despite the availability of the technology. However, they should also note that where electronic methods are superior to paper and books and where the applications developed are simpler to use, computer based technology has prevailed. The examples of electronic mail and computerized literature searches readily come to mind. This author would agree, though, that more widespread acceptance of workstations is dependent on their further evaluation and refinement and that it is the efforts of those who have pioneered electronic imaging in medicine that are enabling this progress.

References

Alter AJ, Kargas GA, Kargas SA et al. The influence of ambient and view box light upon visual detection of low contrast targets in a radiograph. Invest Radiol 1982, 17, 402.

American College of Radiology. ACR Standard for Teleradiology. Reston, VA: American College of Radiology, 1994.

Baxter B, Ravindra H, Norman RA. Changes in lesion detectability caused by light adaptation in retinal photoreceptors. Invest Radiol 1982, 17, 394.

Beard DV. Designing a radiology workstation: a focus on navigation during the interpretation task. J. Digit Imaging 1990, 3(3), 152–163.

Beard DV, Hemminger BM, Perry JR et al. Interpretation of CT studies: single-screen workstation versus film alternator. Radiology 1993, 187(2), 565–569.

Beard DV, Pisano ED, Denelsbeck KM, Johnston RE. Eye movement during computed tomography interpretation: eyetracker results and image display-time implications. J. Digit Imaging 1994, 7 (4), 189–192.

Beard D, Pizer S, Rogers D et al. A prototype single-screen PACs console development using human-computer interaction techniques. Proc SPIE 1987, 767, 646–653.

Beard DV, Walker JGF, Bell I, Cromartie R. Evolved design of a radiology workstation using time-motion analysis and the keystroke model. Proc SPIE 1989, 1091, 121–131.

Belanger G, Robertson J, Coristine M et al. Evaluation of a workstation by clinicians. Proc SPIE 1989, 1093, 214–219.

Braudes RE, Mun SK, Schnizlein J et al. A software development and user interface rapid prototyping environment for picture archiving and communications systems (PACS). Proc SPIE 1989, 1093, 220–229.

Chang PJ, Hoffman E. Multimodality workstation featuring multiband cine mode and real-time distributed interactive consultation. RSNA: infoRAD exhibit 9507WS, 1993.

DeJesus EX. The searchable kingdom. Byte 1997, 22(6), 92NA1–92NA12.

Doi K, Giger ML, MacMahon H et al. Computer-aided diagnosis: development of automated schemes for quantitative analysis of radiographic images. Semin Ultrasound CT MR 1992, 13, 140–152.

Duerinckx AJ, ed. Picture archiving and communications systems for medical applications, Parts I pp. 1–398 and part II pp. 399–490. Proc SPIE 1982, V, 318.

Dwyer III SJ, Templeton AW, Anderson WH et al. Salient characteristics of a distributed diagnostic imaging management system for a radiology department. Proc SPIE 1982, 318, 194–204.

Feingold ER, Grevera GJ, Mezrich RS et al. Web-based radiology applications for clinicians and radiologists. Proc SPIE 1997, 3035, 60–75.

Feingold E, Seshadri SB, Arenson RL. Folder management on a multimodality PACS display station. Proc SPIE 1991, 1446, 211–216.

Gee JC, DeSoto LA, Kim Y. User interface design for a radiological imaging workstation. Proc SPIE 1989, 1093, 122–132.

Giger ML, MacMahon H. Image processing and computer-aided diagnosis. Radiol Clin of North Amer 1996, 34(3), 565–596.

Greenes RA, Bauman RA. The era of health care reform and the information superhighway. Radiol Clin N Am 1996, 34(3), 463–468.

Hafner K, Lyon M. Where Wizards Stay Up Late: the Origins of the Internet. New York: Simon and Schuster, 1996.

Haynor DR, Saarinen AO. The "old study" and the correlative study: implications for PACS. Proc SPIE 1989, 1093, 10–12.

Haskin ME, Haskin PH, Laffey PA et al. Data versus information: which should we exchange? Proc SPIE 1985, 536, 37–42.

Hohman SA, Johnson SJ, Valentino DJ et al. Radiologists' requirements for primary diagnosis workstations: preliminary results of task-based design surveys. Proc SPIE 1994, 2165, 2–7.

Honeyman JC, Arenson RL, Frost MM et al. Functional requirements for diagnostic workstations. Proc SPIE 1993, 1899, 103–109.

Horii SC, Feingold ER, Kundel HL et al. PACS workstation usage differences between radiologists and MICU physicians. Proc SPIE 1996, 2711, 266–271.

Horii SC, Horii HN, Mun SK et al. Environmental designs for reading from imaging workstations: ergonomic and architectural features. J. Dig. Imaging 1989, 2(3), 156–162.

Horii SC, Kishore S, Stevens JF et al. Overlapped image display method: a technique for comparing medical images on a workstation. Proc SPIE 1994, 2164, 456–466.

Horii SC, Schimpf JH, Isles G, Bergeron RT. Digital image viewing stations: radiologist interests and attitudes. Proc SPIE 1994, 454, 224–233.

Huang HK, Mankovitch NJ, Taira RK, Kangarloo H. Implementation of a digital multiple viewing station and early clinical experience. Proc SPIE 1986, 626, 432–440.

Johnston RE, Rogers DC, Creasy JL et al. How to evaluate a medical imaging display workstation. Proc SPIE 1987, 767, 616–621.

Kano A, Doi K, MacMahon H et al. Digital image subtraction of temporally sequential chest images for detection of interval change. Med Phys 1994, 21(3), 453–61.

Kasday LR. Human factors considerations in PACS design. Proc SPIE 1986, 626, 581–592.

Kundel HL. How much spatial resolution is enough? A meta-analysis of observer performance studies comparing plain films and digital hard copy. Proc SPIE 1993, 1899, 86–89.

Krupinski EA, Lund PJ. Comparison of film vs. monitor viewing of CR films using eye-position recording. Proc SCAR '96, 1996, 269–274.

Larsen GN. Interactive image processing for computerized tomography (Ph.D. Thesis). Department of Electronics and Electrical Engineering, University of Missouri at Columbia, 1976.

Lemke HU, Stiehl HS, Scharnweber N, Jackel D. Applications of picture processing, image analysis, and computer graphics techniques to cranial CT scans. Proceedings of the Sixth Conference on Computer Applications in Radiology and Computer/Aided Analysis of Radiological Images 1979, 341–354. IEEE Computer Society Press.

Levin K, Horii S, Mun SK et al. Analysis of data assembling activities for radiologists and its implications for clinical acceptance of PACS. Proc SPIE 1990, 1234, 670–675.

Li X, Valentino DJ, So GJ et al. World Wide Web telemedicine system. Proc SPIE 1995, 2711, 427–439.

Maguire Jr. GQ, Zeleznik MP, Horii SC et al. Image processing requirements in hospitals and an integrated systems approach. Proc SPIE 1982, 318, 206–213.

Mascarini C, Ratib OM, Trayser G et al. In-house access to PACS images and related data through World Wide Web. Proc SPIE 1995, 2711, 531–537.

McNeill KM, Seeley GW, Maloney K et al. Comparison of a digital workstation and film alternator. Proc SPIE 1988, 914, 929–937.

MDIS Technical Development Team. MDIS Medical Diagnostic Imaging Support System Acquisition Document. Huntsville, US Army Engineer Division, C-23 - C-57, 1991.

Meyer-Ebrecht D, Wendler T. Concept of the diagnostic image workstation. Proc SPIE 1983, 418, 180–188.

O'Malley K. An iterative approach to development of a PACS display workstation. Proc SPIE 1989, 1093, 293–300.

Ravindra H, Norman RA, Baxter B. The effect of extraneous light on lesion detectability: a demonstration. Invest Radiol 1983, 18, 105.

Rogers DC, Johnston RE. Effect of ambient light on electronically displayed medical images as measured by luminance-discrimination thresholds. J Opt Soc Am 1987, A4, 976.

Rogers DC, Johnston RE, Brenton B et al. Predicting PACS console requirements from radiologists' reading habits. Proc SPIE 1985, 536, 88–95.

Rossman K. Image quality. Radiol Clin of North Amer 1969, 7(3), 419–433.

Schuttenbeld HHW, ter Haar Romeny BM. Design of a user-interface for a PACS viewing station. Proc SPIE 1987, 767, 844–848.

Scott Jr. WW, Bluemke DA, Mysko WK et al. Interpretation of Emergency Department radiographs by radiologists and emergency medicine physicians: teleradiology workstation versus radiograph readings. Radiology 1995, 195, 223–229.

Sezan MI, Yip KL, Daly SJ. An investigation of the effects of uniform perceptual quantization in the context of digital radiography. Proc SPIE 1987, 767, 622–630

Slasky BS, Gur D, Wood WF et al. Receiver operating characteristic analysis of chest image interpretation with conventional, laser printed, and high-resolution workstation images. Radiology 1990, 174, 775–780.

Steinke JE, Nabijee KH, Freeman R, Prior FW. Operator interface design considerations for a PACS information management system. Proc SPIE 1990, 1234, 444–453.

Taylor JH. Vision. In: Parker JF, West VR, eds. Bioastronautics Data Book, 2nd ed. Washington, DC: NASA, 1973, pp. 611–665.

ter Haar Romeny BM, Raymakers J, van Waes PFGM et al. The Dutch PACS project: philosophy, design of a digital reading room, and first observations in the Utrecht University Hospital in the Netherlands. Proc SPIE 1987, 767, 787–792.

van der Voorde F, Arenson R, Kundel H et al. Development of a physician-friendly digital image display console. Proc SPIE 1986, 626, 541–548.

Vannier MW, Marsh JL. Three-dimensional imaging, surgical planning, and image-guided therapy. Radiol Clin of North Amer 1996, 34(3), 545–56

Section 5

14
Workstation Functions and System Capabilities

STEVEN C. HORII

In a picture archiving and communications system (PACS) design, the function of displaying the images for interpretation and review is handled by the workstation. As such, it serves as the interface between the users and the system and so is placed in a demanding position. Opinions about workstations—how they should be designed and how they should operate—vary widely. On one statement, most of those developing workstations would agree: "There is no single best workstation design." Nonetheless, years of research and development of workstations for medical imaging and other image-related tasks have yielded some principles that serve to guide the engineers and scientists building and evaluating these workstations.

This chapter examines the basic functions performed by a workstation for medical imaging, how overall PACS architecture affects workstations, advances in the various forms of display devices, and the importance of the physical environment in which workstations are used. To help establish what is meant by a workstation, Figure 14.1 shows a block diagram of generic workstation hardware. Although it will not match most designs exactly, the components shown in the figure exist, at least in part, in all imaging workstations.

On a technical level, workstations have some basic functions that need to be supported if users are to be able to gain desired information from the images displayed.

Basic Functions

Speed

A basic requirement for workstations is speed. Some types of film alternators (multiviewers) can move films so fast that they go by in a blur (the transparent band types). Even the slower film alternators can move a four-over-four set of films (amounting to some 96 to 120 images for many of the cross-sectional imaging methods) in some three to five seconds. This is very

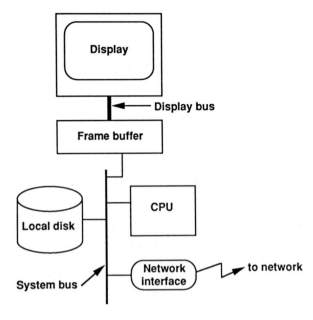

FIGURE 14.1. The major components of a workstation are shown in this diagram. The central processing unit (CPU, for purposes of this illustration) is the collection of microprocessor, random access memory (RAM), manual input devices, and interface components that provide the user interface and image management. Even centralized-archive PACS will have some local disk storage at the workstation if for no other reason than storing the software needed locally. The network interface converts network level signals and messages into those that the CPU can handle. All the components communicate over the system bus. The frame buffer stores the images in fast RAM and provides for conversion of the digital pixel values into analog voltages that drive the display. There may be a display bus to interconnect several frame buffers in multiple-monitor workstations. A separate display bus is used in many cases because of the high speed movement of digital data necessary for displays.

high performance to match in a workstation. For example, moving eight CR films in three to five seconds amounts to a data rate of some 10 to 16 megabytes per second. In general, a desirable target speed is to display an image in less than two seconds from the time the image is selected for display. Most users will not tolerate display times longer than this for routine displays. However, if they understand that an ad hoc request is taking longer because of the time to fetch the study from the archive, they are more willing to tolerate a longer delay. It is desirable to provide either a progress indicator for, or a notice about, how long such a retrieval will take. This avoids the problem of the user not being sure whether or not the system is working. With a multitasking workstation, such a retrieval can be done in the background while other processes (for example, reading another study) can take place in the foreground.

A feature that was implemented on the workstation developed at the University of Pennsylvania (van der Voorde, Arenson, Kundel et al., 1986) took advantage of common user actions. The current examination, plus up to four prior studies, would be kept on local disk. However, icons for up to four studies older than the first four were also displayed. The software automatically displayed the current examination plus the most recent previous study, and users could select older examinations by clicking on the icons. Once a user selected the third prior study, the software would assume that even earlier studies might be desired and would initiate a request from the archive for the older studies. In this way, if the user got to the fifth older examination, it would either have been loaded from the archive or retrieval would be in process. Because most users did not request studies beyond the second or third, this avoided filling local storage with examinations unlikely to be reviewed.

Navigation

Workstations also have to provide a navigation method for finding examinations to be read, comparison studies (older examinations of the same type), and correlation examinations (current or prior examinations of a different type). This navigation process is related closely to the user interface and the mental model assumed. The user interface issues will be discussed subsequently. Table 14.1 lists commonly encountered navigation functions (Arenson, Chakraborty, Seshadri et al., 1990; Feingold, Seshadri, and Arenson, 1991; Greenes, 1984; Jost, Hill, Rodewald et al., 1984; Leung, Ho, Chao et al., 1995).

Image Manipulation

A method for adjusting grayscale is evident from most workstation designs and studies of those designs (Horii, Feingold, Kundel et al., 1996). Adjustment of "window width and level" has been consistently shown to be the most frequently used image manipulation tool. Other image manipulation tools, including some form of magnification (either or both an overall magnify or the analog of a magnifying lens), roaming (either moving around in the magnified image or moving the magnifying window), video inversion ("black bone"), and rotation and flipping of the image, are typical of those provided. Some workstations also perform fast image processing to support edge enhancement, grayscale histogram equalization, and image arithmetic (adding or subtracting images). Specialty workstations may add additional image manipulation functions. Table 14.2 summarizes these image manipulation functions (Arenson, Chakraborty, Seshadri et al., 1990; Feingold, Seshadri and Arenson, 1991; Greenes, 1984; Hohman, Johnson, Valentino et al., 1994; Honeyman, Arenson, Frost et al., 1993; Josh, Hill, Rodewal et al., 1984).

Measuring features on images and calculating pixel statistics are two commonly available functions. These are deemed a necessity for computed tomography (CT) workstations because of the heavy use of these operations on dedicated CT display consoles. Such measurements are diagnostically

TABLE 14.1. Navigation functions.

Worklist	Display a list of examinations to be interpreted (should be reachable by a single keystroke equivalent).
List all	Display a list of all the current day's examinations—the daily list (also reachable by a single keystroke equivalent).
Folder display	For each patient, show the analog of the master jacket.
Next patient (exam)	Moves to the next patient or examination on the worklist.
Previous patient (exam)	Moves to the prior patient or examination on the worklist.
Consult	Interrupts current display, brings up "List all" or "Worklist," and allows selection and display of another patient or examination for consultation purposes.
Consult remote	For consultation between workstations. Invokes the display of the same study on two workstations and two cursors, one controlled by each workstation so that the two users may point to different areas on the image.
Resume last	Returns to exam interrupted by the Consult or Consult remote function (should return to images, format, and grayscale settings as prior to invoking either Consult mode).
Mark as read	Marks the examination as 'read." This should alter the appropriate flag in the image database so that others looking at the worklist or patient list will see the marked examinations displayed as "read." This function should also; (a) by restricted to use by those permitted to read examinations, and (b) prevent others from marking the examinations "read."
Compare	Brings up the patient folder so that a prior exam of the same type or other examination can be displayed for comparison and correlation purposes. Note that some examination types should have a site-configurable automatic display of prior examinations (e.g., chest radiographs will almost always be displayed with the prior examination). Display formats should be both site- and user-configurable.
Stack view/tile view	For cross-sectional and time-sequenced images, allows rapid selection of the stack view (rapid sequential image display in a single image frame) or tile view (images arranged in sequence but spatially separated much as photographed on conventional film). Ideally, stack view should be implementable with a selection on any image in a tile view display; ending the stack view would then return that frame to its original image. Stack view should also be applicable between and within (different series; e.g., noncontrast/contrast, or pulse sequences in MR) examinations for comparison purposes.
Cine loop view	For time-sequenced images, allows variable-speed display of the images to show dynamic phenomena.
Rearrange/save	Allows "drag and drop" rearrangement of the images displayed. While "hanging protocols" should be automated as much as possible, rearrangement is important for comparison purposes. The undo function should return the display to the original configuration. A "Save" function should store the information about the rearranged images so that the next time the same study is called up, it is displayed as rearranged.

See also Table 14.3. There are functions, such as "worklist," that cross boundaries between image navigation and management.

TABLE 14.2. Image manipulation functions.

Window width	Adjusts range of pixel bits sent to the display system. Should always be accessible.
Window level (center)	Sets center of window in pixel bits. Should always be accessible.
Grayscale reset	Resets window width and level settings to initially displayed values.
Zoom/magnify	Invokes an operation that maps the displayed image into a larger area (zoom is typically by pixel replication; magnify uses pixel interpolation).
ROI magnify	Magnifies within a movable region of interest. This should allow for variable degrees of magnification (may be in discrete steps) and should be movable in real time using the manual input control.
Grayscale invert	Reverses the meaning of the highest and lowest pixel values in terms of grayscale; for example, white bones would be displayed as black.
Window width and level presets	Single keystroke equivalent selectable preset WW/WL combinations. For example, lung, mediastinum, and bone for CT.
Image processing	Image processing functions are not commonly used while reading cases; however, access to such functions as edge enhancement, histogram equalization, and application of user-defined filters could be provided through a button that brings up a menu of such functions available.
Undo	At least one level of being able to undo the function just completed. This should be accessible with a single keystroke equivalent. Note: an undo of some image processing functions may be difficult to implement unless a copy of the "original" image is maintained.
Pixel statistics	Reports the number, mean, and standard deviation of pixels in an ROI.
Measure	Provides linear, area, and angle measurements on an image.
Annotate	Allows a user to add text annotation to an image. This function can be used with the display of an ROI or graphics arrows. Users should be able to toggle the annotation on and off. Such annotation should be saved with the image.

important and, in film-based operation, are often filmed as overlays on the image.

Report Display

A method for displaying the radiology reports of the examinations being viewed is also of importance. Although this is often thought of as a feature primarily for review workstations, its utility for radiologists should not be underestimated. In subspecialty radiology practices, it is very useful to know how a correlative study was read when it is being viewed as part of the interpretation of an examination of a different type. In more generalist practices, it is still important to know how a colleague read a prior examination. Display of reports usually requires that some form of interface to the radiology information system (RIS) or hospital information system (HIS) be operational. To a large extent, a successful conversion from film-based reading to the use of workstations for the same work will also involve the replacement of many of the functions now done manually with automated equivalents (Deibel and Greenes, 1996; Horii, Kundel, Feingold et al., 1997). Selection of prior studies to display, arrangement of images when displayed, and clearing of films from the alternator when the readings are done are all examples of image management functions that need to be supported in the workstation environment. If this is not done, the transition to workstations will also mean the migration of support tasks to the radiologist. Although this might seem attractive at first because of potential personnel reductions, the radiologist's time is very expensive and his or her productivity is very dependent on these support functions. Simply moving these operations from clerks and other personnel to the radiologist will have a negative impact on productivity. Table 14.3 lists a set of these image management functions.

System Design Choices

System Architecture

The overall architecture of a PACS will determine the hardware design of the workstations connected to it. There are basically two major PACS designs: the centralized storage version and the distributed storage version (Bell, Ling, and Young, 1992; Glicksman, Prior, and Wilson, 1993; Glicksman et al., 1992; Kishore, Khalsa, Stevens et al., 1994; Stewart and Taira, 1991). The design chosen for the Department of Defense Medical Diagnostic Imaging Support (MDIS) System (Goeringer, 1991; MDIS Technical Development Team, 1991) is the archetype of centralized systems. All images are stored in a very high speed magnetic disk array that is supported by a database management computer and a long-term optical disk archive. The high-speed, wideband nature of the storage system means that workstations do not have to store images locally, and the workstation hardware does not need to include a large-capacity magnetic disk of its own. The MDIS design does include local magnetic disk, but for storage of the workstation software and utilities, not for images. Images are stored locally in the display memory only. The centralized design needs to have the speed and bandwidth necessary to support fast retrieval of images from multiple workstations. In the MDIS system, for example, any workstation can retrieve images from the central storage system at a rate of one second or less per image. This performance

TABLE 14.3. Image management functions.

Delete exam (local)	Provides for deletion of an examination from the local storage (with appropriate warnings).
Autodelete	Provides for automated deletion of examinations from local storage based on user-set criteria.
Mark for teaching file	Flags the examination being read as one useful for teaching purposes.
Mark for nondeletion	Flags the examination being read as one not to be autodeleted. Note that a site-configurable expiration time for this "protection" is useful.
Redirect	Allows sending of an examination to a particular workstation.
Scrapbook	Saves selected images (or pointers to images) in a file. Retrieving this file later would (optionally) first display the scrapbook images while providing access to the full study, if requested.
Print	Provides hardcopy printing of selected images (e.g., the Scrapbook) or a whole study. Print options (film, paper, 35-mm slide) depend on devices in the system. Print function permissions should be configured by class of user.
Local storage statistics	If the system uses local storage for images, this function should display the percentage of capacity currently used.
In progress notice	For time-consuming operations (such as retrieving an archived case) this function should display a progress indicator to give the user some idea when the operation will be completed.
Hanging protocol	Allows for site- and user-customizable arrangements of images, series, etc., as defaults for initial displays. For example, some radiologists prefer to read chest cases with the current films in the center two of four light boxes and the prior study on the outer two light boxes; others prefer the pair of frontal images on two adjacent light boxes and the pair of lateral images on the other two. It should be possible using electronic hanging protocols to support both of these possibilities and others. The arrangement used should be based on user login.
Associate report	If a radiology report is available for an examination on the daily list or for prior studies that will be displayed, a method for displaying that report should be implemented. An entry on the daily list should show report status (none, preliminary, reviewed, finalized or signed, referring physician reviewed). The latter status is one that is being phased in at many institutions.

See Table 14.1. There are functions, such as "worklist," that cross boundaries between image management and navigation.

requires that the network connecting the central storage device and the workstations be very fast; if not, the high speed of the storage is of little advantage.

The alternative design is a distributed system in which there may be one or more short- and long-term storage devices, but the images in current use are stored at the workstation. In this case, the workstation needs to have enough local magnetic disk to store as many images as needed for a typical reading session, including any prior or correlative examinations retrieved from long-term storage. In some senses, this design trades off workstation local storage against network performance. Low-cost local area networks can be used to implement the image transmission network, subject to constraints of the management system. Distributed systems also need to have good image management so that images are moved where they will be needed (workstation local disk) to avoid long transmission delays resulting from network performance. The use of a distributed design with a moderate speed (about 10 megabits per second) LAN is possible with such good image management and also benefits from predictable loads and behaviors. If radiologists and other users tend to view images from the same locations and if the number of ad hoc requests (those not predicted from RIS or HIS information) is low, such designs can work quite well. These considerations also do not include the impact of data compression, particularly lossy compression, that can reduce data per image by a factor of 10 or more. Other chapters in this book will discuss the compression issue in more detail.

The two models are not mutually exclusive; there are designs that are hybrids of both. In particular, there are PACS made up of interconnected smaller systems that may themselves be centralized storage designs. Such designs tend to be those that have "grown" rather than been installed as a single system. In some senses, this is a good, if somewhat engineering intensive, design, as each subsystem can be optimized for its particular tasks.

Local Image Storage

In either the distributed or centralized PACS model, the workstations need some form of storage. In the distributed design, this typically will be magnetic disk. Very fast workstation designs have employed disk arrays (Taira, Simons, Razavi et al., 1990) for local storage rather than single disks because of the gain in speed. Such arrays can transfer multiple bits of the pixel at once rather than a stream of single bits. The diminishing cost of magnetic disk drives is making it possible to provide very large amounts of local disk storage and still meet cost targets for workstations.

For both distributed and centralized PACS models, the workstation has to have storage for the image(s) currently displayed on the monitor(s). Disk transfer speeds and the associated interface and computer bus (the part that interconnects all the workstation central processor components) are not nearly fast enough to keep up with the requirements of the monitors. These typically refresh the image on the screen some 72 to 75 times per second (to avoid flicker). That means all the image pixels have to be displayed in that time, a very high data rate under any circumstances. To meet this requirement, workstations have special fast display memory and digital-to-analog converters to store the pixel data and convert it to the analog form the monitor needs. This memory is usually called a "frame buffer," and its size depends on the monitor resolution. For example, for a 2048×2560 pixel array of 16 bits requires about 10.5 megabytes of such storage. Frame buffers often store more bits than are actually displayed, sometimes as a larger pixel array, but more often as greater bit depth. This allows, in the former instance, for very fast roaming around an image. The latter can provide for fast window width and level adjustments as the whole pixel is stored in the fast storage and window adjustments do not have to rely on moving data from slower system memory to the frame buffer. Fast computer memory chips have followed the trend of other integrated circuit technologies (some would say they lead the trend) of decreasing cost and improving speed and density over time. Such cost reductions have led to some exceptional frame buffer designs, including one of three gigabytes (Shile, Fujii, Ramamurthy et al., 1997).

Workstation Image Processing

Adjustment of image window width and level is one form of image processing. It is necessary because the maximum (completely dark screen to maximum screen luminance) display range of cathode ray tube displays typically means that about eight bits, or 256 gray levels, can be distinctly displayed (Asher and Martin, 1968). Given the 12-bit depth of CT and the ten bits of MRI and CR, there is a large number of images whose grayscale content exceeds that of a CRT. The same is true of film and is, for example, the reason for photographing both lung and mediastinal windows for chest CT.

CRTs require analog voltages to set the luminance of a displayed pixel. This is the reason for the digital-to-analog converter (DAC) as part of the display system. The digital pixel value stored in the frame buffer is sent to the DAC and changed to a voltage. This is then sent to the monitor circuitry where it is amplified and used to modulate the intensity of the CRT beam. Image processing can be accomplished by changing the digital value sent to the DAC or by altering pixel information as it is transferred from local disk or memory to the frame buffer. In either event, image processing can involve changing the value of each displayed pixel based on a mathematical algorithm that uses only the information in that single pixel (window width and level adjustments and video inversion are examples of such processes). More complex algorithms, such as edge enhancement, make use of information in multiple pixels to alter the value of each displayed pixel.

Because CRTs are not usually linear in their display characteristics (Asher and Martin, 1968), doubling the digital pixel value does not necessarily double the displayed luminance, and some adjustment is often needed. Also, human visual perception is far from linear (for example, the same contrast difference is more readily perceptible at higher luminance levels than lower ones) (Fry, 1965; Pizer, Johnston, Zimmerman et al., Chan, 1982), and in some instances it is desirable to compensate for this. Compensation for such nonlinearities is usually accomplished through what are called look-up tables. For CRT linearity, for example, it is simple to imagine a table made up of the input voltages as rows and the output voltages necessary to achieve linearity as columns. For any given input, then, the electronic version of the table would provide the necessary output. Although it may not be obvious, it is simpler to implement such look-up tables in digital, rather than in analog, electronics. The analog version requires nonlinear amplifiers to do this, and they are not always simple to design. In the digital version, a look-up table is exactly that—a matrix of input versus output values. Thus, implementing single-pixel type image processing can then be as simple as modifying the look-up table values.

For more complex multipixel image processing, such as that done for CR images, there is no way to avoid image arithmetic. Such processes require a fast processor, as the number of arithmetic steps increases as the product of the number of image pixel rows and columns. Some display systems make use of separate, dedicated arithmetic processors that are optimized for image processing and can perform these steps more quickly than the workstation central processor.

Workstation Display Devices

Cathode ray tubes have formed the basis of the image workstation since the very earliest such devices (Bell, 1988). As described, CRTs are not linear display devices. Neither is film. CRTs have a relatively lower luminance than film on a lightbox as noted in Figure 14.2. Because CRTs use a filament to generate the electrons needed for the display, they have a limited life. Performance of CRTs varies as they age (Say, Hedler, Maninger et al., 1986), and the amplifier circuitry may drift over time. The physics of CRTs also makes them susceptible to magnetic fields; they will display distorted images in a high magnetic field (as near an MR machine) without special shielding.

Nonetheless, CRTs are capable of quite high performance, displaying perceptually flicker-free images that, unlike film-based ones, can be dynamic and modified in real time. Color CRTs are needed for applications, including nuclear medicine, ultrasound, radiation therapy planning, endoscopic imaging, pathologic imaging, three-dimensional display work, and others that are being added as digital imaging enters the field. Color CRTs are basically the same as black-and-white tubes, but with three guns instead of one. (It should be noted, however, that at least one black-and-white tube design also uses multiple guns to increase luminance.) The phosphor also consists of three primary color phosphorescent substances. A device called a shadow mask allows a particular beam to strike its particular phosphor color. Color CRTs suffer the same problems as black-and-white ones, in some cases worse because of the triple set of electronics. Typically the color phosphors are arranged as either a triad of dots or stripes, making gray scale pixels (all three primary colors involved) larger physically on a color monitor than can be achieved on a corresponding black-and-white monitor. For this reason, it is generally recommended to avoid color monitors for black-and-white image displays unless the color is needed for other parts of the application (nuclear medicine and ultrasound are typical of the mixed-image scenario).

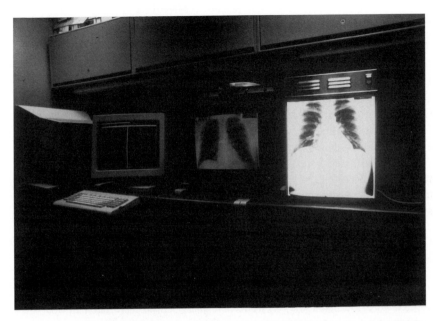

FIGURE 14.2. This photograph shows the same chest image displayed on a workstation monitor (center) and conventional film on a light box (right). The much greater brightness of the conventional light box is evident. While the photographic process exaggerates this difference to some degree, the exposure of the original film nonetheless shows how much more light was received from the light box display. Current high brightness monitors would show a less striking difference.

Color CRTs have a different pixel matrix display capability from black-and-white monitors of the same screen size. Hence black-and-white displays on color monitors have lower spatial resolution than black-and-white monitors.

Given these limitations of CRTs, it is logical to ask if there are any electronic alternatives. The growing popularity of laptop computers and the interest in "next generation" television may provide one answer. Laptops clearly need some form of thin, low-power, high-resolution display. Next generation television could still use a CRT, but the disadvantages of CRTs also plague consumer applications. Laptops use flat panel displays, typically based on liquid crystal technology. Liquid crystals have optical properties of varying degrees of light transmission as voltages are applied to them. Through their optical properties, it is also possible to achieve color displays. In most of the liquid crystal displays (LCDs), an array of cells is formed by depositing transparent conductive films on glass and sandwiching a layer of liquid crystal in between them. Applying voltages to the electrodes will alter the optical properties of the liquid crystal in the cell whose electrodes have been selected. In passive matrix systems, this is what is done. Active matrix systems move the drive circuitry to each cell by creating a transparent array of transistors on the glass. These displays are more costly as they are more expensive to fabricate, but their response is faster (passive matrix displays may suffer from "lag," particularly as high contrast objects are moved on the display). With the drive circuitry at each cell, contrast is also improved. Because the liquid crystals change optical properties but do not fluoresce, LCDs operate by having a light source behind the screen. High luminance is achieved by making this light source bright. However, the liquid crystal optical properties, particularly in the thin layer of liquid used, may not allow for very high luminance without the back light "shining through" the dark areas, so display dynamic range is limited (at present, more so than for CRTs).

Television-sized LCDs have been fabricated, although as of this writing, these are still quite costly. As for other solid-state electronics, however, it is expected that the costs will decline, particularly if the large potential consumer market is realized.

Other flat-panel display technologies that have the potential to replace CRTs include the light emitting class of displays: plasma panels (Say, Hedler, Maninger et al., 1986), field emission displays (Derbyshire, 1994), electroluminescent displays, and light-emitting diode arrays (Sherr, 1993).

Plasma panels operate by having a gas fluoresce when excited by a potential applied across transparent electrodes on glass. These have been in use for a number of years, but are typically monochromatic displays. They can, however, have quite high luminance. Some newer designs can yield color displays.

As shown in Figure 14.3, field emission displays use a series of electron

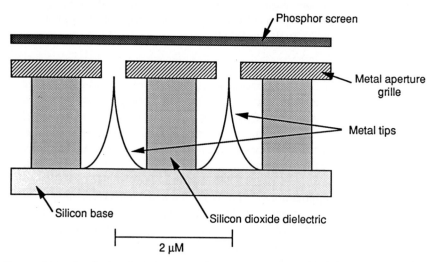

Figure 14.3. The field emission display has a structure shown in this schematic drawing. The device base, metallic tips, and silicon dioxide dielectric (insulating layer) and metal aperture grille are all fabricated using integrated circuit-type techniques. The typical spacing of the tips is about two micrometers center to center. An electric potential and current between the tips and the aperture grille results in emission of a stream of electrons from the tips. The electrons strike the phosphor layer resulting in visible fluorescence. Drawing by the author based on Shyankay 1995/Derbyshire 1996.

emitting points fabricated using integrated circuit technology. These points are surrounded by an aperture grille that serves to accelerate the electrons emitted from the points. Because the electric field intensity around a point increases as the radius of curvature of the point decreases, very high field intensities can be achieved around the points with fairly low potentials applied to them. A phosphorescent screen placed in front of the emitter array serves as the display surface and, like a CRT, it fluoresces in response to the electron bombardment. The integrated circuit fabrication process means that the emitter size can be made very small, and pixel sizes on the order of several micrometers (as opposed to the hundred micrometer size of CRT pixels) have been achieved in the laboratory. Fabrication of these in large scale is a challenge, but no greater than that for active matrix LCDs. Current field emission display technology makes use of diamond, rather than metallic, points as diamond repels electrons, reducing even further the power needed to produce a stream of electrons from the points. Some designs have taken advantage of the ability to micro fabricate thin films of diamond and use diamond patches instead of points (Shyankay, 1995).

Electroluminescent displays have been in use since the 1960s. The Apollo space program made extensive use of electroluminescent (EL) technology both for lighting control panels and numeric displays (Apollo Spacecraft News Reference, not dated). The reasons for this choice were high reliability and low power requirements. Fabricating EL pixel arrays has been done experimentally, but no gray scale devices are in commercial production. Phosphor color is a problem, though some that are closer to white have been developed. EL systems are also very sensitive to moisture and the displays have to be sealed carefully.

Arrays of light-emitting diodes (LEDs) have also been built as laboratory demonstrations for flat panel displays, and large panels for poster-size displays have been tried. The availability of blue LEDs means that full color displays are possible. Making small LEDs with enough luminance is one problem, and for color displays, each pixel would have to have three LEDs. Cost is high for these displays, and although LEDs use far less power than incandescent lamps for the same luminance output, they still use much more power than EL displays or a backlit LCD panel.

Another potential alternative also uses integrated circuit manufacturing techniques. The digital micromirror display (DMD) uses such techniques to produce a panel of small mirrors each with a pivot and drive electrodes (see Fig. 14.4). The drive electrodes are used to produce oscillations of the mirrors that results in a modulation of light reflected from them. These mirrors are also quite small (on the order of 17 micrometers square). This form of display operates by reflecting light rather than emitting it, and laboratory prototypes have been constructed, including some displays that have successfully shown television images with full motion and computer monitor output (Grove, not dated; Sampsell, 1993). Because the DMD uses reflected light, the resulting display is not a flat panel, but more like the size and shape of a projection television system.

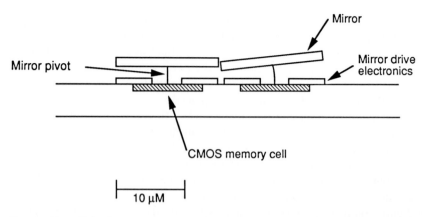

FIGURE 14.4. This diagram shows the schematic structure of a digital micromirror display (DMD). The entire structure is fabricated using integrated circuit-type techniques. The mirrors are quite small—on the order of 15–17 micrometers on a side. The electronics to drive the mirror is fabricated as part of the substrate. The complementary metal oxide semiconductor (CMOS—a type of integrated circuit) memory cell serves to store the mirror's deflection state so that the drive electronics does not have to be refreshed from the frame buffer. In effect, this design has the frame buffer as part of the display. The mirror pivot structure is shown quite simplified for clarity—the actural structure is more complex [See Gove (no date)].

Of these technologies, as of this writing, only the LCD has been manufactured in quantity and at a cost that is potentially competitive with CRTs. Plasma panels have also been made in large sizes and quantities, but the current types are typically monochromatic with either a single bit or very few bits of gray scale. For these reasons, they are not yet competitive with CRTs for medical imaging. There is little doubt that as these alternative display technologies mature, viable replacements for CRTs will emerge. In the past two years, there has been increasing interest in the flat panel for desktop computer displays and there are now several commercial sources of these, all based on the LCD panel.

Workstation Environments

A well-described problem that CRT displays have when compared with film on a lightbox is the much lower luminance of the displayed image on the CRT. Modern CRT designs with features specifically engineered for high luminance have dramatically increased light output, but it is still less than what is achievable with film and lightboxes. What this means in practical terms is that more thought has to go into planning reading rooms and environments than was necessary for film-based working areas. What is the workstation environment?

Since interpreting of radiological images has evolved using film illuminated by light boxes, the reading rooms in which such interpretation is done are also suited to such work. The square footage devoted to film viewers, their spacing, power requirements, heat dissipation, and ambient lighting are all based on devices with high luminance. The "traffic flow" patterns of people to put films on and remove films from these devices, the radiologists who read the cases, and the referring physicians who come to review the images with the radiologist are also part of the reading room design. In many cases, reading rooms are ad hoc affairs, fit in wherever space is left over or can be taken from other departmental functions.

The problem for workstations is that they do not operate like film viewing devices. Their luminance is much lower, as has been discussed. Although personnel do not have to access them to put images up, they still have to be usable for review of studies with referring physicians or with residents who are being trained. Power requirements and heat dissipation may be lower, but the quality of the electrical power often has to be higher. The voltage spikes and sags and the electrical noise that light boxes can tolerate might cause damage to a workstation's electronics. There will be more electrical cables and network wiring to be considered. Work surfaces have to accommodate control panels and other input devices and still have sufficient room for the inevitable manual tasks required, such as reading charts or taking notes.

The workstation environment, then, consists of all of the elements of the reading room plus the heating, ventilation, air conditioning (HVAC), and communications systems and electrical power supplied from outside. Aside from the physical layout, the workstation environment is also dynamic and needs to account for the movement of personnel and access to the workstations and the people using them.

If nothing else, lighting requirements are very different from film-based to workstation reading. The low luminance of workstations compared to light boxes means that the whole of the ambient lighting has to be lower for workstations. The curved surfaces of most CRT monitor screens means that glare lighting sources have to be controlled carefully. The lower overall ambient light may require that task lighting be provided for reading or writing activities. This author has described some guidelines for reading room design for workstations (Horii, Horii, Mun et al., 1989). These include indirect lighting (bounced and diffused from the ceiling or wall), avoiding placement of workstations opposite each other, and the use of partial room partitions or barriers between workstations to control both sound and light spill. If workstations and film viewing have to coexist in a single reading room, then partitions between lightboxes or alternators and workstations are a must and placing alternators and workstations opposite each other is absolutely contraindicated.

Architects familiar with design of radiology departments should be consulted as they have a very good understanding of traffic flow based on room functions. Many architectural offices themselves now use workstations instead of conventional drafting tables, so they have some familiarity with the problems that workstations pose. This author would caution, however, that design principles used for office environments in which workstations are used may not be applied successfully to the medical imaging environment. Many office-based workstation tasks involve very high-contrast subject matter (e.g., text displays) and higher levels of ambient light are not only tolerated but needed. The ideas about imaging workstation furniture, particularly seating and work surfaces, do have some counterpart in office environments and so can be used as guidelines. An architect with a particular interest in healthcare facilities, Rostenberg (1995), has written a book on design of radiology departments that is more up-to-date than other books on such design.

There are anecdotal, but numerous, reports of increased fatigue when reading at workstations compared to film on alternators. The reasons for this are not fully known, but a review of the work of Rogers, Johnston, Brenton et al. (1985) shows that radiologists spend time performing actions that take them away from the alternator or at least serve as a break in the reading process. Examples cited by Rogers include reviewing the patient history including the requisition and other paperwork, sorting through films and hanging them, and removing a film from the viewbox for "hot light" viewing or repositioning. With workstations, particularly those that do support an RIS interface, these tasks are done at the workstation. This author believes that at least some component of the fatigue is a result of the lack of short breaks afforded by the tasks associated with the reading process for film. The increased time spent looking at nonimage areas to perform operations, as noted by Krupinski and Lund (1996) may also contribute to this feeling of fatigue, as the amount of eye movement involved in the reading task is increased.

Better attention to both the ergonomics of the workstation and the workstation environment should help increase acceptance of workstations for primary diagnosis and decrease user physical discomfort while doing so.

Conclusion

Workstations are replacing or will replace conventional film for the diagnostic and review tasks for medical imaging. For this to happen on a large scale, the barriers to acceptance (lack of adaptability, automation, and integration) will have to be overcome. This, in turn, requires that the users of workstations expend more effort in understanding their work in detail, with a knowledge of the human factors involved. Manufacturers need to use this understanding and knowledge in the development of the next generation of workstations. Department administration and the architects who plan departments should learn, preferably by first-hand observation, that the environments into which workstations will be placed are critical to their use and acceptance.

References

Apollo Spacecraft News Reference. New York: Grumman Aircraft Engineering Corporation, L-1 - L-3, no date.

Asher RW, Martin H. Cathode-ray devices. In: Luxenberg, HR, Kuehn, RL, eds. Display Systems Engineering. New York, McGraw-Hill, 1968, pp. 237–276.

Arenson RL, Chakraborty DP, Seshadri SB, Kundel HL. The digital imaging workstation. Radiology 1999, 176, 303–315.

Bell CG. Toward a history of (personal) workstations. In: A Goldberg A, ed. A History of Personal Workstations. New York, ACM Press, 1988, pp. 4–36.

Bell D, Ling DHO, Young IR. Databases. In: Osteaux, M, ed. A Second Generation PACS Concept. Berlin, Springer-Verlag, 1992, pp. 211–293.

Deibel SRA, Greenes RA. Radiology systems architecture. Radiologic Clinics of North America 1996, 34(3), 681–696.

Derbyshire K. Beyond AMLCDs: field emission displays? Electronics Design, October 1994, pp. 56–66.

Feingold E, Seshadri SB, Arenson RL. Folder management on a multimodality PACS display station. Proc SPIE 1991, 1446, 211–216.

Fry GA. The eye and vision. In: Kingslake, R, ed. Applied Optics and Optical Engineering, Vol. II. New York, Academic Press, 1965, pp. 1–76.

Glicksman RA, Prior FW, Wilson DL. Image management within a PACS. Proc SPIE 1993, 1899, 157–164.

Glicksman RA, Wilson DL, Perry JF, Prior FW. Architecture of a high-performance PACS based on a shared file system. Proc SPIE 1992, 1654, 158–168.

Goeringer F. Medical diagnostic imaging support systems for military medicine. In: Huang, HK, Ratib, O, Bakker, AR, Witte, G, eds. Picture Archiving and Communication Systems (PACS) in Medicine. NATO ASI Series F, v 74. Berlin: Springer-Verlag, 1991, 213–230.

Gove RJ. DMD Display systems: the impact of an all-digital display. Web page URL: *www.ti.com/dlp/docs/papers/dmd/dmd.htm.*

Greenes RA. Toward more effective radiologic workstation consultation: design of a desktop workstation to aid in the selection and interpretation of diagnostic procedures. Proceedings of the Eighth Conference of Computer Applications in Radiology; American College of Radiology, 1984, pp. 554–561.

Hohman SA, Johnson SJ, Valentino DJ et al. Radiologists' requirements for primary diagnosis workstations: preliminary results of task-based design surveys. Proc SPIE 1994, 2165, 2–7.

Honeyman JC, Arenson RL, Frost MM et al. Functional requirements for diagnostic workstations. Proc SPIE 1993, 1899, 103–109.

Horii SC, Feingold ER, Kundel HL et al. PACS workstation usage differences between radiologists and MICU physicians. Proc SPIE 1996, 2711, 266–271.

Horii SC, Horii HN, Mun SK et al. Environmental designs for reading from imaging workstations: ergonomic and architectural features. J Dig Imaging 1989, 2(3), 156–162.

Horii SC, Kundel HL, Feingold E et al. What do we need to advance workstations: a critical review with suggestions. Proc SPIE 1997, 3035, 6–14.

Jost RG, Hill RL, Rodewald SS, Rueter AP. An electronic multiviewer. Proceedings of the Eighth Conference of Computer Applications in Radiology; American College of Radiology, 1984, pp. 304–311.

Kishore S, Khalsa SS, Stevens JF et al. On-demand retrieval paradigm. Proc SPIE 1994, 2165, 149–159.

Krupinski EA, Lund PJ. Comparison of film vs. monitor viewing of CR films using eye-position recording. Proc SCAR 1996, 269–274.

Leung KT, Ho BKT, Chao W et al. Image navigation for PACS workstations. Proc SPIE 1995, 2435, 43–49.

MDIS Technical Development Team. Medical diagnostic imaging support system: acquisition document. Huntsville, AL: United States Army Engineer Division, 1991.

Pizer SM, Johnston RE, Zimmerman JB, Chan FH. Contrast perception with video displays. Proc SPIE 1982, 318 (Part I), 223–230.

Rogers DC, Johnston RE, Brenton B et al. Predicting PACS console requirements from radiologists' reading habits. Proc SPIE 1985, 536, 88–95.

Rostenberg B. The Architecture of Imaging. Chicago, American Hospital Publishing, 1995.

Sampsell JB. An overview of the digital micromirror device and its application to projection displays. SID International Symposium Digest of Technical Papers, 1993, 24, p. 1012.

Say DL, Hedler RA, Maninger LL et al. Monochrome and color image-display devices. In: Benson, KB, ed. Television Engineering Handbook. New York, McGraw-Hill, 1986.

Sherr S. Electronic Displays, 2nd ed. New York, John Wiley & Sons, 1993, pp. 201–340.

Shile PE, Fujii T, Ramamurthy V et al. Observer productivity reading full-field-of-view digital mammograms: an evaluation of a softcopy workstation supported by a high-capacity high-performance display buffer. Proc SPIE 1997, 3035, 287–290.

Shyankay J. Diamond films used in flat panel displays. R&D Magazine, April 1995, p. 44.

Stewart BK, Taira RK. Database architecture and design for PACS. In: Huang, HK, Ratib, O, Bakker, AR, Witte, G, eds. Picture Archiving and Communication Systems (PACS) in Medicine. NATO ASI Series F, v 74. Berlin, Springer-Verlag, 1991, pp. 83–89.

Taira RK, Simons M, Razavi M et al. High resolution workstations for primary and secondary radiology readings. Proc SPIE 1990, 1234, 18–25.

van der Voorde F, Arenson R, Kundel H et al. Development of a physician-friendly digital image display console. Proc SPIE 1986, 626, 541–548.

15
Image Compression

MITCHELL GOLDBURGH

The vision of an integrated delivery system includes sharing of clinical data through automating the capture, management, and display of diagnostic information. One of the largest challenges is managing digital images that can account for more than 80 percent of the gross digital data traffic in a hospital or healthcare delivery enterprise.

The term image compression describes a transformation of image data. This operational component plays a vital role in the performance of distributed clinical care systems. Compressed data occupies less storage space, increases the speed at which data can be transferred, and allows for scalability in system components.

Digital imaging and the conversion of analog images to digital records for primary diagnosis in radiology have incited debate on digital image quality and the necessary accuracy of the image representation for clinical and legal purposes. The complexity of validating different compression techniques is extensively discussed in the literature and standards committees. The literature examines both empirical and clinical results with a wide range of results specific to both pathologies and modalities. Specifically, discussions have shown interactions and clinical performance variations based on the image content, the characteristics of the observer and the observer's medium, and the pathology of the image. Studies suggest that artifacts caused by compression schemes and the perceived or real loss of resolution in the images can sometimes be compensated by other image processing techniques. To date, there are few published results from formal multidisciplinary, multi-institutional studies that remove specific institutional or observer issues that validate the use of lossy compression, although several are being formed or are underway.

This chapter surveys the basic definitions associated with image compression. The subject is very broad, and this chapter is not intended to be comprehensive. Rather, the intent is to define terms used to describe compression, highlight currently popular techniques, and review methods of measuring compression's effect on the image for clinical diagnosis.

Definitions of Digital Imaging and Compression

An analog image is defined by continuous shades of gray or grayscale, as found in normal film/screen chest x-rays. A digital image is defined by discontinuous elements of grayscale, as found with digital modalities, such as magnetic resonance imaging. An analog image is converted to a digital image by creating spatially discrete values called pixels. Data processing to enhance or compress images manipulates these pixels to alter the image presentation or size.

For each pixel in a digital image, the optical density is stored as a grayscale value in bytes (eight bits of digital data). These bytes, sometimes two per pixel, are the elements that are manipulated by compression algorithms to store images. One byte represents 256 gray levels (8 bits=2^8), whereas other digital systems use 12 bits to represent 4096 gray levels (12 bits=2^{12}).

Inherent in the conversion to a digital image is a sampling of the original continuous analog image. Thus, the higher the pixel matrix and density of the matrix for a given image, the more representative the digital image is to the original film image and the less that is lost in the sampling of the data.

Digital image compression describes mathematical operations against a single pixel or groups of pixels that result in a smaller representation of the original set. The image compression process has three fundamental steps:

- Modeling of the information in the image.
- A step that introduces controlled error.
- An encoding step to remove redundancy in the transformed data set.

Figure 15.1 shows a block diagram of the compression process.

In its simplest form, compression encodes the raw representation of the data. Encoding describes a process whereby larger sets of information can be represented by smaller codes. The encoding step may be limited to removing redundancy in data by representing series of like values with a single coded value. In radiography, redundant data is exemplified by areas in the image that show consistent optical density, such as the border. An encoding process is considered completely reversible (i.e., bit

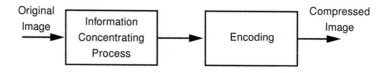

FIGURE 15.1. Model of image compression process.

preserving or lossless) because the image can be decoded to return to the original data set.

If a lossless compressed image is too large to meet speed or storage requirements, then a multistep process that models the original data and quantizes that modeled data precedes an encoding process. This process can remove information that is not required by the receiver of the compressed image or the application of the data. In this format, the original data is not preserved and cannot be restored. The resulting compressed image only represents the original image and cannot be decompressed to exactly match the original image. This defines a compression scheme that is lossy.

Restoring a compressed image is an inverse of the compression process. Simple decoding of lossless compression is often used because this scheme has only one stage of processing and thus is faster than a multiple stage lossy compression scheme. This speed of processing is a trade-off in choosing a compression that must be considered when looking at overall system performance.

The amount of compression created by a coding scheme is defined by the term, compression ratio. The term represents the size of the resulting image compared to the original data. Generally this ratio has units of bytes of data, representing the length of the data stream. By example a lossless original CT image at 512 pixels × 512 pixels (262,144 bytes) can be compressed at 2:1 with the resulting image being only 131,072 bytes.

Speed of transformation, compression ratio outcome and the impact of the compression on the resulting image versus the application or use of the image are measures of performance for compression schemes. This is an area that continues to be the topic of clinical trials and product improvements.

Lossless Compression Techniques

Long used in the data communications field, lossless compression techniques provide a method for compressing data with the ability to reconstruct it exactly. Typical ratios achieved with lossless compression of medical images range from 3:1 to less than 2:1, depending on the content of the image, and the amount of redundant data. This varies according to the modality or image type, because some modality images have information that is more redundant. For example, a CT or ultrasound image have a border (i.e., image mask) that is generally a consistent optical density and contains no clinical information, and thus redundant.

Figure 15.2 illustrates a typical lossless compression technique using adjacent pixels to predict the value of the pixel that is to be encoded. The

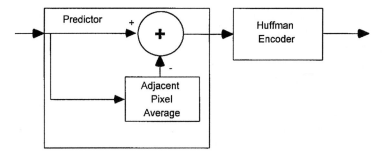

FIGURE 15.2. A simple predictor and encoder.

prediction takes advantage of the fact that the values of the pixels generally do not change quickly in an image. (Sharp edges are not generally associated with natural constructs in the imaging of human anatomy.) The encoder codes difference values that occur often in short bit sequences, and values that occur seldom as long bit sequences. A systematic method for encoding values in this manner is known as Huffman encoding.[1]

Huffman coding measures the number of times each symbol in a file occurs and uses fewer bits to represent the more common symbols. In English text, instead of using 7 bits for each character, E might be stored as 00 and Q might be 10110010. The limitation is that adjacencies, such as Q is usually followed by U, are not used. Huffman works well if there are no such relations, as in medical imaging.

Run-length encoding describes a process whereby strings of the same repeated symbol or pixel are encoded as a count. Delta encoding calculates differences in symbols or pixels as a prestaging to a run-length encoding, whereby the differences are encoded.

Although other schemes operate on specific elements such as pixels, Lempel-Ziv is a compression scheme that codes strings of symbols or pixels. In addition, schemes like Huffman encoding use tables that contain maps used in the encoding scheme that must be transmitted with the data, while Lempel-Ziv does not. However, Lempel-Ziv has poor compression ratios for smaller data files with fewer repeated strings.

Lossy Compression Techniques

Lossy compression by definition is irreversible. It reduces the pixel data set in such a way that restoration to the original data set is impossible. These

---

[1] For a basic understanding of Huffman encoding, the reader is referred to WK Pratt, Digital Image Processing, New York, John Wiley & Sons, 1978.

techniques can result in a loss of spatial and/or contrast information, as well as the introduction of compression noise (i.e., mottle in the image). This difference from the original data may not be noticeable in the case of viewing images—hence the debate on acceptance of this technique for primary diagnosis. The core concern is that the loss of information could lead to misdiagnosis. Studies have shown that perceptually lossless empirically, lossy compression can be used for overreading, comparative studies, and archiving purposes (based on microfilming as the precedent technology). To date, the radiology community limits primary diagnosis to use of mathematically lossless compressed images.

Arithmetic Compression

Arithmetic averaging represents a simple lossy technique in which adjacent pixels are combined into one, using the average of the two adjacent pixels. The simplest compressor uses the last pixel encoded. More complex encoders use a weighted average of the pixels on a row above and adjacent to the pixel to be encoded, along with the last pixel encoded on the row with the pixel to be encoded to take into account the local information. The difference between the prediction and the actual value is passed to the encoder. In its simple form this represents a lossy scheme often used to resize images dynamically at the workstation.

Frequency Domain Transforms

Frequency domain transforms describe processes that convert the pixel data into a spatial frequency map or model. With this transformation, the frequency representations are encoded according to additional input factors, such as a weighting factor or selected frequency filters. This conversion is the fundamental component of the more popular lossy compression techniques.

Large areas where the pixel values change slowly or not at all characterize the structure of a radiological image. For example, in the raw beam surrounding the imaged area, such as the chest, there is a slow change in the pixel value across large areas of the image. When the transform converts the pixel data into a map of frequencies, the energy of the image is displayed. The slow change of the pixel values when transformed concentrates the energy of an image into high amplitude of low frequencies. Generally, however, the sharp details that may be important to a diagnosis are very low amplitude high frequency components.

Tailoring the compression technique to the type of image (i.e., the modality or the anatomy) can give much better results than using a technique uniformly applied to all image types. For plain film images, compression technique uses the fact that most of the energy of the image is in the low frequencies. The energy of the image is also affected by the type of modality, the compression ratio for a radiograph may be higher than the ratio for a CT that has more contrast in the image and thus less redundancy.

Discrete Cosine Transform

The most commonly used frequency domain transform is the Discrete Cosine Transform (DCT). This transform is very closely related to the Fourier transform that decomposes the image into different frequency cells, collecting the energy of the image into discrete bins. Using a cosine transform, the energy at different frequencies can be isolated, and the high compression of the high frequency components can be realized.

The DCT is particularly effective when used as a block transform, because it is even-symmetric (i.e., sampling a square area of pixels). The method first separates the image into small blocks, typically 8 × 8 pixel blocks. The transform is performed on each block independently and then encoded. As a result of the block size, the frequencies represented do not extend to the very low frequencies captured in larger areas across the image. Only the frequencies that can be present in 8 pixels can be represented, frequencies down to 1/8 cycle per pixel. At the same time, the transformed values represent local variations in the image, that is, the variations that occur in that block. Some blocks will have large, high frequency content, but many other blocks will have very little high frequency content. The coding of these differences can result in a high compression ratio. Statistical analysis techniques may be employed to improve the compression further; this process is called adaptive transform coding.

Although the processing speed of the DCT is generally fast (because it has been implemented in hardware), the discrete block transform method can produce blocking artifacts. These artifacts may become increasingly objectionable to the clinician as the compression ratio increases; they may also become more prominent if postprocessing is applied to the image.

Another approach to the DCT is a whole image transform, which addresses the artifact of the smaller blocked DCT. The cosine transform is applied to the whole image at one time. In this case, the mapping of the frequencies produces values that represent the whole image rather than any one area of the image. If the image is generally smooth with only a few areas of activity, this representation may not yield as high a compression ratio for similar image quality (fine detail retention) as does the smaller blocked DCT.

JPEG Transform

The Joint Photographic Experts Group (JPEG) was formed in the late 1980s to consider compression of still images in general electronic photopublishing applications. The JPEG Standard allows for both bit-preserving and lossy compression implementations. The lossless compression is the simple predictor plus an encoder as described above in the discussion of Huffman encoding. For lossy compression, JPEG most often uses an 8 × 8 pixel DCT transform with a Huffman encoding.

Wavelet Transform

Wavelet compression is another digital imaging technique from the photographic and computer graphics industry. Wavelet compression is similar to JPEG in that it applies a transform to the image, quantizes the results of the transform, and applies lossless compression to the quantized results. The major difference is that instead of applying the transform to discrete 8 × 8-pixel blocks, the wavelet transform operates on overlapping areas of an image. As a result, wavelet compression does not produce the blocky artifacts seen at high JPEG compression ratios. Instead, the effect is an overall softening of the image.

The wavelet transform separates an image into down-sampled low frequency and high frequency component images using coefficients. The transform produces a hierarchy of image representations consisting of one low frequency image and a set of iteratively higher frequency add-on pieces. The implementation is often an iterative process that produces very high compression ratios with multiple instances of the image available upon decompression.

Wavelet compression seems to offer around one and a half to three times more compression than JPEG for the same apparent image quality. As always, though, there is a catch. Current wavelet decompression implementations takes one and a half to three times longer than JPEG decompression, so there may be little or no speed difference between the two.

Compression Artifacts

Lossy compression depends on introducing controlled, predictable errors into the image to achieve targeted compression ratios. Each lossy compression technique has its own type of artifacts in the restored image. The ideal compression error is a general random error over the whole image that is not perceptible and does not impact the decision outcome.

Image compression data loss is determined by the quantization stage during the image transformation. This is the stage whereby image error is introduced (see Fig. 15.3).

For lossy compression, arithmetic using floating-point operations contain rounding errors or estimates and mapping of acceptable operations prior to encoding defines the compression performance and amount of data loss. The more coarsely the quantization, the higher the compression ratios that

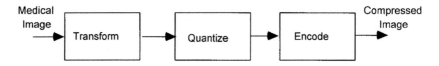

FIGURE 15.3. Lossy compression. Lossy compression uses a quantizer to set the level of compression.

can be achieved, with the consequence being that the compressed image resembles less of the original.

Quantization error appears in a reconstructured image as noise or artifact. In a well-designed compression scheme, the quantization noise is biased toward the higher frequencies, where the higher frequency components are coarser. Alternatively, in the design of a compression scheme, the quantization noise can be spread over the reconstructed image so that the error is less correlated with specific image content.

To achieve higher compression rates, some lossy compression techniques choose to throw away the high frequency components of an image. Because the human visual system is less sensitive to high frequencies, the errors in the image compression can be pushed to the high frequencies with less effect on the perception of the image. If this tendency to limit the high frequencies is carried too far, the details in the image begin to disappear. For example, the details in the bone structure, such as the tribecula, tend to disappear in a radiograph.

Other compression techniques reduce the grayscale levels from the original 12-bits or 10-bits to 8-bits. Reduction beyond this 8-bit level can cause artifacts called contrast stratification. This common artifact is easily perceived and annoying because radiology images are continuous tone images. Moreover, an area where the image is at a single gray level has no frequency detail.

As discussed above, block transforms can produce blocking artifacts. If the transform parameters are not carefully selected against the image content, the edges of the blocks can become quite prominent. This appearance can be masked by the display technique. For an 8×8 block in an image that is 2000×2000 pixels, the blocks are quite small. However, the blocking can be easily seen under magnification and can interfere with the viewing of clinical details such as microcalcifications in a breast image.

JPEG lossy compression, which uses the DCT, has a reputation for producing blocking artifacts on lossy compressed radiology images for compression ratios as low as 10:1. These blocking artifacts can be quite prominent, particularly near sharp edges in an image, such as a staple in a chest x-ray.

Several techniques limit these blocking artifacts. A lapped orthogonal transform is a generalization of the discrete cosine transform used in the

JPEG lossy compression algorithm. When the blocks are overlapped smoothly, the blocking artifacts are essentially eliminated. The result can be a uniform random error spread over the whole image, close to the ideal result.

The artifacts for the wavelet transform tend to be less obtrusive to the observer, since the wavelet transform is also a form of lapped orthogonal transform. The iterative nature of this transform allows the blocking artifact at higher compression ratios to be less apparent than it is under the JPEG method. Studies have shown this to be true at compression levels as high as 100:1 for ultrasound and high contrast CT images.

Postprocessing of digital image data can be adversely affected by error introduced by lossy compression. Edge enhancement, for example, can make subtle fractures more visible; computer-assisted diagnostic tools can high-light attributes of a specific pathology. Compression algorithms do, how-ever, generate edge artifacts that can leave an image vulnerable to postprocessing degradation and to false readings of the image pathology. Whereas evaluation has been based on subjective clinical interpretations, computer-assisted software now offers ways of empirically measuring the effectiveness of the compression algorithm.

Computation Efficiency

Until recently, the application of lossy image compression to PACS has been limited by concerns about cost, performance, and image quality. Expensive, dedicated compression hardware has long been available for specific appli-cations. Only recently has it become possible to implement compression schemes in software or inexpensive hardware that is generally available. This change parallels the development of digital imaging in other professional industries.

Computational comparison is measured by the number of operations per pixel. A fast cosine transform for an 8×8 transform are particularly effi-cient, because many of the arithmetic operations are multiplications by plus or minus 1. Using the fast cosine transform requires on the order of 500 arithmetic computations for an 8×8 block of pixels or about 8 multiplies or adds per pixel. The computation for the lapped orthogonal transform re-quires roughly an additional 100 multiplies or adds, so the lapped orthogo-nal transform is nearly as efficient as the simple discrete cosine transform. The wavelet transform is slightly less efficient, requiring roughly 20 multi-plies or adds for each pixel.

Some hardware arithmetic units are organized to perform a multiply and an add in a sort of arithmetic pipeline. These units reduce the amount of time required for the computation, since many operations can occur in parallel. Today the compression speed of many personal computers (even without augmenting compression processors) is fast enough to minimize the differences among computation times for various compression techniques.

Because it is an established standard, JPEG compression has been commercially available in low cost hardware and software implementations. Used in many imaging applications, JPEG has been shown to be adequate for the lossy compression of medical images. Currently JPEG is the compression technique accomodated by Digital Imaging and Communications in Medicine (DICOM) to illustrate the encoding of compression.[2] The DICOM standard describes a generic method of delineating the methods and tables used to transform an image so it can be decomposed at the receiving end.

What Is an Adequate Compression Technique?

The evaluation of compression techniques for diagnostic imaging is quite complex. Evaluation criteria generally take one of two forms: empirical or clinical. While the empirical evaluation generates statistical differences in the images that are clearly repeatable, the clinical comparison is subjective and has a higher sensitivity.

The mathematical comparison is most often done by compressing an image and then subtracting the restored image from the original. The result describes the absolute differences in the images. By definition, lossless compression results in a difference of zero. The lossy compressed images can have differences in the contrast or spatial domain, or, in some cases, both. In a well-designed compression scheme, these differences will not affect the clinical outcome based on image diagnosis.

Fundamentally, clinical evaluation involves compressing a small number of radiology images and subjectively determining whether the images have suffered clinical loss when compared to the original. The outcomes are judged as aesthetically pleasing or less so, depending on the degradation of the image. Certainly this sort of evaluation is a first step in refining a compression technique.

Clinical evaluation validates a compression technique by measuring its effect on the image as used in the diagnosis of disease. A valid statistical measure of the loss in performance of diagnosis is required to evaluate the compression performance. Statistically, there are two kinds of errors to be evaluated:

- A miss of a pathology (false negative).

---

[2] The current DICOM standard accomodates the JPEG standard descriptions. However, the standard does not endorse JPEG as a medical imaging standard.

- A false alarm that there is pathology present when in fact there is none (false positive).

ROC Study

To determine clinical performance of a compression scheme, radiologists conduct what is known as a Receiver Operating Characteristic (ROC) study.[3] An ROC study evaluates the probability of a miss as a function of the probability of a false alarm by having radiologists view images to find pathology.[4] The pathology they detect on the original film is compared with the pathology found on the image that has been compressed and restored. Several levels of performance are evaluated at one time by asking the viewer to declare with different levels of surety that the pathology is present:

- Possibly present.
- Probably present.
- Surely present.

Declaring the pathology possibly present generates a number of false alarms, because the viewer is trying to find any possible indication of the pathology; at the same time, the probability of a miss is low. Fewer false alarms occur when the viewer is asked to indicate that the pathology is probably present, while the probability of a miss increases. Finally, when the viewer is asked to declare that the pathology is surely present, the number of false alarms is low, but the probability of a miss is higher.

Figure 15.4 shows a ROC curve for a particular set of compressed radiology images compared with the original film image. The ROC curve is generated by the observer viewing images with the selected pathology mixed with other images without the pathology. At a later time, the observer views the restored compressed images with and without pathology. The time difference must be great enough that the observer does not remember the individual cases.

The vertical axis is the probability of detection; the horizontal axis is the probability of false alarm. The probability of detection can be averaged over the probability of false alarm yielding a probability of detection for the pa-

---

[3]The concept of a ROC curve comes from the early days of radio communications. A radio receiver could detect a signal, could miss the detection of signal, or could generate a false alarm. The performance of the receiver was measured by the ROC curve, a plot of the probability of miss versus the probability of false alarm.

[4] Finding a set of images to evaluate compression is a critical first step. The type of pathology can also have an impact on the study since some are more sensitive to compression artifact than others.

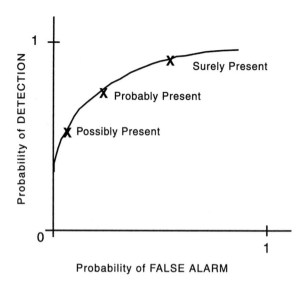

FIGURE 15.4. ROC curve compared to film image. The ROC curve for a selected pathology compared to an original film image.

thology that is independent of the probability of false alarm. This one number is characteristic of the performance in diagnosis of the particular compression technique and level of compression that is being used.

Why not use a simple empirical measure of error like the mean squared error of the restored image compared to the original? The human visual perception does not recognize this error. Restored images from many compression techniques and levels of compression can have almost the same mean squared error, but can have very different observer results. Particularly when the compression tends to cut off the high frequencies, the change in the image can be quite marked while the change in the mean squared error is very small. Increasing the level of compression by a factor of two will have a small effect on the mean squared error.

Levels of Compression: Effect on Outcome

Compression of data can take one of two approaches: (1) fixed compression, variable loss and (2) fixed loss, variable compression. Generally the approach for medical imaging has been to quantify the level of loss and accept a range of resulting compression in deference to the importance of image quality.

Increasing the desired level of compression requires an increase in the amount of data loss; hence, the ROC curve will change. Increased data loss in the image results in the potential for increased errors in the detection of pathology. As a consequence, the ROC curve is applicable only for a particular compression technique at a particular level of compression and for a particular pathology. The complete evaluation of a number of compression techniques at a number of different levels of compression can be a complex task comprising extensive review of different image types, pathologies, and compression ratios. The task complexity is therefore multiplied for each condition added to the study. This need for completeness has been the reason that the studies are slow in being released.

Lossless compression is always acceptable, because the image can be completely restored without error. The observer, the level of compression artifact, the image characteristics, and the clinical application of the image are all relevant factors impacting the acceptance of the lossy compression scheme. Given that the human eye is relatively insensitive to some types of errors and quite sensitive to other types, the data modeling stage of compression is as important as the overall compression (error) level in determining the clinical quality of the resulting compressed image.

The Validity of the ROC Curve

The ROC study discussed above, measures the performance of a compression technique by comparing detection of pathology using compressed and original images. This approach uses the original image and its diagnostic report as the "truth." Unfortunately, however, it has been well established that the performance of radiologists against subtle pathologies is less than perfect. This means that the performance of the radiologist in detecting a pathology using the original image has its own ROC curve. There will be a probability of detection of the pathology for each probability of false alarm with the original image.

The question to be addressed is whether the ROC curve using compressed images differs from the ROC curve using the original images. Because the answer requires a more rigorous determination of truth, the presence or absence of the pathology must be determined by some other means. Evaluation of computed radiology images may require validation by CT examinations for some pathologies and by other means, such as biopsies, for other pathologies. Indeed, some ROC studies cannot be run because there is no way of determining the truth except on a cadaver.

When the truth can be determined by other means, the question is whether the probability of detection for the restored image is different from the probability of detection for the original image. The level of performance can demand a statistical level of confidence, typically 95 percent. With a large enough sample of images with and without the selected pathology, the question cannot be answered. Figure 15.5 illustrates an example ROC test output. The bold line indicates absolute truth from the original data. The ability

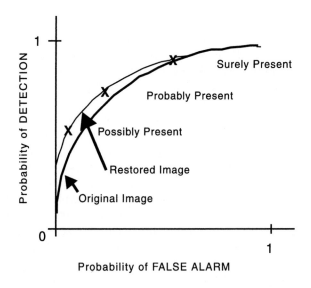

FIGURE 15.5. ROC curve after compression. A ROC study asks the question whether the probability of detection of a pathology has changed after compression.

of the two lines to overlap illustrates the impact of the compression algorithm on clinical performance.

Other Conditions Affecting ROC Study Outcomes

The detection of pathology in an image can be affected by many other things than the compression. The ROC study must take care that the other effects are controlled. Simple things like a higher ambient light level in the viewing room can change the results. The level of activity in the viewing room can also cause changes. One technique to eliminate these extraneous effects is to mix the original and restored versions of different images in any one viewing session. Presumably the environment will have the same effect on the detection of pathology in the original version of some images as it will have on the detection of pathology in the restored version of other images.

In any case, the conditions under which images are viewed for the test should be maintained as consistently as possible and reflect realistic viewing conditions. When the question is whether the detection of pathology is degraded by a move from film to workstation viewing, changes in the viewing conditions are unavoidable and may have as much effect as the compression. In this case it is desirable to separate the question into two parts: the effects of the change in the viewing and the effects of the compression.

Next Steps

Methods of data compression have been studied for almost four decades. Compression is a desired transform for improving the scalability and performance of systems critical technical applications. In the case of medical records, imaging comprises the largest source of data in the patient care environment and thus is one of the larger issues to overcome when converting to an all digital environment.

The use of different compression schemes and algorithms in a PACS affects implementation and results in the power to address mathematical limitations and enhance computational power. To have a positive effect on system performance, the time allotted for the transformation of images should not exceed the uncompressed performance. By choosing compression algorithms from imaging sciences like photography and data communications, medical imaging has been able to utilize the hardware and software from these industries to leverage efficient PACS implementations. The increased use of digital imaging in areas other than medical, combined with increased processing power, have accelerated the deployment of compression in applications like teleradiology and PACS.

Interest in image compression by the radiology community has been heightened by the increased use of digital acquisition and display techniques. Clinicians who have not used compressed images tend to judge any data loss at all unacceptable and may cite medical and legal concerns. Nonetheless, the benefits of teleradiology over low cost, low bandwidth communication lines have caused the community to take a second look. At present, the American College of Radiology recommends only lossless compression for primary diagnosis, but permits lossy compression for overreading and other nondiagnostic applications.

Although more rigorous, large-scale ROC studies are needed to establish definitive guidelines on lossy compression, compression is being used in clincial systems. Techniques for image compression are changing rapidly, and the picture is clear: compression will be implemented to accelerate the inclusion of digital image management into radiology, and the radiology community must continue to face the challenge of validating the clinical use of compression.

Acknowledgments. The author wishes to thank R. Glicksman and D. Wilson, Ph.D., for contributing time and background to support the writing of this chapter.

References

Bentley JL, Sleator DD, Tarjan RE, Wei VK. A locally adaptive data compression scheme. Commun. ACM 1986, 29, 4 (Apr.), 320–330.

Blume H. ACR-NEMA digital imaging and communications standard committee, working group #4, MEDPACS section, Data compression standard #PS2, 1989.

Huang HK. Elements of digital radiology: A professional handbook and guide. New Jersey, Prentice Hall, 1987.

Lou SL, Chan KK. Comparison of interpolative versus full frame cosine transform image compression of digital chest radiographs. In: The UCLA PACS module and related projects. Los Angeles: UCLA Department of Radiology, 1989, pp. 25–33.

Lo SC, Huang HK. Comparison of radiological images with 512, 1024, and 2048 matrices. Radiology, 1986, 161, 519–525.

Metz CE. Basic principles of ROC analysis. In Seminars in Nuclear Medicine, 1978, 8, 282–298.

Pennebaker WB, Mitchell JL. JPEG still image data compression standard. New York, Van Nostrand Reinhold, 1993.

Perlmutter S et al. Measurement accuracy as a measure of image quality in compressed MR chest scans. Proc IEEE Symposium on Image Processing, 1994, 1, 861–865.

Welch TA. A technique for high-performance data compression. Computer, 1984, 17(6), 8–19.

Wen CY et al. Evaluation of the diagnostic quality of chest images compressed with JPEG and wavelet techniques: A preliminary study. Proc SPIE, 1996.

Wilkins LC, Wintz PA. Bibliography on data compression, picture properties and picture coding. IEEE Trans. Inform. Theory, 1971, 17, 2, 180–197.

16
DICOM Standardization

Steven L. Fritz

The DICOM (Digital Imaging Communications in Medicine) standard, published in 1993, is an outgrowth of the standard developed by a joint committee of the American College of Radiology and the National Electrical Manufacturers' Association (ACR/NEMA). Formed in 1983 to develop standards for digital communication of image information, the committee published the first version in 1986 and a second version in 1988. The third version of the standard, renamed DICOM to emphasize its substantially altered content, has addressed some of the problems in the first and second versions and in the process created new issues. It is currently widely accepted within the diagnostic imaging community as the standard on which digital image management systems of the future will be built.

The standard today is essentially complete, although evolutionary changes will still take place. As a stable and mature standard, it is being implemented by a variety of DICOM technology companies and imaging manufacturers. These implementations will bring to light shortcomings in the standard that need correction and will lead to further development. However, the standard is currently adequate to design and implement filmless radiology systems.

This chapter discusses the overall structure of the standard, the models that underlie it, the services it provides, and the support for various networking environments that it encompasses. The objective is to give a clear picture of the content of the DICOM standard, the extent to which it enables multivendor digital image management networks, and the likely developments in the future.

DICOM is an explicitly object oriented standard. It spells out in detail the real-world objects that it models and the information objects by which that modeling is accomplished. It is not specified in terms of any object oriented computer language such as C++ or Smalltalk. The relationship between the models that DICOM does specify and any implementation is left to implementors' discretion.

The most fundamental model contained in DICOM is the DICOM information model, shown in Figure 16.1. It defines the "structure and organization of information related to the communication of medical images." It specifies the content of information objects which, paired with DICOM service requests, form Service Object Pairs (SOPs). Each service is either a network service or a media storage service, such as Store or [Query]. Each

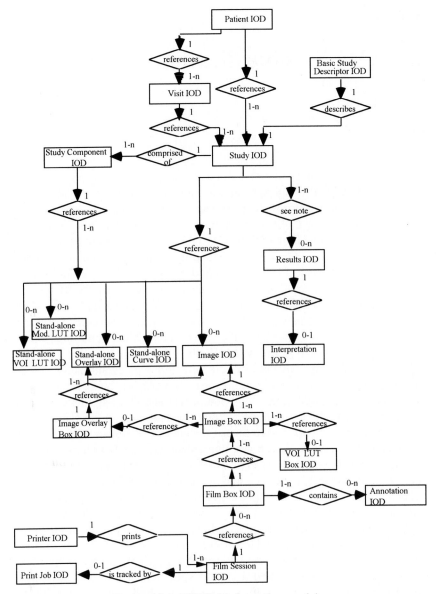

FIGURE 16.1. DICOM information model.

object is specified by an Information Object Definition that defines a related set of attributes of some object in the real world. A SOP Class is a set of services and a set of allowable Information Object Definitions (IODs) to which any of the services may be applied. An example is the Storage Service Class, which specifies application of the Storage service to a CT Image Object.

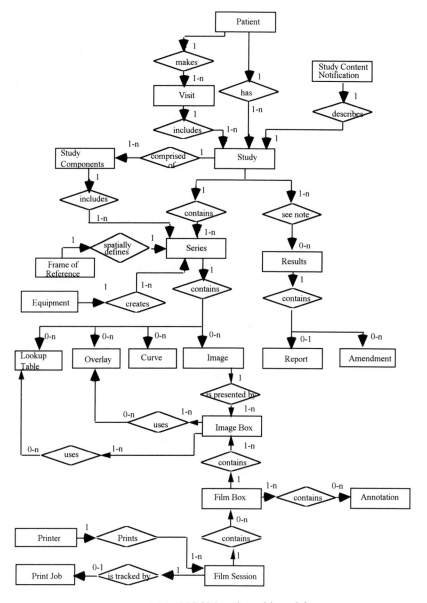

FIGURE 16.2. DICOM real-world model.

The real-world model of DICOM is shown in Figure 16.2. It contains patients, studies, study components, series, and images, as well as familiar tangible objects such as imaging equipment or printers and intangible objects such as look-up tables. The real world model of DICOM was intended to provide a complete set of objects to be managed by a digital image management system. An analogous information model contains an IOD for each of the objects in the real-world model.

There are two different types of IODs: composite and normalized. Composite IODs may contain attributes from more than one kind of real world object. They are restricted to images and a short list of associated objects: standalone overlay, standalone curves, study descriptors, standalone modality and value of interest look-up tables. The CT Image Object IOD is shown in Table 16.1. It is a collection of several modules, each of which contains related attributes of a normalized information object. The modules are further grouped into information entities which describe individual real world objects.

Normalized IODs contain attributes of only one kind of real-world object. An example of a normalized IOD would be the patient module in the CT image object. This module, shown in Table 16.2, contains a number of attributes thought to be important in identifying the patient to whom the image belongs to assist in diagnosis. This information is quite similar to that traditionally imprinted on x-ray films in predigital imaging systems.

By defining each IOD as an explicit set of information attributes that belong to a specific set of real-world objects and that are related to each other in ways that are specified by the DICOM information model, the standard does much of the preliminary design work required for an object oriented implementation of DICOM services. However, several problems remain. One of the principal problems is that several modules contain overlapping sets of attributes of certain real world objects, most importantly patients and studies.

Table 16.3 shows the four modules that make up the Patient information object. While these contain all the defined patient attributes, other collections of these attributes are used in other situations. The composite image object, as indicated above, contains attributes from the Patient Identifica-

TABLE 16.1. Composite image information object description.

Information entity	Module	Usage
Patient	Patient	M
Study	General study	M
	Patient study	U
Series	General series	M
Frame of reference	Frame of reference	M
Equipment	General equipment	M
Image	General image	M
	Image plane	M
	Image pixel	M
	Contrast/bolus	C
	CT image	M
	Overlay plane	U
	Value of interest LUT	U
	SOP common	M

TABLE 16.2. Composite image patient module.

Attribute name	Tag	Type	Attribute description
Patient's name	0010,0010	2	Patient's full legal name
Patient ID	0010,0020	2	Primary hospital identification number or code for the patient
Patient's birth date	0010,0030	2	Birth date of the patient
Patient's sex	0010,0040	2	Sex of the named patient
Referenced patient Sequence	0008,1120	3	A sequence that provides reference to a Patient SOP Class/Instance pair
Patient's birth time	0010,0032	3	Birth time of the patient
Other patient IDs	0010,1000	3	Other identification numbers or codes used to identify the patient
Other patient names	0010,1001	3	Other names used to identify the patient
Ethnic group	0010,2160	3	Ethnic group or race of patient
Patient comments	0010,4000	3	User-defined additional information about the patient

tion and Patient Demographic modules. In addition, the Query/Retrieve defines a set of patient attributes, also overlapping the normalized patient IODs, that is distinct from the patient image module. There are also patient attributes contained in a study query object defined by a Query Model that is a superset of the patient query module attributes. This overlap of the defined IODs and collections of attributes in DICOM means that no one-to-one mapping between IODs and required information objects is feasible.

DICOM Services

The original DICOM standard published in 1993 defined eight service classes:

- Verification.
- Storage.
- Query/Retrieve.
- Study Content Notification.
- Patient Management.
- Study Management.
- Results Management.
- Print Management.

TABLE 16.3. Patient IOD modules.

Module	Reference	Module description
SOP common	C.12.1	Contains SOP common information
Patient relationship	C.2.1	References to related SOPs
Patient identification	C.2.2	Identifies the real world patient
Patient demographic	C.2.3	Describes the patient
Patient medical	C.2.4	Medical information about patient

As shown in Figure 16.3, a service object pair class, an SOP class, is defined by DICOM as "the union of a specific set of DIMSE Services and one related Information Object Definition (as specified by a Service Class Definition) which completely defines a precise context for communication." A Service Group is a set of related SOP Classes. An example of a service class is the Storage service class, in which each SOP class relates a single allowed service, the Storage service, to a single image IOD, a composite image. Thus the storage service class relates the Storage service to all allowable composite image IODs. This service class is the best tested and most widely used DICOM Service Class.

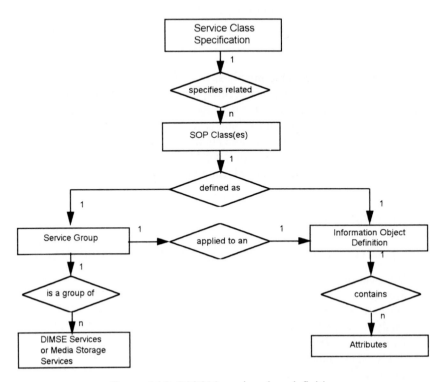

FIGURE 16.3. DICOM service class definition.

There are two types of DICOM Message Service Element (DIMSE) services: DIMSE-C services and DIMSE-N services. DIMSE-C services support operations on composite SOP Instances with peer DIMSE-service-users. DIMSE-N services support operations and notifications on Normalized SOP with peer DIMSE-service-users. Both types of services allow network operations and local media storage operations. This section concentrates on network services.

DIMSE network services operate by exchanging request/response messages between Application Entities (AEs) across a network. Thus a DICOM store from a modality to an archive begins when the modality sends a DICOM Storage request message to the intended destination. The Storage request message is an instance of a specific SOP class. In the case of a CT scanner sending images to an archive, the request messages would be instances of the CT Image Storage SOP class. Each instance would contain a storage service request and the attributes of the composite CT Image IOD. The archive AE, on receipt of the request, would return a response message containing the attributes of the originating service request and a status value. When the status value is Success or an error status, the transaction is complete.

No assumptions may be made about the results of the operation or notification performed, as DICOM does not define the actions to be taken upon receipt of any DICOM SOP Class instance. In the case of the Storage Service Class, the obvious behavior desired is saving the image on a storage device and inserting the query keys of the image into an index for the image store. However, there is no guarantee that the anticipated behavior will in fact occur. To solve the problem of transfer of storage responsibility, a new Service Class, the Storage Commitment service class, has been added to DICOM as an addendum. Receipt of a storage commitment response with a status of Success allows an image source to unambiguously transfer responsibility for storing an image to the destination to which it has been successfully sent. This is the sole instance of a DICOM message exchange resulting in a defined action on the part of the message recipient.

The absence of defined actions in response to all other DICOM messages is problematic. It is possible for an RIS to notify an archive that a new study has been ordered for a particular patient, but as there is no obvious response, it is not clear what is accomplished by the RIS by this message. Further, certain responsibilities are not unambiguously associated with traditional clinical information systems. For instance, an RIS typically maintains a database of patients and studies. When a review workstation needs to determine a list of patients on whom new studies are available, does it query the RIS or the archive to which images would normally be sent? If the archive, should all archives contain databases and be queried independently? If not, how does the archive to which the image is sent for storage communicate the keys and storage location to the central database, and where does that database reside? The absence of obvious answers to these questions suggests that different implementors will arrive at sometimes radically different answers. The difficulties that this presents to the task of finding a multivendor digital image management network based on DICOM are formidable.

Even where the effect of a message may be assumed, the absence of standardized ways of performing certain common image management functions allows multiple, DICOM compliant mechanisms for accomplishing the same purpose. For instance, a fairly common problem addressed using DICOM is transfer of patient and study descriptive attributes from an RIS where they are initially entered when a study is scheduled to a modality on which the study is to be performed. This serves to improve the accuracy of the attributes that are finally associated with the image in a database.

There are several DICOM mechanisms that can and have been utilized to solve this problem. In 1994, the US Army produced a conformance profile for a modality that used the Patient and Study Management service classes in a complex exchange of messages to transfer the attributes required by DICOM for the Image Patient Module of all the image storage SOP classes (Prior, 1994). In 1995, the author described a method implemented at the University of Maryland using the Query/Retrieve service class and a DICOM to HL7 translator (Fritz, Munjal, Connors et al., 1995). In addition, Working Group 6 of the ACR-NEMA committee defined a new service class, Worklist Management, with a Modality Worklist SOP class, to address the same problem. Because the new worklist management class is now part of DICOM, the standard provides at least three ways to handle the same problem. With the advent of the Worklist Management service class came a new set of patient and study identifier objects that again overlap the normalized patient and study IODs.

This duplication of function may finally arrive at a workable solution for every problem, but it handicaps the DICOM implementor by providing multiple choices for the most basic functions of a digital image management system. This, as pointed out, makes it very difficult to achieve true multivendor interoperability for DICOM compliant processes.

DICOM Network Support

The original ACR-NEMA standard defined a single 50-pin parallel interface as the message exchange medium. This limited the standard to point-to-point operations, with a network connecting points left outside the scope of the standard. DICOM introduced for the first time a true network support standard, with a DICOM Upper Layer Service boundary beneath which any of several transfer media were allowed. The most common choice for network support today is TCP/IP, although the 50-pin point to point connection and OSI are also defined. This addition allowed exchange of DICOM messages over readily available network connections without embedding the specifics of the network into the standard. This has resulted in the proliferation of DICOM capability and industry-wide testing sessions sponsored by the Radiological Society of North America at its annual meeting (Moore, 1996). With the addition of network support came new specifications for transfer of messages. The initial DICOM message transfer mechanism specified that DICOM attributes be encoded in a serial stream, in increasing order of the 32-bit tag that identified the attribute, in little-Endian byte ordering. The data encoding of attributes specified one of 24 different value representations also defined in the standard. A data dictionary of DICOM attributes was required to determine the value representation of each attribute. DICOM defined the concept of transfer syntax as a specific encoding of DICOM attributes for transfer between DICOM-compliant systems and specified three allowable transfer syntaxes: little-Endian implicit VR (default), big-Endian implicit VR, and a new big-Endian explicit VR in which the value representation of each attribute is explicitly added to the stream between the attribute tag and the attribute value. This specified in more detail the means of communication between different systems and allowed explicit VR encoding to obviate the overhead of a data dictionary for decoding.

This new flexibility in DICOM was largely instrumental in making it attractive to developers who are now avidly pursuing implementation.

DICOM and Other Standards

In the absence of serious competitors, DICOM remains the standard of choice for medical image exchange. However, its relationship to two other kinds of standards must be assessed. These are the graphics standards developed for graphic image exchange and the HL-7 standard developed for exchange of textual information in medical informatics.

Most of the many graphics standards (GIF, TIFF, etc.) were developed to exchange image data only, without reference to content or the relationship of content to other information objects. Thus a medical informatics standard for image exchange would have to define all related attributes important for diagnosis, such as the resolution of the imaging modality with which the image was made, outside the graphics standard. For historical reasons, this never happened. There was an effort in the ultrasound community to define an expanded version of TIFF called DEFF, but it was never successful in expanding beyond the ultrasound domain. Consequently, the principal connection between DICOM and the graphics standards is in developing translators from DICOM to various standards employed in imaging and graphics software. For instance, transforming a DICOM image to a GIF format image for inclusion in a slide presentation is a frequent task. There is, however, no real use of graphics standards for clinical information management.

HL-7 is a different matter. HL-7 was developed to exchange text information between medical informatics systems for clinical purposes. DICOM was developed to exchange image information without much explicit reference to HL-7. As a consequence, the two standards developed differing approaches to many of the same issues. To take a single example, HL-7 defined a six-component Person Name attribute type, valid only with ASCII encoding, while DICOM defined a five-component name. DICOM also allowed non-ASCII encoding but restricted the mechanism by which components could be encoded in a message stream.

The HL-7 and DICOM organizations are currently working to merge the data definitions of the standards, at least to the extent required to support interoperability. Currently the focus of much attention for providing RIS data to modalities, the DICOM Worklist Management Service Class uses joint DICOM/HL-7 concepts such as a Facility Episode instead of a Visit to describe an encounter of a patient with a healthcare provider. Because these are new attributes, modules and IODs, they do not fit into the preexisting framework of the Query/Retrieve and Patient Management service classes. This is part of the reason behind the appearance of new service classes. Eventually DICOM and HL-7 will have a common data dictionary sufficient to mediate interactions between HL-7-based HIS systems and DICOM-based DIMS networks. Still to come is application semantics standardization to mediate merging of RIS and DIMS systems into a single information manager for radiology applications.

The Future of DICOM

DICOM is moving steadily into the future as the standard of choice for DIMS design. The merging of DICOM and HL-7 models and data dictionaries will make possible DICOM to HL-7 gateways and eventually integrated DICOM/HL-7 radiology information networks. Several steps remain before this goal is reached.

The first step will be widespread availability of DICOM compatible DIMS networks. These will be single-vendor networks linking modalities, archives, image review workstations, and image printers into a comprehensive network. HL-7 interfaces will allow access to RIS systems that are operated independently of DIMS networks and DICOM Storage Class SCP capability will allow most modalities to send images into the DIMS archive and/or to DIMS workstations. Most vendors now offer DICOM compatibility or plan to do so in the immediate future. This will make possible multivendor image management systems in which the basic network components are produced by a single vendor and modalities and printers from multiple vendors may be attached.

The next logical step is to determine semantic definitions of DIMS functions so that the basic network can be a mosaic of components from multiple vendors. The vendors may not be motivated to determine common semantics because this will in principle reduce the sales of their integrated networks. Only if they see a market opportunity by opening the system will such common semantic models originate from the vendors. However, university research groups can and should work on developing such reference architectures to lead the way.

Ultimately RIS systems will become DICOM-compatible components of DIMS networks, with HL-7 interfaces to other components of the overall Healthcare Organization Information System. DICOM workstation application functionality will migrate to clinical information workstations. At this point those systems that need to manage clinical imaging studies or reports that incorporate clinical images will support DICOM functionality as part of their basic suite of capabilities.

Beyond that integration of DIMS into HIS networks, additional functionality and services to support it will continue to be defined. For example, as functional MRI studies become more common, new services to support image management and display functions specific to this extremely high volume service may be added. As the overall HIS definition evolves, DICOM too will evolve to keep pace.

PACS researchers have been working since the mid-1970s to see this goal achieved. The advance of technology in modalities, workstations, networks, printers, and archives have finally made it possible for the millenium of medical image management to coincide with the millenium of the calendar. Just as diagnostic imaging technology in CT, MR, ultrasound, and angiography blossomed in the 1970s and 1980s, and DIMS technology came to fruition in the 1990s, imaging researchers will discover new imaging technologies such as functional MRI and other, as yet undiscovered, modalities. The vision that drives the technology community in the latter half of the twentieth century is the futuristic vision of the sickbay of the Starship Enterprise. It has yet to be achieved, but remains as tantalizing a picture as ever of what yet may be.

References

Fritz SL, Munjal S, Connors J, Csipo D. Implementing a DICOM-HL-7 interface application. Proc SPIE 1995, 2435:100–107.

Moore SM. Observations on DICOM demonstrations at the RSNA annual meetings. Proc SPIE 1996, 2711:89–97.

Prior FW. DICOM 3.0: Digital imaging communications in medicine, User conformance profile for modality interfacing, version 1.5. Penn State University, 1994.

17
Enabling Technology: DICOM in the VA's Hospital Information System

Peter M. Kuzmak and Ruth E. Dayhoff

Medical systems can provide better services if they work cooperatively, sharing data with each other as needed. Patient identification information is a critical piece of data that must be identical in all systems in order to link result data to the correct patient. Standards have been defined to provide this data in a vendor-independent fashion. However, only one standard, Digital Imaging and Communications in Medicine (DICOM), is specifically designed to handle text, images, and binary data.

The DICOM Standard brings open systems technology to the medical imaging marketplace. The Department of Veterans Affairs (VA) has incorporated DICOM capabilities into its VISTA* hospital/radiology information system (HIS/RIS) architecture in order to be able to interface with commercial medical imaging products. Image management is integrated into the VISTA HIS software and clinical database. Radiology images are acquired through DICOM and stored directly in the HIS database. Images can be displayed on low-cost clinician workstations throughout the medical center. High-resolution diagnostic quality multimonitor VISTA workstations with specialized viewing software can be used for reading radiology images.

Two approaches are used to acquire and handle images within the radiology department. Some sites have a commercial Picture Archiving and Communications System (PACS) interfaced to the VISTA HIS, whereas other sites use the direct image acquisition and integrated diagnostic display capabilities of VISTA itself. A small set of DICOM services has been implemented by VISTA to allow patient and study text data to be transmitted to image producing modalities and the commercial PACS, and to enable images and study data to be transferred back.

---

*VISTA is the new name for the overall hospital information system architecture for the VA, and consists of several components, including its HIS (previously known as the Decentralized Hospital Computer Program, or DHCP), its imaging system, DICOM, client workstation technologies, server technologies, and the network infrastructure.

DICOM has been the cornerstone in the ability to integrate imaging functionality into the healthcare enterprise. Because of its openness, it allows the integration of system components from commercial and noncommercial sources to work together to provide functional cost-effective solutions. This could result in quicker deployment of digital imaging in the field and significant cost savings.

This chapter describes the VA's first 5 years of experiences with DICOM, in the belief that they offer guidance to other institutions working to establish interfaces between their HIS/RIS, PACS, and image producing modalities. Throughout the chapter, the term HIS is used to refer to the VA's HIS/RIS and to the larger information architecture known as V*IST*A.

The VA Experience

Architecture

The VA currently implements two different architectures with regard to radiology device interfaces, depending on whether a commercial PACS or the VA internally developed V*IST*A PACS solution is used.

The architecture for a commercial PACS, depicted in Figure 17.1, has three high-level components—the modality itself, the V*IST*A HIS, and a commercial PACS. In this scenario, the modality will interface to the V*IST*A HIS for the patient demographic information and to a commercial PACS for exchanging images and image management information.

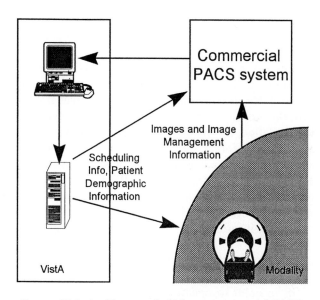

FIGURE 17.1. Architecture 1: Using a commercial PACS.

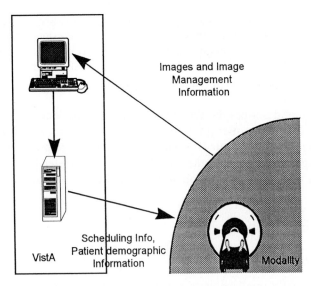

Figure 17.2. Architecture 2: Using the V*IST*A Imaging System as a PACS.

In the second architecture, the PACS is incorporated within the V*IST*A HIS, as illustrated in Figure 17.2. Note that from a modality functional perspective there is no real difference between scenario 1 and 2. The interface from the modality to a commercial PACS is now used between the modality and the V*IST*A imaging system.

Data Requirements

Any PACS needs several different kinds of text data from its associated HIS in order to operate properly. The HIS sends current patient identification and order entry information to the PACS so that it can register patients and process orders. All patient demographic changes are sent to the PACS to prevent patient mismatch and avoid duplicate patient registration. Examination progress information is sent to the PACS to trigger event processing, such as printing labels when the patient arrives. Radiology reports are entered on the HIS and are passed to the PACS, so that they can be displayed on the PACS in conjunction with the images. Clinical scheduling information is needed for prefetching images from the storage archive, and patient tracking information is necessary for display of patient information by ward.

The PACS must supply the HIS with information about examinations that have been performed. Notification of completion of an examination must be sent to the HIS in order to update the order status and to identify which examinations have digitized images. Where image transfer is required, the PACS must also send the HIS a list of the images associated with each completed order. The PACS images are transferred across the interface and stored in the HIS image file servers. They are then retrieved from the HIS file servers and displayed on the imaging workstations. In similar fashion, in the future, HIS images must be able to be transferred to the PACS and stored, and then retrieved and displayed on PACS workstations.

Each image producing modality should be supplied with a common set of patient and study information originating from the HIS. The modality should select the applicable set of data for the study and place it in the header of each image that it produces. This simple procedure not only alleviates the need for the data to be manually reentered at the modality (and the associated errors), but it also standardizes the data that is placed in the image header. The modality should send its image to a storage provider and furnish notification when all the images in a study have been successfully transmitted. This "image transfer complete" notification allows the study to be placed on a "to-be-read" worklist on a PACS. A modality requires patient demographic and study information, as follows:

- *Patient Information:* Patient name, date of birth, patient ID, patient sex, other patient/study IDs, allergies, patient race, pregnancy status, patient comments (e.g., lab data, problem list, most recent discharge summary, progress notes), patient location, primary care provider (referring physician), attending physician (physician of record).
- *Study Information:* Study SOP instance unique identifier (UID), case number (a radiology number that is reused on a weekly basis), accession number, ordered procedure (both a CPT code and locally used code), modality, reason for study, technologist performing the study, room location for study, requesting physician.

All of the data requirements for the modality can be satisfied with DICOM services.

Interface Development

First Generation: ACR-NEMA Version 2.0

When the Baltimore VA Medical Center (VAMC) purchased a commercial PACS in 1991 from Siemens Gammasonics, Inc. (which has now become a General Electric product), the agreement stipulated that the vendor would support a "bidirectional ACR-NEMA Version 2.0 text and image interface to DHCP which would be upgraded to DICOM Version 3.0, once that standard had been approved." This interface turned out to be critical to the success of filmless radiology at the Baltimore VAMC. Detailed interface specifications were developed jointly by the VA and vendor technical staff; in October

1993, following several months of VA and vendor testing, the interface was certified as operational by the chief of radiology and was placed into production. This interface is now operational at six VA medical centers and one Indian Health Service GE PACS site.

A text-only portion of the interface was subsequently created and modified to work with the Comprehensive Health Care System (CHCS), the HIS of the Department of Defense (DOD), and the Medical Diagnostic Imaging System (MDIS), the military version of the GE PACS. This configuration is now operational at 14 DOD medical centers.

These interfaces have been successful, with several million text messages exchanged at the various sites and over 2 million images transmitted from the PACS to the HIS at the Baltimore VAMC.

Second Generation: DICOM

While the VA's ACR-NEMA Version 2.0 interface was being designed and installed, the ACR-NEMA Committee developed Version 3.0 of their standard and renamed it DICOM (NEMA, 1994). DICOM differs from ACR-NEMA in four major ways:

- DICOM is object oriented. All of the data elements are collected together into standard information object definitions, which are communicated by a standard set of services.
- DICOM has a standard communications mechanism, using generally available TCP/IP.
- DICOM brings open systems technology to the previously proprietary medical imaging marketplace. DICOM can be used to interface PACS not only to HIS but also to image producing modalities, storage servers, workstations, laser camera printers, and other devices.
- DICOM is not "just for radiology" anymore. The American Society for Gastrointestinal Endoscopy, College of American Pathologists, American Dental Association, and American College of Cardiology are all involved in DICOM related standards activities.

In December 1994, the VA began the task of converting the PACS interface from ACR-NEMA Version 2.0 to DICOM. The scope of the DICOM interface project was widened to include handling the image producing modalities as well, with the intent of having them use DICOM to feed diagnostic quality radiology images directly into the VA's own imaging system.

In the past 3 years, the VA has made considerable progress on the development of their DICOM capabilities. Interfaces to seven different commercial PACS implementations and twenty different modalities have been placed into operation. Still, the VA is just beginning to deploy DICOM within their overall information system; efforts over the next few years will determine how successful this project is.

ACR-NEMA Interface Methodology

Requirements

"A PACS is an information system. It may include or be interfaced to a Radiology Information System and in addition may be interfaced to a Hospital Information System. Data integrity and consistency between and among these interconnected information systems is critical for the functioning of a medical treatment facility" (Prior, 1994).

The Baltimore VAMC, which opened in January 1993, has both the VISTA Imaging System and the GE PACS. To avoid double entry of data, a bidirectional text and image interface was provided between the two systems. The HIS supplies patient event data to the PACS, while the PACS sends downsample images (8-bit, 1k × 1k maximum size) to the HIS for incorporation into patient medical record along with the associated report text.

Architecture

The architecture of the PACS at Baltimore has been described elsewhere (Kuzmak and Dayhoff, 1994). As shown in Figure 17.3, the first generation PACS interface consists of three components: a text gateway, an image gateway, and a shared file server. ACR-NEMA Version 2.0 defines a message format, but no communications mechanism. A shared file server accessible to both the HIS and PACS is provided for the exchange of the messages. Each message is stored in a separate file on the server. There are separate high, medium, and low priority message queues for the HIS and PACS. The files are processed in a sequential first-in-first-out order. After each request message is processed, the response message is stored on the file server in a similar manner. The queue input and output pointers are stored on the file server and are accessible to all systems. There is also an image directory on the file server where the PACS places the images it sends to the HIS.

(The original shared file server used Novell NetWare 3.12 and Novell NFS 1.2c. The files on the server were accessible to the HIS interface gateway running DOS via IPX/SPX and the vendor PACS gateway running VMS via TGV NFS or MacIntosh via IPX/SPX. This was upgraded in October 1996 to used Microsoft NT Server 4.0 with AppleTalk and Hummingbird NFS.)

Messages

As shown in Table 17.1, several types of messages are sent across the interface. Some of the messages to PACS originate from HIS event-driven Health Level 7 (HL-7) transactions. There is a one-to-one mapping of HL-7 text transactions to ACR-NEMA messages. All HL-7 transactions contain redundant patient identification information that is passed with each ACR-NEMA message. The ACR-NEMA image transfer messages have no HL-7

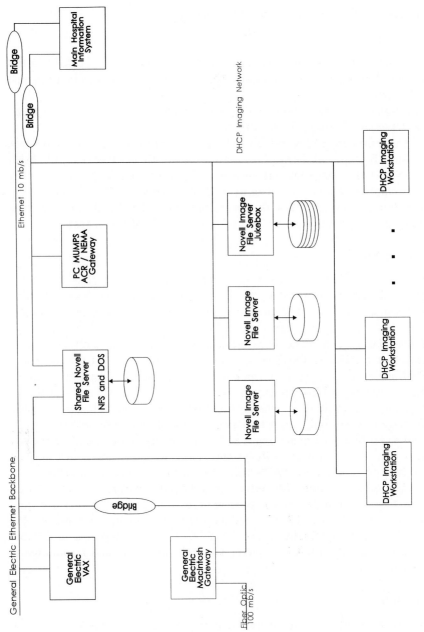

FIGURE 17.3. DHCP/PACS Interface.

TABLE 17.1. V*IST*A - PACS DICOM message flow.

Interface message	Direction
Patient demographic change	→PACS
ADT (admission)	→PACS
Order entry	→PACS
Examination change	→PACS
PACS acquires images	
Examination verification	→PACS
Examination complete	→V*IST*A
Get PACS image request	→PACS
Get PACS image data	→V*IST*A
Get PACS image response	→V*IST*A
Report transfer (preliminary)	→PACS
Report transfer (final)	→PACS
ADT discharge	→PACS

counterparts. The interface processes these messages by directly accessing the HIS database.

A patient admission or a change in demographic data triggers an admission/discharge/transfer (ADT) message or a patient demographic message to be sent to the PACS. An order entry message is sent to the PACS when the HIS processes a request for an examination. This may be done at the time the order is scheduled or when the patient arrives in radiology. In the former case, an examination change message is sent when the patient arrives in radiology. The order entry message contains all of the essential patient demographic and radiology order information, and triggers the examination processing on the PACS.

When the images have been acquired by the PACS, an examination completion message is sent back to the HIS. This message contains all the information needed by HIS to retrieve the images, including status information and a list of the image identifiers that are part of the examination. The status information and list of image identifiers are associated in the HIS with the radiology exam. The inhouse-developed imaging system uses the image identifiers to retrieve images from the PACS so that they can be moved to and viewed at the V*IST*A imaging workstations. The *Get PACS Image Request, Get PACS Image Data,* and *Get PACS Image Reply* messages are used to retrieve images from the PACS.

The radiology report is entered and edited on the HIS. Released and verified reports are sent to the PACS via a report transfer message.

ACR-NEMA Operational Rollout

The original bidirectional text and image ACR-NEMA Version 2.0 interface became operational with the GE PACS at the Baltimore VAMC in October 1993. Shortly thereafter, the DOD Medical Diagnostic Imaging System (MDIS) Project Office requested that the text-only interface be modified to support for its HIS (CHCS). These changes were completed, and DOD placed its first HIS-PACS interface into production at Madigan Army Medical Center (Ft. Lewis, Washington) in July 1994. The ACR-NEMA Version 2.0 interface is currently installed at 21 government sites using the GE PACS.

Benefits

The common benefit experienced at all the VA and DOD sites is that passing patient, order, and report information directly from the HIS to the PACS greatly improves the flow of work in the radiology department (Siegel, 1995). The presence of the interface allows continuous flow of information between these systems. The process is automated from the time the order is placed until the report is completed. Since radiology orders are transferred to PACS almost immediately, duplicate patient registration and the associated transcription errors are eliminated.

Image transfer to the inhouse-developed imaging system at the Baltimore VAMC demonstrated the advantage of providing "reference quality" (1k × 1k × 8-bit) radiology images to treating clinicians throughout the hospital.

Transaction Volumes

An earlier study details transaction volumes (Kuzmak, Norton, and Dayhoff, 1995). The Baltimore VAMC is a 327-bed hospital that in 1994 performed approximately 45,000 radiology procedures and had approximately 245,000 outpatient visits. The Madigan Army Medical Center (AMC) is a 400-bed hospital that performed approximately 145,000 radiology procedures in 1994 and had approximately a 900,000 outpatient visits.

As shown in Table 17.2, the Baltimore VAMC performed approximately 220 radiology procedures per day. More than 95 percent of those studies were digital. Most of those images were transmitted to the inhouse-developed imaging system. Each study received two reports, a preliminary copy and a final version.

The Madigan AMC performed approximately 475 radiology procedures per day. Each order transaction was initially generated when the order was scheduled and updated when the patient arrived. Registration for each outpatient visit triggered a patient demographic change transaction on the HIS, approximately

TABLE 17.2. Approximate number of ACR-NEMA messages per day (Baltimore VAMC and Madigan AMC, January 1995).

Message type	Baltimore VAMC number per day	Madigan AMC number per day
ADT	70	150
Patient demographic change	110	3000
Order entry	220	475
Examination change	10	475
Examination complete	187	—
Get images (image transfer)	187	—
Report transfer	440	475
Total	1224	4575

3000 per day. Only final patient reports were transmitted. At Madigan, the 3000 patient demographic change transactions per day slowed the PACS so much that orders could not be processed in a timely fashion. Temporarily disabling the patient demographic change transaction on the HIS improved performance.

Shared File Server Architecture

The high volume of HIS-PACS transactions requires the interface to be fast. Our experience is that the time for the text gateway to process a HL-7 transaction and generate the ACR-NEMA message is on the order of one second or less. The time for the commercial PACS to process the ACR-NEMA message is between 5 and 10 seconds or more. When there are numerous messages coming from the HIS, the queues back up and the PACS falls behind.

Because the commercial PACS was slow at processing messages and HIS events tend to occur in bursts, a three-tier message prioritization mechanism had to be implemented. Time-critical events like new orders are processed first, before reports, which are processed second. Nontime critical events, such as examination-pull-messages, are processed last.

PACS support personnel requested that formatted ASCII listings of the binary ACR-NEMA messages be generated so that text file searches can be used to find problematic transactions.

DICOM Interface Methodology

In September 1994, encouraged by the success of the ACR-NEMA Version 2.0 HIS-PACS interface and based upon the multiple potential uses for DICOM, the VA made the decision to develop comprehensive support for DICOM. This capability is now used to interface with commercial PACS, and for interfacing directly to the image producing modalities and other DICOM devices as shown in Figure 17.4.

In designing the general-purpose DICOM interface, the VA staff incorporated some of the characteristics of the previous interface and added new capabilities to support new features. The DICOM design uses similar methods for message encoding and decoding. The priority message queues of the previous interface are retained. Support for TCP/IP communications and DICOM message exchange has been added, replacing the shared file server approach of the previous interface. Standard service classes and information object definitions are used, replacing the ad hoc private elements (i.e., shadow groups) and ad hoc message composition previously used. DICOM image transfer mechanisms are now supported.

The interface design is intended to be general enough to be used for the full spectrum of current applications and to be extensible enough to be able to handle future applications that will go beyond radiology.

PACS Interface Integration Components

The integration of the VistA HIS and a commercial PACS involves several separate components: VistA, the commercial PACS, the provider(s) of the

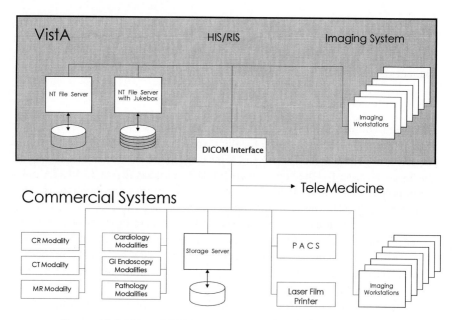

FIGURE 17.4. V*IST*A DICOM —Commercial system connectivity.

DICOM Modality Worklist service, and the image producing modalities as shown in Figure 17.5.

The following series of events occurs as each study is processed:

1. The V*IST*A HIS initiates the examination process by passing new patient and study event data to both the commercial PACS and the modality worklist provider. The same data stream is used for both the PACS and the modality worklist provider(s). (Figure 17.5, #1 and #2). The unique

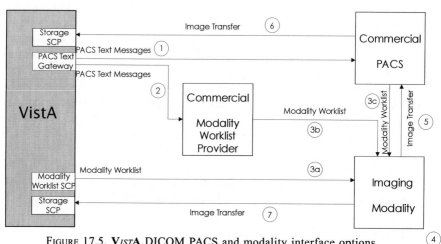

FIGURE 17.5. V*IST*A DICOM PACS and modality interface options.

identifiers (UIDs) for the patient, visit, study, report, and interpretation are included in this data, allowing these entities to be correctly identified by all of the various systems.

2. The image producing modality system queries the modality worklist provider to obtain a current list of patients and studies to be performed at that station (Figure 17.5, #3a, #3b, or #3c,).

3. The image producing modality system acquires the images and places the VIST A patient/study data in the image headers (Figure 17.5, #4).

4. The image producing modality system sends the images to the commercial PACS (Figure 17.5, #5).

5. The PACS sends the images to VIST A to be added to the HIS database (Figure 17.5, #6).

6. Nonradiology "visible light" images may be transferred directly from the modality to VIST A, bypassing the PACS (Figure 17.5, #7).

Components of the VIST A Modality Interface

Four separate components are required for the VIST A modality interface: the VIST A HIS, the modality worklist provider(s), the image producing modalities, and one or more VIST A storage providers. The VIST A modality interface presently supports both the DICOM modality worklist service and the DICOM storage services, shown in Figure 17.6.

The modality worklist service supplies new HIS patient and study information directly to the modality so that it does not have to be manually entered. The storage service is used to transmit a set of images from the modality to the HIS. The information supplied by the modality worklist service is incorporated into the image headers, making them easier to identify when they are processed on the HIS.

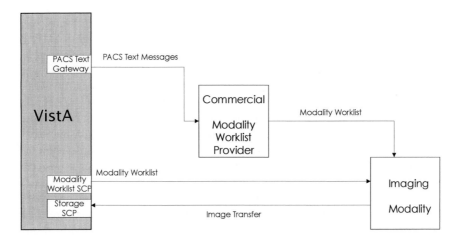

FIGURE 17.6. VIST A DICOM modality interface options.

In the future, the DICOM storage commitment and performed procedure step services will be added to V*IST*A, to notify the recipient of the images at the completion of the study.

V*IST*A DICOM Implementation Details

Architecture

The majority of the V*IST*A DICOM application is written in MUMPS, the same language as the V*IST*A HIS (Kuzmak and Dayhoff, 1995). MUMPS handles DICOM communications, DICOM association negotiation, reading and writing DICOM datasets, access to the V*IST*A database, interfaces to the HIS, and higher level applications. The communications portion of the image transfer application (i.e., the DICOM C-STORE service) and image processing functions are written in C for the sake of speed. The V*IST*A DICOM application runs on top of the Microsoft Windows NT Workstation, Version 4.0 operating system. The Micronetics MSM-NT Version 4.3.2 of MUMPS is currently used for the V*IST*A DICOM application (MSM-NT, 1997).

Message Dataset Files

Each DICOM message dataset transfer requires a message processing step and a message communication step. DICOM message datasets are stored in NT operating system files between these two steps. An incoming message dataset is placed into a file as it is received, and is read out of the file as it is processed. An outgoing message dataset is placed into a file as it is generated, and is read out of the file as it is sent. These two steps are performed in different ways in order to support the synchronous and asynchronous modes of operation of DICOM.

The synchronous mode of DICOM operation requires completing one message request on an association at a time. As shown in Figure 17.7, a single system task performs both the message processing step and the message communications step. This facility is used to handle DICOM query requests (e.g., from modality worklist users). The query service provider uses a single port for handling requests. A direct text process is spawned in the background for each DICOM association. The process negotiates the association, handles the query request, and then terminates when the association is taken down. This architecture can easily handle multiple simultaneous query requests. The request and response message datasets are stored in files between the two steps.

The asynchronous mode of DICOM operation requires handling any number of message requests on an association at a time. Separate tasks are used to perform the message processing step and the message communications step. As illustrated in Figure 17.8, the asynchronous interface consists of

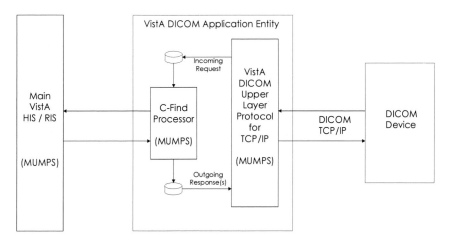

FIGURE 17.7. V*IST*A DICOM architecture (Worklist Management Service Class).

three components: a DICOM Application Entity (AE) message handler, a file server with a set of prioritized sequential first-in-first-out message queues, and a DICOM Upper Level (DUL) communications facility operating on top of TCP/IP. The queue architecture was retained from the first generation PACS interface to handle the "bursty" nature of transactions in a hospital information system, in which there are a large number of different types of messages with different priorities.

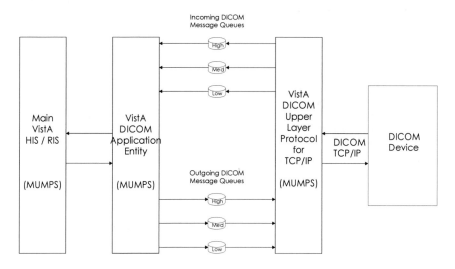

FIGURE 17.8. V*IST*A DICOM architecture (excluding the Storage Service Class).

The message dataset files are organized into first-in-first-out queues, which form a buffer between the task performing the processing and the task performing the communications. Incoming messages are stored in the queue and are processed in the order they were received. Outgoing messages are stored in the queue and are sent in the order they were generated.

DICOM requires supporting three levels of priority: high, medium, and low. Different messages may be assigned different levels of priority. To ensure prompt notification of time-critical events, the V*IST*A application code gives orders and changes to orders top priority, patient demographic changes and radiology reports medium priority, and examination pull requests low priority. Three sets of first-in-first-out queues are used, one set for high priority messages, one set for medium priority messages, and one set for low priority messages. All the messages in the high priority queue are processed first, those in the medium priority queue are processed second, and those in the low priority queue are processed last. DICOM messages are typically kept on the file server for a minimum of 1 week, in order to be available to diagnose system failures.

DICOM Message Handler and Communication Facility Implementation

Both synchronous and asynchronous modes share the same message handler and communications facility. The message handler is layered between the HIS and the DICOM message dataset, and supports the DICOM Message Service Element (DIMSE) and the service classes. The message handler obtains data from the HIS and generates outgoing DICOM messages writing them to the file system; it also parses incoming DICOM messages and passes the data to the HIS. The message handler can output ASCII formatted DICOM dumps of all the incoming and outgoing messages that it processes. (This is another feature that was retained from the first generation PACS interface.) Formatted ASCII listings of the DICOM messages may be kept on the file server along with the original DICOM messages. This feature may be used as an aid to support personnel, so that text file searches can be used to find problematic transactions.

The communications facility handles the association negotiation (Association Control Service Element or ACSE) and the Upper Layer Presentation Data Service (Protocol Data Unit/Presentation Data Value or PDU/PDV encapsulation). It is responsible for the transmission of DICOM message datasets between other DICOM devices over TCP/IP.

Commercial PACS Interface Messages

Interface Message Issues

Experience with the ACR-NEMA interface suggested that a similar message scheme should be used to implement the DICOM interface. The ACR-NEMA

Version 2.0 interface used a notification message (i.e., a push mechanism) to send event information from one side to the other. All the information for each event was conveyed in a single message. A query capability (i.e., a pull mechanism) was not incorporated into the Version 2.0 interface design.

Removal of the Requirement for the N-GET Mechanism

Standard normalized DICOM services are designed to operate on a single information object definition (IOD) at a time, and require a combination of notification (N-EVENT-REPORT) and query (N-GET) services to get all the related data. A notification message contains the data for a single IOD. Other related IODs may be referenced in the notification message, but additional query requests are needed to access their data.

The VISTA DICOM interface was designed differently from the outset for several reasons. The N-GET, it was thought, would introduce unnecessary complexity and delay into the interface design. Supporting a useful N-GET service would be difficult because the underlying HIS HL-7 transaction mechanism does not provide a query capability and the VISTA PACS interface was by design to be stateless. Further justifying the VA's decision were subsequent concerns from PACS vendors about their difficulties issuing the N-GET request for additional information (e.g., the requirement for multiple associations, the need for roll-back on incomplete transactions).

The removal of the requirement for the N-GET mechanism was accomplished simply by sending redundant study and/or patient information with every message.

Mapping Events to DICOM Messages

A related interface design goal is that there be a one-to-one mapping of real-world events to the DICOM messages. Every event maps to a single DICOM N-EVENT-REPORT request message. Each applicable data field is translated into its corresponding DICOM element. All of the patient information from each event transaction is included in each DICOM request message. The redundant patient information allows the PACS to create the patient database entry if necessary.

The interface takes full advantage of the fact that the HIS HL-7 transaction mechanism sends redundant study and/or patient information for each event. The VA has created specializations of the standard Detached Visit, Study, Interpretation, and Study Component Management SOP Class. These specializations provide complete redundant study and/or patient information with each message, so that the PACS can process each message without requiring additional information. This technique entirely alleviates the need for the use of the N-GET service.

Consolidating all the information in one transaction has a number of merits. Because there are fewer messages and no N-GET query issues, the design provides benefits of simplicity, performance, and robustness. Another advantage is that the messages provide the complete set of information for the site personnel who have to maintain the interface.

Passing Redundant Patient Identification Information

The interface uses a single N-EVENT-REPORT transaction to communicate the each event and includes the redundant patient identification information. For example, the Order Entry HL-7 transaction is mapped to a Create Study event type of VA Detached Study Management SOP Class. The PACS receives the order information in the message and checks if the patient with the UID existed. If the patient is already on file, the redundant patient data is ignored. (The PACS vendors have the option of using this information to update their systems, if necessary.) If the patient is new, the information in the redundant patient data is used to create the patient in its database; the study is then be created.

Report Transfer Issues

The default report transfer technique for DICOM is to send reports to a PACS using two N-EVENT-REPORT messages: one to create the result object and a second to create the interpretation object. The VA has one-to-one-to-one mapping between studies, reports, and interpretations, and prefers sending one transaction rather than two. The updated event type of the VA Detached Interpretation Management SOP Class Interpretation Updated is used and provided with enough information in specializations to create the result object, if necessary. There are three specializations: the referenced patient sequence, the referenced study sequence, and the redundant patient data.

Examination Completion Issues

A further specialization for maintainability is that redundant patient data is added to the N-CREATE of the study component management for the examination complete transaction. This is needed both for processing the message on the HIS and for maintenance.

Lack of Standard Masterfile Dictionary Communications

One common shortcoming of the PACS is the way it maintains the masterfile dictionary data, the importance of which the PACS community has underestimated. The DICOM standard fails to address the need to propagate institutional masterfile information. Rather than assign this task to their software developers, PACS vendors have delegated it to their site support staff. Without current masterfile dictionary data, the PACS cannot correctly maintain its own copies of the institutional masterfiles and cannot use this data in messages sent from the PACS to the HIS. The masterfile dictionary maintenance task needs to be automated; institutional entity dictionaries should be added to DICOM and maintained in a standard way.

Additional Specializations: Physicians and Institutional Locations

DICOM does not treat physicians or institutional locations as entities. Without codes, it is difficult to differentiate between two providers with the same name, and particularly difficult for the PACS to send messages to the HIS that require the code. Additional specializations are needed to be able to assign a code to each physician or institutional location to uniquely identify them. These specializations follow the model used for the *Procedure Code Sequence* (0008,1032).

String/Text Length Restrictions of DICOM

DICOM imposes length limitations on string and text data that are too restrictive. This is a fundamental property of the DICOM information object definition. As shown in Table 17.3, the value representation of each DICOM attribute defines the communication format and the maximum length.

Most HIS do not use the DICOM information model and are not bound by these restrictions. The VA has uncovered several instances in which either not enough characters are permitted by DICOM for an element value, or there is a value representation mismatch. Clearly, longer lengths or possibly removal of length restrictions entirely are needed in these instances.

The reason why the study was ordered is one of the most important pieces of clinical information that the radiologist receives about the patient. It typically includes a short medical history, followed by a request to look for a specific finding. On the HIS, this data is entered into an arbitrary-length multiple line free text field. This is an example of value representation mismatch between the HIS and DICOM.

The standard data element *Reason for the Study* (0032,1030) has a DICOM Value Representation (VR) of Long String (LO), which has a maximum length of 64 characters. Many of the reasons entered by VA physicians for the study exceed this length. (The same is true for the new Modality Worklist Module elements *Reason of the Requested Procedure* (0040,1002), and *Reason for the Imaging Service Request* (0040,2001).) The VISTA DICOM PACS interface has a private short text data element for the Reason for the Study with a maximum length of 1024 characters. (We have seen instances where even that is not long enough.)

TABLE 17.3. Attribute value representation (VR).

VR name	Definition	Length of value
SH	Short string	16 characters maximum
LO	Long string	64 characters maximum
ST	Short text	1024 characters maximum
LT	Long text	10240 characters maximum

The *Patient's Address* (0010,1040) has a DICOM Value Representation (VR) of Long String (LO), which has a maximum length of 64 characters. If the Patient's Address exceeds 64 characters, it is truncated.

The *Ethnic Group* (0010,2160) has a DICOM Value Representation (VR) of Short String (LO), which has a maximum length of 16 characters. The VA standard values for this field exceed this limit. Special short values are sent instead.

The *Interpretation Text* (4008,010B) has a DICOM VR of Short Text (ST), which has a maximum length of 1024 characters. The *Interpretation Diagnosis Description* (4008,0115) has a DICOM VR of Long Text (LT), which has a maximum length of 10240 characters. The normal practice at the VA is to use Interpretation Text and Interpretation Diagnosis Description interchangeably. As a result, the Interpretation Text length (1024 characters) is frequently exceeded. To solve this problem, both the Interpretation Text and the Diagnosis Description are concatenated together and sent as the longer Interpretation Diagnosis Description.

VISTA Commerical PACS Interface Messages

The VISTA HIS is designed to acquire data about patient care events and to "push" this data to external systems. The asynchronous mode of operations is used to queue and prioritize the DICOM messages that are sent to the commercial PACS· VA-specific SOP Classes were created for the event transactions. These are listed in Table 17.4.

Modality Worklist Provider

The Modality Worklist Service is the DICOM service that obtains patient and study information from the hospital radiology information system and supplies it to the image producing modalities. This service is designed to

TABLE 17.4. VISTA DICOM PACS interface messages.

Real-world event	Direction	Detached VA SOP class and event type
Patient demographic change	VistA→PACS	Patient management, patient updated
ADT	VistA→PACS	Visit management, visit updated
Examination pull	VistA→PACS	Visit management, visit scheduled
Order entry	VistA→PACS	Study management, study created
Examination change (cancel)	VistA→PACS	Study management, study updated
Examination verification	VistA→PACS	Study management, study updated
Examination complete	VistA←PACS	N-CREATE of the study component management
Get image request	VistA→PACS	C-MOVE request of query/retrieve
Get image data	VistA←PACS	C-STORE of storage service
Get image response	VistA←PACS	C-MOVE response of query/retrieve
Report transfer	VistA→PACS	Interpretation management, interpretation updated

operate around a query mechanism that allows the modality to "pull" selected patient and study information on demand. The VISTA HIS can function as the provider of the Modality Worklist service. The VISTA Modality Worklist provider maintains a database of active studies. The Order Entry (OE) transaction causes a new study record to be added to the active study database, while the Examination Verification or the Examination Change (cancel) transaction causes the records for study to be deleted from the active study database. A query from the modality (i.e., a C-FIND Request) causes VISTA to return data from one or more records in the database. The VISTA Modality Worklist provider is implemented using the synchronous mode of operation. Each query request is handled by a separate spawned task that interrogates the database and transmits the results. The synchronous mode lets VISTA process multiple simultaneous query requests on different associations at the same time.

A commercial Modality Worklist provider may be furnished as part of a modality package. VISTA can send the DICOM HIS patient/study event data stream (described in the above section) to one or more commercial providers of the Modality Worklist service. The commercial service providers can then handle their respective modalities. Although the Modality Worklist service is generally used to convey information about current studies to the modality, an important feature of the VISTA Modality Worklist service provider is that it can also supply information about old studies as well. If the requested study is not in the active database, the information will be obtained from the long-term HIS database. This is particularly useful for film digitizing when old films are being scanned and is a capability not found in most of the commercial products.

VISTA Storage Class Provider—Image Acquisition

The VISTA storage class provider acquires the images from the modalities and temporarily stores them until they can be matched with the proper patient and study in the HIS database. The VISTA storage class provider consists of a C process and a MUMPS process. The C process functions at a low level and transfers image datasets from the network to files on magnetic disk. The MUMPS process performs all of the housekeeping chores required for image acquisition. It negotiates the association, handles the C-STORE request, accesses the VISTA database, determines where to store the image, stores a pointer to the image file in the VISTA database, and generates the C-STORE response, as shown in Figure 17.9. VISTA DICOM storage has been verified with twelve commercial modalities.

A single VISTA DICOM storage class provider can support several modalities simultaneously. Mouse clicking on a modality icon starts a modality storage provider process. This launches the C process, which then starts the MUMPS process, communicating with it via TCP/IP as shown in Figure 19.10.

VISTA obtains images from a commercial PACS using the DICOM Query/ Retrieve service. The PACS sends the Study UID to VISTA in the Examina-

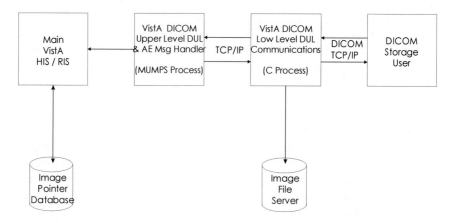

FIGURE 17.9. VISTA DICOM architecture: Storage Service SOP Class Provider.

tion Complete message. VISTA then issues a C-MOVE request to copy all the images to the VISTA storage provider.

Image Processing

After the DICOM images have been acquired by the VISTA storage class provider, they must be correctly matched to the proper patient and study in the HIS database. Matching the image to the original study requires correct patient and study identification to be present in the DICOM image header. Since the usage and format of the DICOM fields containing this information is not yet uniform in the industry, manufacturer/model specific techniques

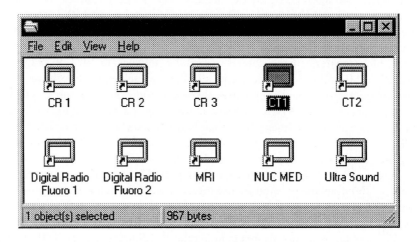

FIGURE 17.10. Modality folder.

are used to extract and process the data. The identification information can either be automatically acquired through the Modality Worklist Service, or it can be manually entered at the modality console. Because manual data entry is chronically error prone, however, additional manual procedures are then needed to link incorrectly identified images to the proper patients and studies. The VA has issued a specification listing the data items that are required to be placed into the image headers by the modality.

Once the images are properly identified, they are converted into a format that can be rapidly displayed on V*IST*A workstations. The DICOM Standard accommodates a variety of formats for expressing image data. First, multiframe DICOM objects are converted into a set of single image files. Second, the DICOM image headers are stripped off, converted to ASCII, and stored in text files. Then, the images in different formats are converted into a "normalized" form, where all adjustments have been made to the data prior to the viewing. The V*IST*A display workstation uses an 8- to 12-bit unsigned integer monochrome pixel format, where zero is intended to be displayed as black. Raw DICOM pixel values are converted into this format using modality manufacturer/model specific filtering to adjust the pixel values and remove hardware generated artifacts. V*IST*A also generates separate down-sampled computed radiography images for use at reference-quality clinician's workstations.

In the future, V*IST*A will incorporate commercial DICOM display toolkits capable of showing DICOM images directly, without requiring this image normalization step.

Image Display

The general-purpose V*IST*A Clinician Workstation can display images on a VGA monitor. These are currently available with up to 1600 × 1200 pixel resolution.

The special-purpose V*IST*A Radiologist Workstation features up to four 2k x 2k portrait mode monochrome monitors for diagnostic quality viewing. The software is written using the DOME DimplX toolkit.

*V*IST*A Storage User – Image Transmission*

The V*IST*A storage user is currently manually invoked to transmit DICOM images. Shortly, a V*IST*A Query/Retrieve Provider will be included to permit DICOM workstations to access the image database directly. As shown in Figure 17.11, the V*IST*A Query/Retrieve Provider is split into two processes. The MUMPS process is the provider for the Query/Retrieve SOP Class, and the C process is the user of the Storage SOP Class. The MUMPS process entirely handles the query C-FIND request, looking up the records in the database and returning the matches. The MUMPS process performs all the house keeping chores for the retrieve C-MOVE request. The MUMPS process negotiates the association, handles the C-MOVE request, accesses the image pointer in HIS database, determines the location of the image, spawns

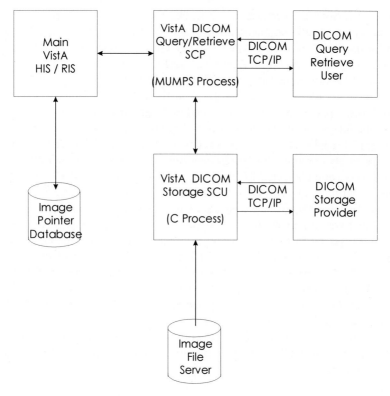

FIGURE 17.11. V*IST*A DICOM architecture: Query/retrieve SOP Class Provider, Storage Service SOP Class Provider.

the C process (once for each image transfer), and generates the C-MOVE response. The C process issues the C-STORE request and transfers the image dataset from the file server disk over the network.

To send an image to a DICOM storage provider, the image has to be reconstituted in DICOM format from the processed normalized image and its ASCII text header. Once done, a utility transfers the DICOM image over the network to the storage provider.

Examples of Operational Systems

Commercial PACS Interfaces

EMED PACS—Boston, MA VAMC

The first DICOM text interface with a commercial PACS was with EMED E-Systems Raytheon at the Boston VAMC in late 1996. In April 1997, the DICOM Query/Retrieve service became operational for image transfer from the EMED PACS to V*IST*A. Six thousand images a day are being sent to V*IST*A across this interface and can be seen on V*IST*A workstations throughout the medical center.

GE PACS – Baltimore, MD VAMC

As mentioned, the Baltimore VAMC was the original site of the first VA HIS-PACS interface. In October 1997, the Baltimore GE PACS to V*IST*A image transfer was upgraded to use the DICOM Query/Retrieve service. Several other VA GE PACS sites are planned to use the DICOM Query/Retrieve service in 1998. The GE PACS continues to use ACR-NEMA Version 2.0 and the shared file server for text transfer.

Additional DICOM PACS Text-Only Interfaces

In January 1997, the Agfa PACS at the Los Angeles VAMC became the second facility in the VA to become operational with the DICOM text interface, followed by the Agfa PACS at Leavenworth, Kansas, in late spring. In the summer of 1997, the interface with Parameter Development's PACS at the Houston VAMC became operational. Late in 1997, the interface with IBM/ BRIT's PACS at the Dallas VAMC became operational. Interfaces are also operational with Cemax-Icon at the Palo Alto VAMC and other sites. It is also anticipated that the Query/Retrieve service will become operational at some of these sites in 1998.

Modality Interface Projects

Direct Image Capture

Image transfer in DICOM is handled by the Storage Service SOP Class. The VA information systems architecture supports the Storage Service SOP Class both as a user and as a provider, meaning that V*IST*A can both send and receive images. The Storage Service user and provider application entities were originally tested with the public domain Mallinckrodt simple storage and send image routines (Moore, Beecher, and Hoffman, 1994). Interfaces are currently operational with the GE and EMED PACS, and with the following image producing modalities: Picker CT, MR, and NM, General Electric CT, DRS (digital radio fluoroscopy), LCA DLX (digital x-ray angiography), and Advantage Workstation, ATL Ultrasound, Fuji CR (DeJarnette), Fuji CR (Analogics), and the Lumisys Film Scanner (Mitra).

Several sites are now operational with direct modality image acquisition (see Wilmington and Washington below). All the DICOM image producing modalities at the Baltimore VAMC were connected to V*IST*A Storage Providers to acquire test images for the DOD DIN-PACS evaluation suite.

DICOM TCP/IP Messages

The Baltimore and Perry Point VAMCs have been consolidated and now share a single HIS and a single PACS at the Baltimore location. A joint VA/DeJarnette/Fuji/GE project was initiated to establish a bidirectional image and text link between a CR modality at Perry Point and the information systems at Baltimore, a distance of about 40 miles. Perry Point patient and study data are entered into the HIS at Baltimore and are sent to DeJarnette at Perry Point. Computed Radiography (CR) images acquired on the Fuji at Perry Point are sent by DeJarnette to the GE PACS in Baltimore for reading. V*IST*A sends the DICOM HIS patient/study event data stream to a commerical modality worklist provider (DeJarnette Medishare) located at the Perry Point VAMC. The DeJarnette Medishare creates a database and provides a worklist facility at the Fuji CR modality. This link has been in continuous operation since March 1996. A second similar interface is now operational between the Baltimore and Ft. Howard VAMCs.

Modality Worklist SOP Class

The VA is working with DeJarnette, Mitra, and Picker Magnetic Resonance (MR) Division to test the capabilities for the Fuji Computed Radiography system. The Picker MR Division used the V*IST*A DICOM Simulator to aid their development work and testing. Picker publicly demonstrated their interface working with the V*IST*A DICOM Modality Worklist Simulator at the 1996 Annual Meeting of the (1998) Radiological Society of North America. Interfaces are now operational with six products.

V*IST*A Diagnostic Radiology Image Management

There is a current ongoing development effort that extends the capabilities of the windows-based V*IST*A imaging system to support radiology applications.

Wilmington, DE VAMC

The Wilmington VAMC is the first facility to use the capabilities of V*IST*A for diagnostic reading with a goal of becoming completely digital. Although it was able to purchase digital image producing modalities, budgetary constraints ruled out obtaining a commercial PACS. The Wilmington staff decided to provide diagnostic radiology image management using V*IST*A Imaging components.

The Wilmington VAMC has an inpatient capacity of 78 hospital beds and has 114,000 outpatient visits per year. The radiology department performs approximately 26,000 studies annually. The network architecture of the Wilmington system is shown in Figure 17.12. There are three V*IST*A DICOM Storage providers for eleven modalities shown in Table 17.5. Processed images are placed on one of two 40-gigabyte Digital Alpha NT file servers, and are then immediately copied to a two-terabyte jukebox. Three four-monitor diagnostic quality workstations are used for reading the images. Over 125

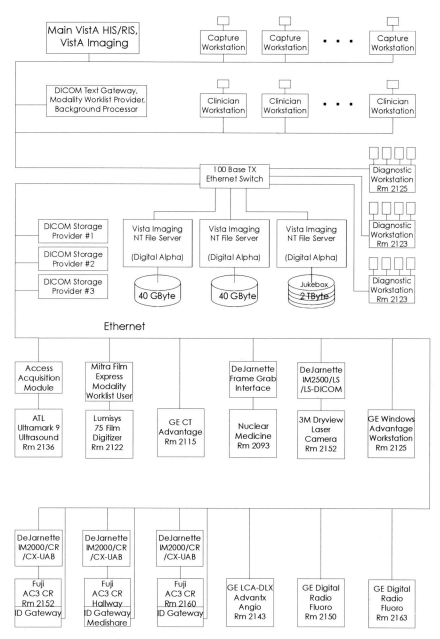

FIGURE 17.12. Wilmington VAMC V*IST*A Imaging Network

clinical workstations are installed throughout the medical center, each with a 17-inch (1280 × 1024) color VGA monitor.

All digital modalities are operational, and images are acquired for all studies. When the system was still quite new and the radiology staff was in a

TABLE 17.5. DICOM devices at the Wilmington VAMC.

Quantity	Manufacturer/model	DICOM interface
3	Fuji AC3 Computed Radiography	DeJarnette
1	GE LCA DLX Advantx Angioiography	GEMS
2	GE Digital Radio Fluoroscopy	GEMS
1	ATL Ultramark 9 Ultrasound	ATL/ACCESS
1	Lumiscan 75 Film Digitizer	Mitra
1	GE CT Advantage	GEMS
1	Siemens Nuclear Medicine (ICON)	DeJarnette
1	3M Dryview Laser Camera	DeJarnette
1	GE Windows Advantage Workstation	GEMS

learning mode, film was printed for all studies. Now that system verification has been completed and confidence in the digital capabilities has been established, the film printing has been discontinued.

The system is being very well received by the radiology staff, the medical staff, and the administration. There is a very high level of enthusiasm and acceptance surrounding the project. The radiologists are excited by being able to see more detail in the digital images than film and by the potential for making more accurate diagnoses. The medical staff enjoys being able to see reference quality CR images and full resolution CT images on its PC workstations. The administration likes the fact that the newly constructed facility is functioning well, that VIsTA PACS is totally integrated within the HIS, and that quality of service and productivity seem to be improving.

Washington, DC VAMC

The Washington VAMC is the second pilot site for VIsTA diagnostic radiology image management. The Washington VAMC has an inpatient capacity of 376 beds and has 305,000 outpatient visits per year. The radiology department performs approximately 73,000 studies annually.

All digital images from three Fuji CR AC3, two Picker PQ2000 CT's, and a Picker Edge MRI are already being sent to the VIsTA system. These images are being read by the radiologists on eight diagnostic quality workstations. The Washington VAMC has just undergone a complete upgrade of its digital network infrastructure, with new vertical fiber optic cable, wire closet hubs, and horizontal Category 5 unshielded twisted pair installed everywhere. A total of 450 clinical imaging workstations have been installed, so that images can be seen by clinicians throughout the medical center.

Experiences with DICOM

Overall, the VA experience with DICOM has been very favorable. An unprecedented degree of interoperability has already been achieved, along with new levels of operational reliability and robustness.

DICOM has enabled the V*IST*A Imaging System to interface directly with the image producing modalities, and this is an extremely useful capability. DICOM is also being used to interface with vendor-supplied PACS. The commercial DICOM offerings that we have tested and interfaced with were developed using toolkits that are quite mature, and interfacing to them has been fairly easy.

The DICOM unique identification scheme for the patient and study form the information structure necessary for teleradiology. This is a great benefit of DICOM. We expect this to be widely used within the federal government in the future.

Needed Improvements

There are several parts of the DICOM standard that we would like to see changed (Kuzmak and Dayhoff, 1997). More interoperability is possible—and necessary. We found DICOM-imposed length limitations on string and text data to be far too restrictive. Our HIS was written well before DICOM and supports unlimited length free-text data fields. We found fields containing string data on our HIS that were longer than the corresponding DICOM allotment. We also found value representation mismatches between the free-text fields on our HIS and the corresponding DICOM string elements. The DICOM Committee is actively working to improve this situation.

The lack of a standard DICOM facility for communication of institutional master file data is another concern for us. We would like to see a DICOM standard produced for the propagation of master file data.

A related issue is that DICOM does not treat physicians or institutional locations as entities. DICOM does not support the unique identification codes for physicians and locations. Without them, it is difficult to differentiate between two providers with the same name. This becomes particularly troublesome when a commercial PACS must send provider information in messages to a HIS that requires such codes.

We encountered several difficulties interfacing DICOM to the VA's existing HIS. The original DIMSE-N normalized message scheme was found to be poorly suited for use with the existing VA HIS. This was replaced with a VA-designed specialization, which did not require the N-GET service.

Modality Implementations

Current modality implementations of DICOM are too diverse and lack certain capabilities. In spite of the fact that for the last ten years the DICOM Accession Number element (0008,0050) has been required to be in every image header (and is needed by all PACS to identify the study), most modality implementers have not provided a mechanism for entering it. Of the dozen or so modalities that we have in production, there are seven different ways to pass the accession number. Six of these ways require transferring it from some other field. One cannot pass it at all.

There appears to be an inconstant usage of the Photometric Interpretation element (0028,0004). The values MONOCHROME1 and MONOCHROME2 seem have opposite meaning between digital radiofluoroscopy and the other x-ray modalities. In digital radiofluoroscopy, black bone is MONOCHROME2 and white bone is MONOCHROME1, while in the other x-ray modalities, it is the other way around. It is also difficult to determine when the PACS has received all the images from the modality so that the study can be placed on an "Unread Study Worklist."

Clearly, the PACS industry would greatly benefit by having a uniform, proper, and consistent usage of the DICOM standard by the modality industry.

VA DICOM Compliance Requirement for Modalities

The VA has writen a national modality DICOM compliance requirement document to address these problems (Oooeterwijk, Kuzmak, Dayhoff et al., 1998). This document includes a standard list of data elements that are required to be in every image header. It states that the modality shall obtain these data items through the Modality Worklist Service Class. Rules are included on the Photometric Interpretation element's usage. The modality is required to provide a notification mechanism as to when all the images have been sent to the storage provider. All modality manufacturers must use a uniform, consistent core subset of DICOM services to satisfy these requirements.

V*IST*A DICOM Simulator

The V*IST*A DICOM applications are constructed so that they can run in simulator mode without an actual connection to the HIS. The VA provides a V*IST*A DICOM simulator to their DICOM vendors so that they can do all of their testing inhouse. A set of real patient data (sanitized to protect confidentiality) is supplied with the simulator to mimic as closely as possible the actual events. Further testing can be performed across the Internet between the vendor site and our software development facility. Final testing is performed on-site with test data before live operation.

The presence of the simulator at vendor sites has been a major factor contributing to the initial overall success of the project. Several vendors have stated that providing them with our V*IST*A DICOM simulator has greatly facilitated their development work and improved the reliability and quality of their product when installed on site.

Conclusion

The VA experience with DICOM has been very favorable, despite some minor limitations of the standard. An unprecedented degree of interoperability has been achieved, along with new levels of operational reliability and robustness.

By enabling the inhouse developed imaging system to interface directly with the image producing modalities, DICOM provides an extremely useful capability. DICOM is also being used to interface with vendor-supplied PACS. Commercial DICOM offerings tested by the VA were developed using mature toolkits; interfacing to them has been fairly easy. Providing the VA's DICOM simulator to the vendors facilitated their development work and improved the reliability and quality of their products when installed on site. With the growth of telemedicine in the federal sector and elsewhere, DICOM's unique identification scheme for the patient and study will form the information stucture necessary for teleradiology.

The DICOM standard did have some shortcomings that created difficulties in interfacing to the VA's existing HIS, including its RIS component. As a result, DICOM's original normalized message scheme was replaced with a VA-designed specialization, which did not require the N-GET service. Several difficulties remain to be resolved. DICOM-imposed length limitations on string and text data are far too restrictive. Written well before DICOM, the VA's HIS supports arbitrary length free-text data fields, some containing string data longer than the corresponding DICOM allotment. In addition, the VA has found value representation mismatches between the free-text fields on the HIS and the corresponding DICOM string elements. The VA is working with the DICOM Committee to improve this situation.

The VA has achieved significant success in its attempt thus far to support DICOM capabilities with its V*IST*A HIS. Overall, the VA's experience is that DICOM truly is fulfilling its promise to bring open system technology to the medical imaging marketplace. By capitalizing on the success of the DICOM standard and the resulting opens systems environment, the VA expects significant cost benefits that will accelerate deployment of digital imaging nationally within its medical centers. The VA hopes to deploy many DICOM applications on a large scale across its entire hospital system in the future.

Acknowledgments. The authors would like to thank Dr. Eliot Siegel and the Radiology Department at the Baltimore VAMC and Dr. M. Elon Gale and the Radiology Department at the Boston VAMC for the opportunity to develop the initial commercial PACS interfaces; Gerald Perry and Maryann Shovestul of the Radiology Department of the Wilmington VAM&ROC; Drs. Ross Fletcher and Daniel Fernicola of the Washington VAMC for permitting their sites to be used as the pilots for V*IST*A PACS; Herman Oosterwijk, President of Otech, for his assistance in the development of the VA's Modality Interface DICOM Conformance Requirements; Fred Goeringer, formerly Director of the MDIS Project Office, for the opportunity to gain experience with the interface at the Department of Defense sites; and Dr. Fred Prior, then at Pennsylvania State University, for advice about DICOM.

References

Kuzmak PM, Dayhoff RE. A bidirectional ACR-NEMA interface between the VA's DHCP integrated imaging system and the Siemens-Loral PACS. Proc SPIE 1994, 2165, 387–394.

Kuzmak PM, Dayhoff RE. Implementing the digital image and communications for medicine (DICOM) protocol. M Computing 1995, 3(3), 33–40.

Kuzmak PM, Dayhoff RE. DHCP modality interface, DICOM conformance statement (draft). Washington DC: US Department of Veterans Affairs, February 28, 1996.

Kuzmak PM, Dayhoff RE. Experience with MUMPS-based DICOM interfaces between the Department of Veterans Affairs HIS/RIS and commercial vendors. Proc SPIE 1997, 3035, 134–145.

Kuzmak PM, Dayhoff RE. VISTA PACS interface, DICOM conformance statement (draft). Washington DC: US Department of Veterans Affairs. January 10, 1997.

Kuzmak PM, Norton GS, Dayhoff RE. Using experience with bidirectional HL7-ACR-NEMA interfaces between the federal government HIS/RIS and commercial PACS to plan for DICOM. Proc SPIE, 1995, 2435, 132–143.

MSM-NT. Micronetics Design Corporation, 1375 Piccard Drive, Suite 300, Rockville, MD 20850, 1997, (301), 358–2605.

Moore SM, Beecher DE, Hoffman SA. DICOM shareware: A public implementation of the DICOM standard. Proc SPIE, 1994, 2165, 772–781.

National Electrical Manufacturers Association (NEMA). Digital Imaging and Communications in Medicine (DICOM), standards publication PS 3. Washington DC, NEMA, 1994.

Oosterwijk H, Kuzmak PM, Dayhoff RE, Carozza DN, Siegel EL. Request for Comment, Modality Interface DICOM Conformance Requirements, Version 1.0. Department of Veterans Affairs, Washington, DC, 1998. http://www.va.gov/oa&mm/busopp/formats.htm

Prior FW. DICOM 3.0 user conformance profile for modality interfacing, version 1.5. Hershey, PA, The Pennsylvania State University College of Medicine, 1994.

Siegel EL, Diaconis JN, Pomorantz S, Allman RM, Briscoe B. Making Filmless Radiology Work. J Digital Imaging 1995, 8, 151–155.

Section 6

18
PACS and Telemedicine in the VA

REBECCA L. KELLEY AND ROBERT M. KOLODNER

Telemedicine and healthcare informatics are increasingly recognized as critical components in sustaining quality clinical care. As the largest integrated healthcare provider in the United States, the Department of Veterans Affairs (VA) is changing its focus from individual hospitals to an integrated, networked healthcare delivery model that covers the entire continuum, from in-home services to tertiary care. Advances in telecommunications and the use of telemedicine will play an essential role in improving patient/clinician access, education, and satisfaction, and in reducing costs associated with duplicative clinical resources.

As shown in Table 18,1, there are hundreds of telemedicine applications within VA, with some form of telemedicine at every VAMC in every state. A current listing of VA active and planned telemedicine activities is available at http://www.va.gov. These applications support VA staff in providing high-quality, cost realistic patient care and carry forth the vision expressed by the VA Task Force on Telemedicine.

Consistent with the definition adopted by the Task Force, the VA concept of telemedicine "encompasses everything from the use of standard telephone service through high-speed, wide bandwidth transmission of digitized signals in conjunction with computers, fiber optics, satellites, and other sophisticated peripheral equipment and software" (Dunn, Almagro, Choi et al., 1997). VA Medical Centers (VAMCs) are finding uses for the full range of telemedicine applications, from "low tech" to "high tech." For example, low-cost automated response systems, accessed by telephone, have been enthusiastically accepted by patients and staff at many sites.

PACS and Teleradiology in VA

Filmless radiology offers one of the most compelling "high-tech" models for telemedicine. Although VA has been using telemedicine in some modes for more than 14 years, the VA radiology projects are in some ways the farthest reaching and most transformational, even though they have been operational for only three years or less. Their experiences to date offer lessons learned for telemedicine in general. Despite steep learning curves,

355

TABLE 18.1. Telemedicine applications now used in VA.

Clinical	Administrative
Teleimaging, including teleradiology, telepathology, nuclear medicine interpretation, and dental imaging	Hospital inquiry to the national Veterans Benefits Administration eligibility database
Remote cardiac pacemaker monitoring and evaluation	Continuing medical education, including satellite TV distance education
Electrocardiogram interpretation	National data reports
Exchange of patient specific data among hospital information systems	Patient dial-up access to scheduling and pharmacy information
Multimedia patient data	Remote dial-up access for staff into the hospital information system
Nurse teletriage systems	Networked e-mail
Videoteleconferencing	Videoteleconferencing

filmless radiology appears to be having successes in clinical and economic terms, as discussed elsewhere in this volume. The widening use of digital radiology today will foster telemedicine, specifically teleradiology, and nuture the move beyond institutional boundaries to multi-institutional networks.

Most teleradiology applications have built on conventional film-based radiology programs (Institute of Medicine, 1996). These programs have faciliated the growth of telemedicine by taking advantage of three characteristics of radiology:

- Its well-established consulting infrastructure based on mail and courier services.
- Its early use of digital imaging technologies.
- The availability of Medicare payment for teleradiology consultations.

The Baltimore Model

The teleradiology program developed at the Baltimore VAMC illustrates these three characteristics, but boasts a distinctive evolution. It was the outgrowth of the decision to adopt a filmless system for a new facility constructed in the early 1990s. Only mammography was to be film based. The Baltimore VAMC used the ACR-NEMA standard to interface a commercial PACS with its HIS named V*IST*A (Veterans Health Information System and Technology Architecture). In place since 1994, this bidirectional interface passes images and text data (e.g., patient demographics, orders, and reports) between the two systems. Considered a critical component to the operation of the radiology department and hospital in a filmless environment, the interface has benefited the radiology department and the hospital as a whole. Currently, this interface is upgraded to DICOM version 3 (Kaplan, 1995).

The interface is able to maintain a high level of consistency between the Radiology Information System (RIS) contained in V*IST*A and the commercial PACS databases (NEMA, 1994). The teleradiology system uses a DICOM interface to send patient demographic and order information from the V*IST*A HIS to the computed tomography (CT) scanner and computed radiography (CR) systems at the remote sites. The images are then sent back to the PACS at the Baltimore VAMC for reading.

With the interface between the PACS and the HIS/RIS, physician orders placed on V*IST*A serve as a "trigger" for transfer of relevant historic images from long-term storage on the optical jukebox to short-term storage. This makes the images more quickly available for review and decreases the time radiologists and clinicians must spend waiting for images to be retrieved from the optical jukebox, significantly their productivity. This has resulted in paperless, in addition to filmless, operation for the radiologists.

Imaging reports are entered into the V*IST*A system and transferred to the PACS though the interface. As reports are edited and verified on the HIS/RIS system, changes are transmitted to update the commercial PACS database. This mechanism prevents double entry of reports and makes all radiology reports available to users of both the PACS and the HIS/RIS.

In addition to the integrated text interface, there is an interface that moves images between the PACS and the V*IST*A imaging database. This permits the HIS/RIS to retrieve each image generated on the PACS for display using the V*IST*A imaging workstation. These workstations are used at VAMC Baltimore for integrated display of all imaging modalities including dermatology, bronchoscopy, gastroenterology, surgical pathology, ENT, vascular, orthopedics, neurology, cystoscopy, radiology, and nuclear medicine.

The use of the text and image interfaces to the commercial PACS has resulted in substantial improvements in data accuracy and integrity, efficient use of personnel, and economic savings. The experience at the Baltimore VAMC suggests that a robust bidirectional interface between a commercial PACS and the HIS/RIS, and complete automation of the data transfer are essential for successful operation of the system (Kolodner, 1997).

An outstanding example of telemedicine, the Baltimore model includes the Picture Archiving and Communications System (PACS) and teleradiology network located in the Capitol Network Veterans Integrated Service Network (VISN) 5. Recently three VAMCs in Maryland (Baltimore, Perry Point, and Ft. Howard) combined to form a single institution under a single director. Clinical services are integrated for all locations, with one result being the combination of three radiology and nuclear medicine departments into a single service. Teleradiology is used to support this new organization.

Lessons Learned

The implementation of the PACS at VAMC Baltimore has resulted in a number of operational improvements in the radiology service and the medical center in general, as shown in Table 18.2 (Lowitt, Kauffman, Hooper et al., 1996; Pomerantz, Siegel, Protopapas et al., 1995; Siegel, 1995; Siegel and Brown, 1994; Siegel, Denner, Pomerantz et al., 1995). The average time from when a study is performed to when it is read dropped from about one day to less than one hour. The "lost" image rate, defined as the number of studies not interpreted within 48 hours of being performed, dropped an order of magnitude of approximately eight percent to approximately 0.6 percent. The "film" retake rate dropped from approximately 5 percent to less than one percent.

In addition, the PACS has resulted in productivity gains. Radiologist productivity increased by more than 20 percent. Technologist productivity also increased. For example, CT technologist productivity increased by approximately 35 percent after the transition to filmless operation.

Although the average length of stay and the average daily census dropped by more than 10 percent after introduction of the PACS, it was difficult to determine the extent to which these decreases were the result of the PACS or to the many other external forces acting to decrease these parameters.

Clinician surveys indicated a high level of satisfaction with the filmless operation, with 93 percent preferring the PACS to film and only three percent preferring film to digital operation. Most clinicians indicated that the PACS resulted in substantial savings in the use of their time.

A preliminary economic analysis of PACS at the Baltimore VAMC suggests that the major savings are obtained through elimination of film and related supplies and file room personnel, as well as by improved productivity by technologists and radiologists. However, these savings are roughly equivalent to the additional expenses incurred from PACS equipment capital depreciation and the service contract on the system, and equipment upgrades are likely to increase expenses over time. Thus, at the radiology departmental level, the PACS appears to pay for itself, but probably does not result in significant savings given the costs of the equipment and service.

At the hospital level, however, there may be substantial savings associated with the use of the PACS. Clinicians at the Baltimore VAMC estimate

TABLE 18.2. Radiology imaging system benefits: Baltimore VAMC.

- Allows real-time interpretation of studies
- Process automated from order to report
- Decrease in lost films
- Film retake rate decreased
- Radiology utilization increased
- Film room workload decreased dramatically
- Allows more specialization by radiologists
- Some decrease in radiation dosage to patients

time savings using the PACS to be approximately 30 to 60 minutes per day. Even a more conservative 10 to 12 minutes per day could result in yearly savings from $.25 million to $1 million for a medium to large medical center. Hospitals with PACS have reported decreases in length of stay, yet the impact of PACS overall on the cost of stay has proven very difficult to estimate. It has been suggested that PACS improves patient throughput in outpatient areas or the emergency room with a PACS; this too must to be rigorously evaluated.

In a multihospital network, PACS could result in savings significantly greater than those achieved at the hospital level. Using high-speed telecommunications, a single PACS can support multiple medical care facilities in either a central location where studies are interpreted or over a distributed architecture, where the image interpretation workload is spread out. Thus, the overall cost of the PACS can be shared by multiple medical facilities, reducing the cost of the digital imaging system at each facility. Preliminary experience with large-scale, filmless radiology operations suggests there will be major socioeconomic impact on radiologists at the departmental, hospital, and network level. Understanding these socioeconomic changes will help administrators and radiologists maximize the benefits of the technology while minimizing the pitfalls that might occur with the inevitable transition to a filmless environment.

VA's VISTA Imaging

With today's technology, it is possible to digitize and store medical images in networked computer systems. These images can be viewed on workstations located throughout a hospital, along with patient record text. The Department of Veterans Affairs (VA) has implemented such an imaging system as a component of its nationwide healthcare information system, the Veterans Health Information Systems and Technology Architecture (VISTA).

The VAMC in Washington, DC, has been operating the VISTA Imaging System for more than seven years, capturing images in cardiology, gastroenterology, pulmonary, hematology, surgery, podiatry, dentistry, and selected scanned radiology films. As shown in Table 18.3, a study done on the VISTA Imaging System at the Washington, DC VA Medical Center found that the

TABLE 18.3. Imaging system benefits: Washington DC VAMC.

- Complete patient data allows better care.
- Simultaneous availability of images.
- Increased communication among clinicians.
- Fewer repeat procedures.
- Important role in conferences.
- Continuing medical education on-the-job.
- Patients can see their condition and participate in treatment decisions.
- Automatic peer review.

system "was changing clinical work in ways that physicians considered beneficial" (Joint Working Group, 1996). Clinical users felt that the system improved patient care because images were always available. It augmented other clinical information and improved communication among specialists. It decreased the time required to reach consensus at conferences because everyone was referencing the same images.

Through VistA, all VA medical facilities are electronically interconnected and can exchange information for administrative and clinical purposes. VA facilities are connected to each other by a wide area packet-switched network consisting of 23,000 miles of fully digital optical fiber network, with four backbone nodes and 22 tributary nodes. Most VA medical facilities use frame relay running at 1.544 megabits/second; some medical facilities have upgraded to the Automatic Transfer Mode (ATM) functions. In addition, T1 tie-lines have been installed among centers that share a large amount of data. This is necessary because VA has reorganized its healthcare system from over 170 independent medical centers in 22 patient healthcare networks across the country. As a result, each network is in the process of consolidating medical services across its facilities. Thus, a surgical subspecialty unit located at one facility might provide the patient care services for all patients within its network requiring that treatment.

Through VistA, increased emphasis is placed on complete and accurate computer-based patient information at the point of care. Practitioners need immediate access to patients' medical records to make well-informed, safe judgments and recommendations and to avoid unnecessary visits and procedures. VistA is focused on clinical applications that provide patient-oriented data views and allow providers rapid access to clinically relevant data during all phases of the patient's care. The VistA integrated database, designed for a multiuser, interactive environment, optimizes data entry and access while minimizing redundancy. The database management system, VA FileMan, gives nonprogrammers the ability to retrieve and display data for locally tailored reports. By adhering to national VistA programming standards, facilities may also develop software solutions for local needs. VistA uses standard reference datasets, including ICD-9, CPT, and DSM-IV codes; SNOMED codes; RDA nutrient data; drug nomenclature, trade names, and strength; states, counties, and zip codes; medical serial titles; APA psychological instruments; and standard laboratory test names. Integral to VistA is an electronic mail system (MailMan) that functions in the local environment and provides linkages to other facilities and to the Internet.

The imaging capability of VA's VistA is unique because of the variety of data types supported and its integration with an existing hospital information system. Medical images and other data, such as x-rays, pathology slides, endoscopy views, electrocardiograms, and images of lesions, can be viewed by clinicians at workstations located throughout the VA health care system network. Viewing of clinical images on workstations serves two major purposes. First, images are examined to make medical diagnoses, for example by a radiologist, pathologist, or dermatologist. Second, images are also referred to when making medical decisions, such as when a clinician examines all aspects of the patient's condition to select a treatment regimen. The image quality required for these two types of processes may be different. The radiologist interpreting a diagnostic imaging study needs to detect or exclude all abnormalities. The treating clinician may need to view a particular lesion described in the radiology report to evaluate the degree of abnormality, determine the impacts of the lesion on the patient, and select a treatment strategy.

Some specialties have defined a minimum resolution and required number of digitized bits for diagnosis. The requirements that radiologists have for computer workstations are somewhat different from those of other users. Radiologists have medical requirements for spatial resolution and brightness for the image display and an operational requirement for retrieval and display speed which are directly related to performance.

The American College of Radiology (ACR) Standard for Teleradiology (1994, pp. 168–173) stipulates that it is the responsibility of the radiologist to "provide images of sufficient quality to perform the indicated task" and to "satisfy the needs of the clinical circumstance." The ACR standards stipulate that the "display system" should be 2K × 2K × 8-bits or better and that it should support tools to perform window/level (contrast/brightness), magnification, image invert, image rotate, and linear measurement. The monitor is required to have a brightness of "at least fifty foot lamberts." This suggested standard for teleradiology can be met with a PACS workstation using a monitor that can display a 2K × 2K image. Alternatively, the requirement that the "display system be 2K by 2K × 8-bits or better" could be fulfilled using a video buffer that could hold an eight megabyte image and a lower resolution monitor such as a 1.6K × 1.2K pixel display. This would require that the physician viewing the image use the workstation's magnification tools to review the full image dataset.

In addition to the medical requirements for a very high level of image quality, a radiology workstation must offer similar or faster image throughput and handling than a conventional film viewbox or alternator. A four-monitor workstation is required for review of most conventional radiographs and cross-sectional studies to permit rapid review of current and reference images from previous examinations. A workstation with fewer monitors requires many more keystrokes and more time and consequently constrains productivity of the radiologists. Images as large as 8 megabytes (a typical chest radiograph) should be available in fewer than three seconds, and it should be easy for the user to arrange these images for comparative purposes. The database structure should be hierarchical, and all imaging studies should be accessible on all workstations.

These "special" requirements for image quality and throughput by the radiology department currently can only be met with relatively costly workstations that would be prohibitively expensive as generic imaging workstations throughout a medical center. The solution to this constraint is the use of multiple types of workstations. The VA has mixed subspecialty workstations, such as the commercial PACS at the Baltimore VA, with the V$_{IST}$A imaging workstations. These standard off-the-shelf workstations can be modified to include multiple 2,000 pixel monitors rather than the usual single less expensive 1,200 pixel monitor.

The quality of data required for diagnosis and treatment varies by specialty, and many specialties have not performed studies to determine the image quality required. Additional variables are important in other specialties. For example, in pathology, important variables include color quantization, spatial resolution, brightness, contrast, gamma, focus, convergence, and color balance (Black-Schaffer and Flotte, 1995). The issue may be further obscured because the necessary image quality will vary with the types of abnormalities being distinguished. Telemedicine makes requirements more complicated, as there may be a need for video teleconferencing for patient interaction and identification of significant lesions, and still image transmission for diagnosis at a higher resolution. At the present time, there are no defined requirements for "reference" quality images used by treating clinicians.

Digitized medical images can require particularly large computer files. A number of systems use image compression, with or without irreversible loss of data, to reduce image storage and transmission requirements. Some studies have been done to measure the ability to make diagnoses using various modes of image compression.

The ability to transmit images among institutions can meet a variety of existing staffing and consultation needs, as well as reduce the cost of outside review. It allows subspeciality physicians to provide consultation to sites lacking specialists. Image transmission offers a promising extension to quality control procedures. Sites where one or two physicians must cover night and weekend call schedules can use teleconsultation to reach on-call physicians at their residences, allowing staff to provide rapid response at lower cost. Teleconsultation can also serve as a tool to facilitate "peer review" or the provision of a second opinion for imaging studies as is required in most hospitals (Kolodner, 1997).

Other VA Initiatives

In 1996, a telepathology project to transmit live images of microscope slides and other specimens visualized in real time using a robotically controlled microscope linked pathologists at the VAMC in Milwaukee, a large facility, with the VA in Iron Mountain, where there were fewer and less complex surgical cases. Pathologists at both sites reported a low rate of diagnosis deferral and a high rate of intraobserver concordance between telepathologic and conventional light microscopic diagnosis for surgical pathology. Moreover, the system allowed pathologists to review peripheral blood smears, microbiology preparations, and other specimens for microscopic examination almost as rapidly as if they were located at the host site (VA, 1996).

More than 200 locations within the VA healthcare system provide dental care, with the majority using film-based imaging. A project at the VAMC in Washington, DC, has incorporated dental images into the electronic medical record using *Dental Link* software and a V*IST*A *Cam* Escort Portable video camera. Analysis showed that the application effectively reduced

- Image sending time from 2 to 7 days if mailed to less than 10 minutes
- A large part of the need for infection control procedures in the x-ray image development process
- The need for conventional dental x-ray storage space
- The time needed to obtain films for use at the time of dental appointment.

By making images available in the dental operatory, the project eliminated the need to move patients in and out of the dental radiology suite. It was also expected to eliminate construction and maintenance costs associated with the dental clinic darkroom (Dayhoff, 1995).

A study of dermatological imaging at the Baltimore VAMC compared exams performed in-person with exams conducted over a live two-way video link with a dermatologist. Patient acceptance was high, and clinical agreement between physicians conducting live and video exams was measured at 80 percent. Although physicians reported high satisfaction, their responses varied greatly when bandwidth differences were also considered. At T1 speeds, 7 percent of physicians said that they had difficulty examining the skin, but at one-quarter T1, about 40 percent reported difficulty. Overall, physicians expressed confidence in the diagnoses in 98 percent of live exams compared to 85 percent of video sessions (Kuzmak and Dayhoff, 1996). Dermatology is a promising telemedical application because skin disorders are common, primary care physicians have relatively little training in dermatology, and dermatologists tend to be concentrated in urban areas.

As VA continues to move toward service networks, other innovative techniques will be developed and piloted to determine whether they can be used cost effectively in the VA healthcare setting. Many are being validated in radiology applications that are able to advance because of the VA's unique nature.

Infrastructure, Policy Issues, and Barriers to Telemedicine

As in other areas of health services management and clinical practice, VA has a wealth of experience to offer with regard to telemedicine in a managed care environment. Healthcare reforms within both the public and private sectors have resulted in concerted efforts to apply tools that might help to increase access to quality and result in more cost-effective service. New information technologies, including telemedicine, are viewed as tools toward the successful implementation of health maintenance organizations, strategic alliances, and new joint venture arrangements. These tools will serve as mechanisms for increased patient participation and shared decision making.

Cross State Licensure and Liability

Telemedicine raises a number of legal concerns with regard to licensure and clinician accountability, particularly relating to cross-state practice. Although interstate telemedicine is not currently widespread, state licensure laws are perceived as a barrier to the expansion of this type of health care practice in many parts of the county. Recent state action, such as that by Kansas, to tighten current licensure laws in response to telemedicine, have further raised concerns about state licensure. Congressional interest in the licensure of telemedicine providers has taken the form of requests for information and proposed legislation anticipated for 1997.

In contrast to the state healthcare sector, VA has benefited by not being limited by individual state licensure regulations. VA staff are salaried and licensed throughout the VA medical system. VA staff licensed in one state are able to practice in any VA facility nationwide. This enables clinicians with specialized expertise to be consulted regardless of their physical location.

Third-Party Reimbursement

The current lack of third-party reimbursement for telemedicine services is considered to be one of the major barriers to telemedicine's rapid deployment. Many third-party payers have taken a "wait and see" approach toward telemedicine reimbursement. On the federal government side, Medicare and Medicaid, which are wholly or partly administered by the Health Care Financing Administration (HCFA), have varying policies covering telemedicine. Under Medicare, if standard medical practice does not require face-to-face contact between patient and health professional, then it will cover the service, as in the case of teleradiology or telepathology (Institute of Medicine, 1996). Medicaid coverage for telemedicine varies from state to state. Thus, coverage of health professionals and services also vary greatly.

On the private sector side, very little information exists on private payer coverage of telemedicine. Evidence to date, however, suggests that few private payers cover telemedicine consultation services, although most cover radiology and similar imaging services. Regardless of the payers involved, the major issue is whether any additional benefits provided to patients and healthcare professionals by telemedicine are worth the potential additional costs. This is particularly of concern to the Medicare and Medicaid programs, which are facing constant threats to their financial solvency.

The lack of reimbursement of a telemedicine application from a third party does not prevent VA's use of a telemedicine system, because VA medical centers and VISNs are self-determining based on the application's value to the strategic healthcare goals of VA as a whole, and the availability of funds. As VA's regional VISN concept takes hold, individual VA Medical Center telemedicine programs could serve as functional test laboratories where at least two of the major barriers to private sector implementation (cross-state licensure/liability and reimbursement) are not barriers to implementation.

Safety and Standards

The use of advanced telecommunications technology to deliver health care brings with it a host of concerns about safety and effectiveness. Many of the telemedicine systems in use today are adaptations of existing teleconferencing or desktop computer systems which were originally designed for purposes other than healthcare delivery. Clinicians express some discomfort with the lack of established practice standards for telemedicine consultations and equipment for any range of potential specialty applications, and the lack of large published trials demonstrating efficacy. Without any appropriate sources as back up, the clinician's exposure to litigation is increased.

It is, however, important to note that these sources do exist for teleradiology. Although there is some criticism that the American College of Radiology (ACR) standards require "high-end" equipment even when it is not needed, programs and specialists gain considerable reassurance from the standards and the aura of acceptability that widely accepted standards convey (Abt Associates, 1996).

Both the American Medical Association, which has endorsed telemedicine as a solution to access-to-care problems, and the American Telemedicine Association have studied a number of issues related to telemedicine and have urged medical specialty societies to develop appropriate practice parameters (Grigsby, Barton, Kaehny et al., 1993). Except for the ACR standards, there appear, as yet, to be no published professional standards or practice guidelines developed by the physician community. A wide range of technologies and applications falls under the umbrella of telemedicine. This diversity poses a significant challenge to establishing standards for safe or efficacious practice, especially in light of the paucity of objective evaluative studies. The lack of technical, educational, and clinical practice standards in telemedicine could lead to practices or situations that could adversely affect patient safety. For example, the lack of standards can lead to the purchase of equipment that not only cannot communicate with one another, but does not provide adequate images for clinical decision-making. Without standards, the accuracy of data that is compressed and decompressed in transmission may be compromised. Inadequate standards can also result in poor training of practitioners, in whom the grasp of modern information and telecommunication technologies is essential to quality care.

The U.S. Federal Food and Drug Administration (FDA) is the leading federal agency with responsibility for protecting the public against unsafe devices. With the exception of mammography, however, FDA does not set overall policies about safety, but determines the safety of specific devices for which a manufacturer has applied for market approval. The advent of telemedicine has created new challenges for the FDA. As a first step in addressing telemedicine issues, the FDA has recently designated the Division of Reproductive, Abdominal, Ear, Nose, Throat and Radiological Devices to take the lead role in reviewing telemedicine devices. The FDA is nearing completion on a specific classification for medical imaging management devices. This regulation avoids setting any specific resolution requirements, but offers a starting point for the agency in dealing with some of the questions created by this technology (Siegel, Pomerantz, Reiner et al., 1995).

Another relatively new and increasingly important area of potential FDA oversight is new software applications for telemedicine equipment. Of particular interest are PACS. Although most frequently associated with teleradiology, PACS have functions that are often the linchpin of most clinical telemedicine systems. PACS software organizes data files and provides image processing functions such as filtering (e.g., edge enhancement), measurement (e.g., distance, area and volume determinations), and special image displays (3D surface and volume rendering). These technical capabilities lie at the heart of most telemedicine systems (USDA, no date).

The FDA's Center for Devices and Radiological Health has convened a task force to look at the many issues involved in software policy. These workshop proceedings will be available on the FDA Internet World Wide Web (WWW) site in the future, along with more focused discussions concerning the regulatory status of software devices and any proposed federal software policy.

Privacy, Security, and Confidentiality

Clearly, privacy and security concerns are not unique to telemedicine. Because of the unique combination of the live interactive video of patient data, video imaging, and electronic clinical information that is generated between two distant sites during a telemedicine encounter, privacy concerns that normally pertain to patient medical records may be magnified within the telemedicine arena. Lack of privacy and security standards play an important role in the legal challenges facing telemedicine (e.g., malpractice) and have profound implications for the acceptance of telemedicine services.

In dealing with these issues, understanding the meaning of these terms is important. According to the U.S. Information Infrastructure Task Force on the National Information Infrastructure, "Information Privacy" is the ability of an individual to control the use and dissemination of information that relates to him/herself. "Confidentiality" is a tool for protecting privacy. Sensitive information is accorded a confidential status that mandates specific controls, including strict limitations on access and disclosure. "Security" is all the safeguards in a computer-based information system. Security protects both the system and the information contained within it from unauthorized access and misuse, and accidental damage. Security also includes training policy and training, not just technologies.

There are several federal initiatives on health care and patient privacy currently underway. The Department of Health and Human Services (HHS) has several initiatives relating to the privacy and security of health information through the interagency Health Privacy Working Group, as well as the HHS Data Council and its Privacy Working Group. The National Library of Medicine has asked the Computer Science and Telecommunications Board of the National Academy of Sciences to examine social and technical means for protecting privacy and security and to identify areas for future developing and testing; its report was published in early 1997 (Institute of Medicine, 1997). The Health Insurance Portability and Accountability Act of 1996 (Public Law No. 104.191, the Kennedy-Kassebaum bill) directs the secretary of HHS to make detailed recommendations to Congress "with respect to the privacy of individually identifiable health information" (Institute of Medicine, 1996).

Telemedicine Evaluation

Despite the growing interest in telemedicine and the need for "hard data," little is currently known about the extent of telemedicine in the United States. Detailed studies are underway to begin to collect better clinical and cost data from various federal agency demonstrations. Results from these studies, however, will take time to prepare. The vast majority of current telemedicine projects are just beginning to emerge from the proof of concept state, and it will take time to gather a critical volume of experience and data to answer many of the questions posed regarding telemedicine. According to the Federal Joint Working Group on Telemedicine (Institute of Medicine, 1996), some of the first steps for the global evaluation of telemedicine include:

- Development of a uniform evaluation tool for telemedicine projects/ applications.
- Evaluation of Medicaid telemedicine programs. Currently nine states offer some telemedicine coverage under their Medicaid programs, but there is no general evaluation effort for them to share their experiences, successes, failures, etc.
- Evaluation of telemedicine in managed care settings.
- Evaluation studies of telemedicine need to be expanded to managed care settings, and in particular, to rural managed care settings. Currently there is very little penetration of managed care in rural settings, but several managed care plans personal, most notably in Minnesota and California, believe that telemedicine might provide a more cost-effective way for the plans to reach rural communities.
- Quality and efficacy of care. Very little of current research is systematically evaluating quality and efficacy of telemedicine services.

- Evaluation of telemedicine in postacute care (home and long-term care). One study in Ohio suggests that more than 30 percent of emergency hospital readmission of Medicaid patients from nursing homes might be prevented by timely teleconsulting triage with the patient's primary care practitioners.

Early efforts to evaluate the impact of PACS, such as Flagle's analysis in this book, can serve as a guide to evaluating telemedicine applications. Improvements in the field will depend on agreement by those interested in telemedicine that it is important to invest in systematic evaluation of telemedicine's effects on the quality, accessibility, cost and acceptability of health care. The following elements to be considered in planning and reporting an evaluation have been published by the Institute of Medicine (Telemedicine, 1996, p. 102):

Elements of a Telemedicine Project Evaluation

Project description and research question(s)
Strategic objectives
  Examine how the project is intended to affect the organization's goals.
Clinical objectives
  State how the project is intended to affect individual or population health by changing the quality, accessibility, or cost of care.
Business plan or project management plan
  Specify the test of concept for a telemedicine application and/or financial analysis.
Level and perspective of evaluation
  Clinical, institutional, system, or societal level
Research design and analysis plan
Strategy and steps for developing valid comparative information
  Characteristics of experimental and comparison groups
    Patients, providers, geographic, organizational, and so on.
  Technical, clinical, and administrative processes of the organization(s) involved.
Measurable outcomes
  Identify the variables and the data to be collected.
Sensitivity analysis
  The extent to which conclusions may change if values of key variables or assumptions change.
Documentation of methods and results
  Formal documentation or publication of evaluation

In some cases, rigorous evaluations of telemedicine applications will result in positive findings that will, in turn, encourage wider adoption of these applications. In other cases, the results may be disappointing, yet they may also stimulate further technical innovation and more attention to user needs and circumstances. Thus, even negative results can viewed as opportunities. The task for evaluators is not to justify telemedicine as such, but to provide the credible and relevant information that people need to make immediate decisions and plans for the future.

References

Abt Associates. Exploratory evaluation of rural applications of telemedicine: Final report, October 23, 1996.

Center for Devices and Radiological Health. Telemedicine related activities: a white paper. CITY: US Food and Drug Administration.

Kolodner RM. Computerizing large integrated health networks: the VA success. New York, Springer-Verlag, 1997.

Dayhoff RE. Integration of medical imaging into a multi-institutional hospital information system structure. Proc Medinfo, 1995.

Dunn BE, Almagro UA, Choi H et al. Summary of first 200 cases diagnosed using real-time dynamic-robotic telepathology. In press.

Grigsby J, Barton PL, Kaehny MM et al. Analysis of expansion of access to care through use of telemedicine and mobile health services: Report 1, literature review and analytic framework. Denver: Center for Health Policy Research, 1993.

Institute of Medicine. Telemedicine: a guide to assessing telecommunications in health care. MJ Field, Ed. Washington DC: National Academy Press, 1996.

Joint Working Group on Telemedicine Report to Congress (White Paper). December, 1996

Kaplan PM. Information technology and three studies of clinical work. ACM SIGBIO Newsletter 1995, 15(2), 2–5.

Kuzmak PM, Dayhoff RE. An architecture for MUMPS-based DICOM interfaces between the Department of Veterans Affairs HIS/RIS and commercial vendors. Proc SPIE 1996.

Lowitt MH, Kauffman CL, Hooper FJ et al. Patient and physician perceptions of teledermatology: a pilot study in the Baltimore Veterans Affairs Medical Center. AMIA Spring Congress Abstract Book, 1996.

National Electrical Manufacturers Association (NEMA). Digital Imaging Communication in Medicine (DICOM): NEMA Standards Publication PS 3. Washington DC, NEMA, 1994.

Pomerantz SM, Siegel EL, Protopapas Z et al. Experience with PACS in the operating room in a filmless hospital. In the Proceedings of the 1995 Image Management and Communications Conference. IEEE Computer Society Press, 1995.

Siegel EL. Impact of filmless radiology on the Baltimore VA Medical Center. Military Telemedicine On-Line Today. IEEE Computer Society Press, 1995.

Siegel EL, Brown A. Preliminary impacts of PACS technology on radiology department operations. Proc SCAMC, 1994.

Siegel EL, Denner J, Pomerantz SM et al. PACS and medical media in a filmless hospital. In the Proceedings of the 1995 Image Management and Communications Conference. IEEE Computer Society Press, 1995.

The Federal Food, Drug, and Cosmetic Act, Sec. 201. [32 of US Code title 21] (h) (1996). Regulation of Medical Devices et al. III-5.

Veterans Administration. Dental HOST project: HOST final report. Washington, DC, VA, October 31, 1996.

19

VA's Integrated Imaging System: A Multispecialty, Hospital-Wide Image Storage, Retrieval and Communication System

RUTH E. DAYHOFF

Image storage and communication is very important in the practice of medicine. A wide variety of images are used in treating patients, including drawings, photographs, images such as x-rays and endoscopic pictures, and graphical data such as electrocardiograms. Images are an important part of the medical record of the patient, but they are not normally stored in the patient's chart because of their awkward size or nonpaper media. Rather, they are stored throughout hospitals by the various medical departments that collected them. Typically, text is used to describe and interpret images in the chart, but nonstandard terminology and the inherent difficulty in describing a complex image with words prevent full data communication.

With today's technology, it is possible to digitize, store, and distribute medical images in networked computer systems. The images can be viewed on workstations, as shown in Figure 19.1, located throughout a hospital, along with patient record text (Dayhoff, 1993; Dayhoff and Maloney, 1993). The Department of Veterans Affairs (VA) developed the first multispecialty, integrated Imaging System. Originally, it was called the DHCP Imaging System because it was an integral part of the Decentralized Hospital Computer Program (DHCP), the hospital information system developed by the VA. More recently, it has been called the V*IST*A Imaging System. The VA's Imaging System has been operating at the Washington VA Medical Center since 1990. It is also operating at the Baltimore VA Medical Center where it is interfaced to a commercial radiology picture archiving and communications system (PACS) (Kuzmak and Dayhoff, 1994). It is currently being installed at a number of other VA medical centers.

The major goal of the VA's Integrated Imaging System is to provide complete patient data in an integrated manner that facilitates the clinician's decision-making. Data are available to clinicians at any workstation at any time. The system handles high-quality image data from many specialties, including cardiology, pulmonary and gastrointestinal medicine, pathology,

370

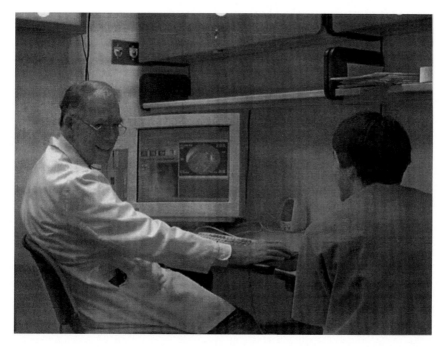

FIGURE 19.1. Clinicians view images and reports on workstations located throughout a hospital.

radiology, hematology, and nuclear medicine, as well as textual reports from the hospital information system and scanned documents. Images and associated text data are available to clinicians throughout the hospital on high-resolution windows-based workstations which are interfaced to the main hospital system in a client–server architecture. The Imaging System improves the quality of patient care, enhances clinician communication, and is used routinely at conferences, morning report, and during ward rounds.

The Imaging System also meets the needs of specialists performing clinical procedures and providing consultations. These users capture images during medical procedures such as bronchoscopies (see Fig. 19.2), endoscopies, or cardiac catheterizations and associate these with procedure reports. They identify clinically significant images, those that contribute to diagnostic or treatment decisions, for viewing by clinicians. They tend to view a larger quantity of images per procedure and have more need to enhance images during interpretation and comparison.

In addition, the Imaging System provides an excellent infrastructure to support the transmission of images among medical facilities for remote consultation. The ability to transmit images among institutions can meet a variety of staffing and consultation needs, as well as reduce the cost of outside review. It allows subspecialty clinicians to provide consultations for sites lacking specialists. Image transmission offers a promising extension to quality

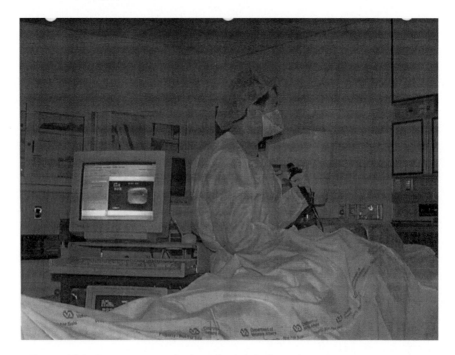

FIGURE 19.2. Images are routinely collected during a bronchoscopy procedure.

control procedures. Sites where one or two physicians must cover night and weekend call schedules can use teleconsultation to reach on-call physicians at their residences, allowing staff to provide rapid response at lower cost. Teleconsultation can also provide a tool to facilitate peer review or the provision of a second opinion for imaging studies as is required in most hospitals.

A clinical imaging system with workstations and servers provides a number of benefits for medical facilities that own commercial PACS systems. It allows the use of low-cost, off-the-shelf workstations throughout the medical center for viewing of images and medical record data. The higher availability of workstations makes it possible to operate a filmless hospital. The interface between the HIS and PACS system provides critical data to both systems to reduce double entry of data, allows the logical association of data from both systems, and enhances the information available to users. Vendor independence provided by compliance with the Digital Image and Communications for Medicine (DICOM) standard is key to making the systems work together and providing all data on any workstation.

System Architecture

The VA has implemented a unique distributed system that manages medical images as an integral part of its hospital information system (HIS) (Dayhoff and Maloney, 1993). Imaging workstations located throughout the hospital capture and display a wide variety of medical images, including cardiology, bronchoscopy, gastrointestinal endoscopy, hematology, surgical pathology, surgery, dermatology, and radiology images. Interfaces to commercial imaging systems provide additional image input. A complete image management infrastructure is provided including image database, magnetic and optical disk image storage devices, automatic image file migration among servers, image capture and display, and usage tracking.

As illustrated in Figure 19.3, the VA's Imaging System integrates data from a variety of sources, such as the hospital information system, various image sources within the hospital, and commercial image systems. Integration occurs at several different levels: the network level, the information management level, and the user interface on the workstation.

Standards are especially important for integration of systems. Standards allow systems to communicate with any other standard system, not just those purchased at the same time or from the same vendor. Developed by the National Electrical Manufacturers Association (NEMA), Digital Imaging Communication in Medicine (DICOM) is the key standard for medical imaging. It is being used not only for radiology imaging, but also for cardiology, gastroendoscopy, pathology, and dentistry. This standard describes all communication aspects of digital image production, storage, retrieval, transmission, and display in a medical environment, and how these functions are related to various information systems (NEMA, 1994).

Several other technology developments are also helping in system integration. For example, published Application Programmer Interfaces (APIs) and remote procedure calls allow one software developer to incorporate soft-

	Hospital Information System (HIS)	VA's Imaging System	Commercial Image Systems
User Interface	Multimedia Workstation with Multimedia Patient Record Software		
Data Capture	Keyboard, Pen, Instrument Interfaces	Workstation Image Frame Grab, DICOM, TWAIN, SCSI, other interfaces	Data acquisition devices, device interfaces, etc.
Data Contents	Textual Patient Information	Images, objects	Images, graphics objects, etc.
Information Management	HIS Image Management Module		
Data Storage and Access	M, RPC Broker	Windows NT/ DICOM	DICOM, SQL, Proprietary, etc.
Network	Ethernet and TCP/IP over Local and Wide Area Networks		

FIGURE 19.3. VA's Imaging System integrates data from a variety of sources at several different levels: network level, information management level, and user interface level.

ware written by others. The ability to mount servers across wide area networks allows integration of data storage. Internet communications allow broad access to data and service sources based on standards.

Network

The network infrastructure within the VA includes local area networks at individual medical facilities and a wide area network connecting all facilities.

A local area network is used to connect imaging workstations to multiple magnetic and optical disk image file servers, to the VA's hospital information system, and to commercial systems. The local area network uses Ethernet (10 or 100 megabits/second) in a star concentrator/hub topology. All of the workstations on a floor are connected to a concentrator located in the floor's wiring closet. The concentrators/switches are connected by fiber optic cable run vertically in the wiring closets to the switch located in the computer room. Each concentrator and each server is connected to a separate port on the hub.

All VA facilities are connected by a wide area packet-switched network consisting of 23,000 miles of fully digital optical fiber network with four backbone nodes and 22 tributary nodes (Dayhoff and Maloney, 1993). Frame relay running at 1.544 megabits/second connects all VA medical centers; efforts are currently underway to increase this bandwidth. Additional T1 or ATM communications lines have been installed between centers that share a large amount of data.

The VA is now organizing patient care subnetworks across the country and is beginning to consolidate medical services within the networks. Thus, a medical department, such as radiology, laboratory, or dermatology, located at one facility will provide patient care services for all locations within its network. Three medical centers in the Baltimore area have consolidated recently. This reengineered patient care process depends on high-quality communications between locations, with transmission of text, images, and other multimedia data.

Information Management

The HIS software plays a critical role in providing integrated information to the clinical user. It maintains reports for all procedures and examinations, as well as information about all images. Associations for images and corresponding reports are stored in its image management module. In addition, it tracks image accesses and handles the automatic migration of image files between rapid magnetic and slower optical storage devices.

Hospital Information System

The VA uses a hospital information system, the V*IST*A, developed and maintained by its own staff. V*IST*A is written in the ANSI standard M (MUMPS) programming language and runs on a variety of hardware platforms. V*ISTA* is in the public domain and is used in all 170 VA Medical Centers, as well as in a derivative form by the Department of Defense, the Indian Health Service, other government agencies, and private hospitals worldwide. This internal system development approach provides compatibility among systems in all of the VA facilities and allows the VA to enhance its HIS to meet constantly changing user and administrative requirements.

The VA's V*ISTA* system is different from multivendor systems in that it is an integrated system based on a central set of software development tools. All of V*ISTA*'s many software modules, such as the laboratory, pharmacy, radiology information system (RIS), surgery, medicine, health summary, clinical record, and local and regional registry modules, are based on the VA toolkit and adhere to its rules. Thus interfacing is simplified by the commonality of structure, programming language, and communications.

Image Management

Image management is performed by a software module of the HIS. Every image known to the system has an entry in the image object database file of the HIS. This file contains information about the image object, including control information about the imaging software, the list of components making up the object, the location of the object and its access method, the image attributes, and association information for report data. The imaging workstation software uses this information to access the image file servers and to control the image display. All images and patient text data are available from any workstation in the medical center to users with security access. Images are accessed in three different ways:

- Directly from a file server using its file and print services.
- From a commercial system using a standard protocol such as DICOM.
- From a vendor-supplied Application Programmer Interface (API).

Images acquired by commercial systems may be duplicated on the VA's imaging servers or accessed directly from the source system.

User Interface

The multimedia workstation platform used in the VA is based on PCI-bus Pentium systems containing a video display board with at least four megabytes of memory. The windows-based workstation meets clinicians' needs for displays of:

- True color images of up to 16 million colors per pixel as required by pathology, dermatology, and endoscopy.
- 12- or 16-bit grayscale images for radiology and cardiology.
- Other multimedia data, such as motion video and audio data.

- Graphical data such as electrocardiograms.
- Hospital information system textual data.

Digital image capture may be performed directly using the workstations. Multimedia electronic record software will be discussed in detail below.

Workstations are located in a number of departments and patient care areas. There are image display workstations in patient treatment and conference areas, including the clinical wards, emergency room, outpatient clinics, intensive care units, auditorium, and medical and surgical conference rooms. An image printer is located in the medical media department and other network printer locations. Multimedia workstations are also capable of image capture, as will be discussed later.

The VA uses a client server architecture to allow its clinical workstation clients to communicate with its hospital information system servers. TCP/IP messages are used for communications between VA developed Remote Procedure Call (RPC) Broker software located on the HIS and the windows-based software on the workstations. All messages are processed through the broker software that performs the requested operations on the HIS and returns the results to the workstation via a TCP/IP message. Security logon and server connection is also handled by the broker software. With the proper security privileges, a workstation user may connect to any HIS server on the wide area network. Workstations currently run the Microsoft Windows 95 or NT operating system. Software running on the workstations is written in Borland's Delphi or Microsoft Visual Basic, except for integrated off-the-shelf products. The use of the VA toolkit and the broker software allows the integration of multimedia data.

Images are accessed and displayed on the workstation client from Windows NT servers, DICOM servers (near future), or through API calls for electrocardiogram waveforms. First, the HIS image management module provides access information to the workstation software. Then, the workstation software performs the correct access procedure, depending on the object type. Servers may be off-the-shelf commodity items, or they may be provided by medical equipment vendors. Magnetic and optical disk storage is automatically handled by the HIS image management software and is indistinguishable to the user except for differences in image display times.

There are legal requirements for long-term storage of images. Images stored digitally must be read throughout the required time period. Practically, changes in technology may require copying of images from one long-term storage device to a newer one when technology upgrades are made. Clinical requirements for rapid access may be stricter than legal requirements.

Multimedia Electronic Patient Record

The online electronic patient record goes beyond the paper chart in functionality and readily available information. Treating clinicians use images, reports, and other patient data to make patient care decisions. They need a variety of patient information provided by many specialists in many formats. Using paper charts, clinicians experience difficulties in assembling complete patient information because much of the data is stored elsewhere or is missing. Online medical records have helped this problem by providing simultaneous access by multiple users to a record that cannot be misplaced. Its accessibility is improved by automated retrieval techniques. As image and other multimedia data are added to the online medical record, its completeness and depth of information far surpass that provided by any paper chart.

Information integration is important to the success of the online medical record. The clinical users want to be able to access all data from any workstation at their facility. It is important that access to related information of all kinds is available without numerous manual operations. Users need to access all this information with a single logon and a single patient lookup.

The workstation user interface must integrate data from different sources, including:

- HIS components such as laboratory, radiology, pharmacy.
- HIS patient record components such as problem list, progress notes, discharge summary.
- Image systems such as PACS.
- Other multimedia systems such as electrocardiogram systems.

It must serve both treating clinicians and consulting specialists, and provide display, capture, and telemedicine functionality.

A variety of views should be available for information display. The user needs access to data by patient, by procedure, by date of procedure, by report status, and by provider. In addition, specialists need to retrieve studies based on their reporting status, and on patient problem or diagnostic codes associated with the study.

Finally, patients may be seen at multiple facilities. It is necessary to access patient data from another site. This can be done with the multimedia workstation software using the wide area network.

Capture of Image Data
for the Electronic Medical Record

Data entry has always been the most difficult and time-consuming aspect of electronic medical records. However, the capture of images can be a relatively easy procedure (Dayhoff, 1993), often easier than entry of text descriptions. VA's imaging workstations are used during medical procedures, such as endoscopic, surgical, or physical examinations, to digitize images from a video source. The user identifies the patient and enters any pertinent descriptive information related to the images. This simple procedure takes less than 30 seconds; the result is more informative than providing a textual

TABLE 19.1 Image input workstation location.

Cardiology
Gastrointestinal endoscopy
Bronchoscopy examination room
Surgical pathology reading room
Hematology laboratory
Dermatology clinic
Emergency room
Rheumatology clinic
Operating room
Cystoscopy suite
Radiology department
Nuclear medicine department
Dental clinics
Ophthalmology clinic

description of the image. Typically, the clinician selects images that are significant to the patient's diagnosis or treatment course, or otherwise document the procedure performed.

Images may be captured using workstation hardware (via frame grab, TWAIN, or SCSI interface), they may be transmitted from independent systems (via a DICOM or other interface), or they may be accessed via a vendor-provided API. Workstation image capture within the VA is done in a number of locations, as shown in Table 19.1. Images are generally collected by consulting services to meet diagnostic and follow-up needs, as well as the needs of the treating physicians. Radiology and nuclear medicine images are best provided across DICOM standard interfaces in digital form (NEMA, 1994).

The number of images captured per procedure varies by the specialty. This is determined by the users themselves. Table 19.2 indicates the average number of images captured per procedure for the most common procedures.

Images may be captured directly from a medical device, such as a CT or MRI scanner, a PACS system, or an electrocardiography system. If the device has a standard DICOM Modality Worklist interface, image capture may be done automatically, requiring little or no human intervention other than

TABLE 19.2. Users have determined how many images should be captured per procedure.

Procedure	Images/procedure
Bronchoscopy	3.0
Cardiac cath	9.5
Echocardiography	3.7
GI endoscopy	2.9
Hematology	2.7
Surgical pathology	3.6
Dermatology	3.1
Neurosurgery	2.0
Urology	2.8

identifying the exam that is being performed. With such an automatic interface, generally all images are captured, including negative exams and those images that may not be clinically significant.

The VA has interfaced several commercial radiology PACS systems with its hospital information system using the DICOM standard. This interface was originally DICOM (ACR-NEMA) Version 2.0 but has been upgraded to DICOM Version 3 (Kuzmak and Dayhoff, 1996).

Images are generally collected during a medical procedure, such as an endoscopy, surgery, or radiological examination. Therefore, most images are linked to the procedure report in the hospital information system. This means that the user may easily display the report when viewing the image or vice versa. Images may be sorted by the data elements stored as part of the report, such as diagnosis, complications, and so on. The image and the report provide the data and the interpretation to the treating clinician.

Image Quality and Display Requirements

Viewing of clinical images on workstations serves two major purposes. Images are examined to determine medical diagnoses, such as those done by a radiologist, pathologist, or dermatologist. Images are also viewed during medical decision-making, when a treating clinician reviews all aspects of the patient's condition to choose a treatment regimen. The quality and quantity of images required for these two processes are often different. The specialist interpreting a diagnostic imaging study needs to detect or exclude all abnormalities. The treating clinician may need to view a particular lesion described in the specialist's report to evaluate the degree of abnormality, determine the impacts of the lesion on the patient and the relatedness of the lesion to the patient's symptoms and other problems, and to select a treatment strategy.

The image quality required for diagnosis varies by specialty. As the required horizontal and vertical resolution and pixel depth increase, the size of the digital file that represents the image increases. This means that images for different specialties from different sources require varying amounts of storage space. Some digitized medical images require particularly large computer files. A number of systems use image compression, with or without irreversible loss of data, to reduce image storage and transmission requirements. However, compression can reduce quality by introducing artifacts that interfere with diagnosis. Some studies have been done to measure the ability to make diagnoses using various modes of image compression.

Some specialties have defined a minimum image resolution and required number of digitized bits for diagnosis. Different variables are important to various specialties. Radiologists have medical requirements for the spatial resolution and brightness of the image display and an operational requirement for retrieval and display speed that are directly related to performance. The American College of Radiology (ACR) has developed a standard for teleradiology that addresses image display quality (1994). It requires the display system to be 2K× 2K × 8 bits or better and to support tools to perform window/level (contrast/brightness), magnification, image invert, image rotate, and linear measurement. In pathology, important variables include color quantization, spatial resolution, brightness, contrast, gamma, focus, convergence, and color balance (Black-Schaffer and Flotte, 1995). The issue may be further obscured because the necessary image quality will vary with the types of abnormalities being distinguished. Generally, capture resolution is held constant, so the highest resolution is required for all images. At the present time, there are no defined requirements for reference quality images used by treating clinicians.

Telemedicine complicates image quality requirements because video conferencing may be used to interact with the patient and identify significant lesions, while transmission of higher resolution still images is used for diagnosis. Slower communications lines can be used for the conference if high-resolution still images are available (Lowett, 1996).

In most specialties, captured images are selected by specialists as providing significant input to diagnostic or treatment decisions. A small number of images are stored for each procedure. Storing the full diagnostic resolution image does not require excessive storage space. However, this is not the case when automatic interfaces are used to capture high-volume, high spatial resolution images, such as those produced for radiology examinations. In this case, images have not been selected by the radiologist as being clinically significant. Viewing clinicians must select the images they wish to view. If full resolution images (2K × 2K × 12 bits) are used for all clinical viewing, the system speed will be adversely affected. An alternative approach is to create a downsampled or compressed version of these images for reference viewing at clinical workstations; the radiologists still read the full diagnostic resolution images. Another option is to allow the radiologists to select the clinically important images; this has, however, been operationally difficult with currently available commercial PACS offerings. Clinicians will need to establish image quality requirements for reference quality imaging.

Specialists view images more intensively, more rapidly, or using more image manipulation than do generalists. To address differences in manipulation and speed requirements, the VA's imaging system provides two sets of radiology viewing software, one for the specialist and one for the treating clinician. The radiologist's reading workstation supports up to four 2K × 2K monitors, uses a fast Ethernet (100 megabits/second) connection to the servers, and is based on a Pentium Pro II processor with a large amount of memory in the workstation. Interfaces to PACS systems or DICOM workstations allow the use of commercial workstations for the interpretation of radiology studies.

User Access to Information

The multimedia workstation allows clinicians to view the multimedia electronic medical record. Users sign onto the workstation with their hospital information system security logon codes. The patient is identified once, in the same manner as on hospital information system terminals. A user may access data by patient, viewing all of the patient's image and text data; this "visual chart" capability is generally used by treating clinicians. A user may also view data related to a clinical procedure, including images and report, as seen in Figure 19.4. This mode is generally used by specialists, such as radiologists, pathologists or cardiologists, when producing procedure reports. The VA's multimedia workstation allows both modes of access.

Experience

Hospital-Wide Multispecialty Imaging System

The Washington DC VA Medical Center has been operating the VA's Imaging System for 6 years, capturing more than 200,000 images in cardiology, gastroenterology, pulmonary endoscopy, hematology, surgery, vascular studies, podiatry, dentistry, and selected scanned radiology films.

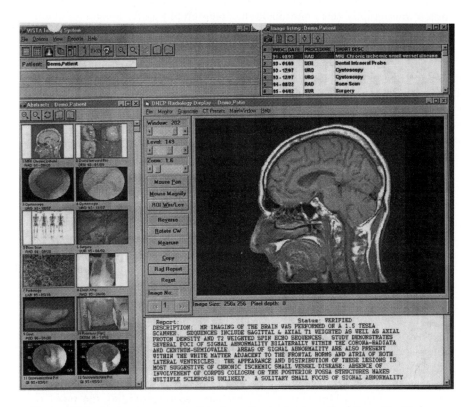

FIGURE 19.4. A user may access data by patient, viewing all of the patient's image and text data on the "visual chart" interface.

TABLE 19.3. Imaging system benefits found at Washington, DC, VAMC.

Complete patient data allows better care.
Simultaneous availability of images.
Increased communication among clinicians.
Fewer repeat procedures.
Important role in conferences.
Continuing medical education on the job.
Patients can see their condition and participate in treatment decisions.
Automatic peer review.

Five image capture workstations were initially installed. Additional workstations were added as physicians requested them. There are presently approximately 20 capture workstations in use. The number of images captured has steadily increased since the initial system implementation, both because of the increase in the number of specialties using capture workstations and because of increased intensity of use. Currently, approximately 5,000 images are captured per month. Over the 6 year period, approximately 7,500 patients have had images captured, averaging 20 images/patient. Images are typically captured to illustrate abnormal or unexpected findings, to document procedures, or to record a snapshot of the patient's condition for use in continuing care. Implementation of direct DICOM digital acquisition of computed tomography (CT) and computed radiography (CR) images is underway. This is expected to increase the number of images captured dramatically.

There are approximately 300 display workstations in the medical center. Images are routinely viewed by clinicians during conferences, rounds, medical procedures, and follow-up care. It was originally expected that clinicians would review cases individually. In fact, there is much more group viewing than was anticipated, resulting in requests for installation of workstations in most conference rooms. In the near future, the medical center will be installing 900 workstations, allowing access from clinic exam rooms and clinician's desks. This may change the viewing patterns, but group viewing will most likely continue to be very important.

A study done on the VISTA Imaging System at the Washington VAMC found that the system "was changing clinical work in ways that physicians considered beneficial" (Kaplan, 1995; Kaplan and Lundsgaarde, 1996). Clinical users felt that the system improved patient care because images were always available. It conveyed clinical information better than written reports, improved communication among specialists, and decreased the time required to reach consensus at conferences because everyone saw the same images, as shown in Table 19.3.

The growing use of the system and its integration into clinicians' processes of providing patient care has created an institutional dependency on the system. Image capture occurs during patient procedures, and image display often takes place during conferences. This means that there is an immediate need for support when a problem occurs on a workstation. Information resources organizations may not be accustomed to providing the rapid response required by a large number of workstations. Although workstations and networks have become more reliable over the past years, organizations should not underestimate the staffing requirements to support clinical workstations.

Interface to a Large-Scale Commercial Imaging System

The VA's Imaging System was enhanced for use at the Baltimore VA Medical Center by adding an interface to a commercial radiology PACS system. The commercial PACS system acquires radiology images and supports filmless operation. An ACR-NEMA standard bidirectional interface passes both images and text data between the PACS and VISTA Imaging System (see Kuzmak). Text data includes patient demographics, orders, and reports needed by the PACS system. All radiology images are transferred from the commercial radiology PACS system to the VISTA Imaging System after being downsampled. Approximately 45,000 images come across the interface per month. Both clinical multimedia workstations and radiology PACS workstations are located throughout the hospital for display of the more than 2,000,000 images that are available online. The interface has resulted in several major benefits to the hospital and radiology department and is considered to be a critical component in the ability to operate the radiology department and hospital in a filmless environment (Dayhoff and Siegel, 1997).

The major benefit of this interface is the ability to maintain a high level of consistency between the HIS/RIS and commercial PACS databases. Additionally, the interface prevents double entry of patient demographics and ordering information which results in savings in time and personnel resources. Because all orders are placed on the HIS/RIS and transferred to the PACS database and workstation, radiologists are able to view requests for new imaging studies as well as old images and reports. This has resulted in paperless, in addition to filmless, operation for the radiologists. Imaging reports are entered into the HIS/RIS system and then transferred to the PACS via the interface. This mechanism prevents double entry of reports and makes all radiology reports available to all users of both the PACS and the HIS/RIS.

The use of the text and image interface to the commercial PACS has consequently resulted in substantial improvements in data accuracy and integrity, efficient use of personnel, and economic savings. The experience at the Baltimore VA Medical Center suggests that a robust bidirectional interface from a commercial PACS to the hospital information system and complete automation of the data transfer is essential for successful operation of the system (Dayhoff, 1995).

Telemedicine: An Extension of Digital Imaging Systems

With incremental investment, digital images and other patient record data may be communicated between medical facilities to assist in patient care. Digital imaging systems within hospitals provide a firm foundation for telemedicine. Telemedicine may be based on point-to-point communication, where two facilities share patients and data. In a networked group of hospitals, such as the VA medical care system, it is important that care providers be able to communicate with all other medical centers through the network. Sites that work more closely together may run point-to-point communication lines for special purposes. Compliance with standards is particularly important as more components are added to such a complex system.

An example of telemedicine between medical facilities is the PACS and teleradiology network at the Baltimore VA Medical Center. Three VA medical centers in Maryland recently combined to form a single institution under a single director with clinical services that serve all locations. This integration resulted in the combination of the three radiology and nuclear medicine departments into a single service. In addition, a single hospital information system now serves all locations. Teleradiology is being used to support this new organization.

The PACS System at Baltimore VA Medical Center is used to read radiology studies produced at the other sites. DICOM is used for communication between the HIS and the radiology image acquisition devices. For each radiology order, the hospital information system located in Baltimore sends three separate DICOM messages containing demographic and order information. The receiving interface at the remote site places the information in a local database and provides worklist information to an image acquisition device (Kuzmak and Dayhoff, 1996). Computed tomography and computed radiolography images are acquired at the remote sites and sent over the high-speed T1 line to the Baltimore VA Medical Center hospital information system, approximately 40 miles away. In the near future, the images will be simultaneously stored at the sending site on local DICOM servers to minimize subsequent traffic on the T1 lines. The images are interpreted using the commercial PACS and then sent to the VISTA Imaging System at Baltimore. Here they flow into the integrated patient medical record to be associated with other images and patient data. The full electronic patient record is then available to multimedia workstations at all sites over the wide area network. Image transfer is somewhat slower than over the local area network, but transmission speeds are fast enough that prefetching is not necessary for clinical use. Clinicians can browse the patient's record and access images on an ad hoc basis.

The Palo Alto VA Medical Center is using the VA's imaging system in a somewhat different way for telemedicine. Dermatology image capture workstations are located at remote sites connected via the VA's wide area network to the Palo Alto facility. Images captured on the workstation are saved on the image server located in Palo Alto. These images are then visible using the VA's multimedia patient record software at any of the consolidated VA facilities.

Future Plans

Extensions are being added to the VA's imaging system to provide further support for radiology. A diagnostic quality reading station is under development. This station can support four 2K × 2K radiology display monitors on a

Microsoft Windows 95 or Windows NT client. The user can select images by study and view hundreds of images at a time. Image manipulation capabilities such as window, level, zoom, pan, sharpen, smooth, and cine views are provided. Actions can be initiated by mouse or keyboard.

Several types of DICOM interfaces are being completed, including an HIS-to-PACS interface, a worklist modality interface, and a storage provider interface. These will allow medical centers to build systems by combining DICOM components provided commercially and developed inhouse. The VA's experience with DICOM interfaces thus far has been encouraging. The success rate in interfacing is very high, with relatively short periods of time required to rectify any discrepancies in implementation.

Conclusions

Systems integration is a key factor in system efficiency (Kaplan and Lundsgaarde, 1996), capability, and user acceptance. Integration may require system architectures that provide interfaces to standalone systems. Information available in one system can be employed to assist the users of another system. From the user's perspective, all data are available from a single source: the workstation. Because of integration, data that are entered into any of the systems serve all users. This results in the availability of a critical mass of information for the users. Because users are more likely to find what they need from the system, they look first to the system and find it cost effective to place information in the system. Reaching this critical mass is essential to achieve the maximum benefits from an online integrated patient record system.

The VA has built its information systems in progressive steps. It extended its hospital information system to produce an imaging system and used its imaging systems as a foundation for telemedicine. External systems were integrated as necessary. This progressive approach avoids redundancy and lowers costs. It also allows process reengineering to take place in steps.

Many institutions today are undergoing reengineering to improve cost effectiveness. System implementation and reengineering often proceed in concert. To obtain optimal benefits from a new technology such as digital imaging, telemedicine, and the electronic patient record, some changes are required to the processes involved in providing medical care. Additional staff time may be necessary during the adjustment period to achieve savings later. Users require easy-to-use systems that facilitate their workflow and patient relationship, maintain completeness of patient information, deliver high-quality data, and protect privacy and the security of patient information.

After the initial adjustment period, users become familiar with the capabilities of a new technology. At this point, they can rethink their requirements that were initially based on manual processes. For example, radiology reading stations are modeled after alternators where four to eight films can be viewed at once. It may be possible in the future to substitute reading techniques supported by the workstation, such as the use of stacks of CT or MR images which can be flipped through or viewed as a motion image. The ability to reorganize the layout of MR images on the workstation offers advantages over fixed layouts on films. With innovative manipulation techniques, radiologists are noticing the advantages that the workstation can provide over techniques that currently imitate manual processes.

It is important to look beyond the immediate benefits when assessing cost effectiveness of systems. Often automated systems have far-reaching effects and broad benefits that may not be easy to measure. Assessments may need to wait until the system is fully integrated with the medical care processes. Reaching a critical mass of online information can take one to several years after operation begins. Premature evaluation may produce misleading results.

Integrated systems benefit the entire healthcare organization. Implementation decisions must consider organizational as well as economic and technological issues (Kaplan and Lundsgaarde, 1996). A broad group of individuals must work together at many phases to achieve systems integration. However, the value of the resulting integrated system can be far greater than the sum of the individual systems.

References

American College of Radiology. (ACR). Standard for teleradiology. Digest of Council Actions, Section Iiw, 1994, pp. 168–173.

Black-Schaffer S, Flotte TJ. Current issues in telepathology. Telemed J 1995, 2, 1.

Dayhoff R. Integration of medical imaging into a multi-institutional hospital information system structure. Proc MEDINFO, 1995.

Dayhoff RE. The electronic medical record: Data capture and display methods for images, electrocardiograms, scanned documents, and text. Proc Image Management and Communications Conf, IEEE, Berlin, June 1993.

Dayhoff RE, Maloney DL. Exchange of VA medical data using national and local networks. Annals of the NY Acad Sci 1993, 670, 62–63.

Dayhoff RE, Siegel E. Digital imaging within and among medical facilities. In: Kolodner RM (ed). Computerizing Large Integrated Health Networks: the VA Success. New York: Springer-Verlag, 1997, pp. 473–490.

Kaplan B. Information Technology and three studies of clinical work. ACM SIGBIO Newsletter 1995, 15(2), 2–5.

Kaplan B, Lundsgaarde HP. Toward an evaluation of an integrated clinical imaging system: identifying clinical benefits. Meth Inform Med 1996, 35, 221–229.

Kuzmak PM, Dayhoff RE. A bidirectional ACR-NEMA interface between the VA's DHCP integrated imaging system and the Siemens-Loral PACS. Proc SPIE 1994, 2165, 387–394.

Kuzmak PM, Dayhoff RE. An architecture for MUMPS-based DICOM interfaces between the Department of Veterans Affairs HIS/RIS and commercial vendors, Proc. SPIE Medical Imaging 1996.

Lowett M. Tele-dermatology, AMIA Spring Conference, 1996.

National Electrical Manufacturers Association (NEMA). Digital Imaging Communication in Medicine (DICOM), NEMA Standards Publication PS 3 (1994). Washington, DC, NEMA, 1994.

20
Hospital-Wide PACS: The Hammersmith Solution

Nicola H. Strickland

Concept

The Hammersmith Picture Archiving and Communication System (PACS) project was conceived in 1985, when an application was made to the British Department of Health for the Hammersmith Hospital to be considered as a research and development site for a major hospital-wide PACS project. This initiative demonstrated considerable foresight because, in those days, the technology was not available to institute a clinically usable PACS of this size. However, by the time the hospital went out to tender for commercial bids for the PACS project, it was technically possible to implement a hospital-wide PACS with sufficiently fast transmission and adequate image display to meet the needs of the clinical user. Detailed preliminary studies were made of the hospital imaging workload and its distribution (Glass, Reynolds, and Allison, 1993). For example, records were kept not only of the number of radiological examinations performed each year, but also of the proportion of examinations in the various imaging modalities, body parts imaged, the number of radiological examinations for each outpatient visit, the average number of images for each exam for plain film radiography, and so on. All this detailed information enabled us better to define the exact requirements that would need to be fulfilled by a PACS tailored to suit our precise needs at Hammersmith Hospital.

The tendering process resulted in the PACS contract being awarded to a consortium of Loral Western Development Laboratories and Siemens Gammasonics, Incorporated. This partnership was then bought out by Loral Medical Imaging Systems, then became part of the Lockheed-Martin Corporation and is now owned by General Electric Medical Systems. The results of these preliminary studies were used to draw up a very detailed legal document, the memorandum of specification, specifying the exact attributes of the PACS required and thus contractually committing the vendors to meeting the hospital's needs. Staged payments were made following conformance testing at each milestone of the installation process.

The PACS project at Hammersmith Hospital has achieved its goal of hospital-wide completely filmless operation over two years ago (1st April 1996), and since then all clinical specialties in the hospital have been using the PACS for all their inpatient and outpatient work. Hard copy film is produced only in the following circumstances:

- Cases where there is to be an outside referral or transfer of a patient to another hospital.
- Magnetic resonance (MR) reporting (while awaiting a further software development providing a reporting display protocol), although MR images are acquired onto PACS for review purposes.
- For teaching sessions held at other institutions.

Mammography is not performed at Hammersmith Hospital.

Architecture and Organization

The Hammersmith Hospital PACS is based upon centralized storage, with the images stored separately from the image information (e.g., overlays) and patient demographics (Glicksman, Wilson, Perry et al., 1992). No images are stored locally at the display workstations. The system architecture is centered on the short-term image storage device, the information storage unit (ISU), and a fast shared file system, which is a redundant array of inexpensive disks (RAID). This RAID device is connected to all the input modalities and all the hospital workstations by fast optical fibers. The ISU has a 256 gigabyte capacity, (upgraded from a 40 gigabyte RAID, which was the largest available at the time the PACS was purchased), and can hold online one week's worth of all the images needed by the hospital, using a lossless 2:1 compressed format. This allows all images to be reported by a radiologist before any lossy compression is applied to the data.

The ISU RAID can achieve sustained transfer rates of 40 megabytes per second over multiple channels. Each image fiber to each workstation is capable of transferring data at 12.5 megabytes per second. The images are written directly into the local workstation random access memory and not onto local disk. Thus the image network functions with a star topology that has potential for future upgrade to a switched technology using asynchronous transfer mode (ATM). The shared file server architecture means that all workstations can access the same image pool with the same speed, so that the ISU acts as a very fast apparent local disk to every workstation and every imaging modality in the hospital. Display of images from the ISU is accomplished in under 2 seconds.

Long-term archival storage of images is provided by two 1-terabyte optical disk jukeboxes (ODJs), which archive computed radiography (CR) image data at 10:1 irreversible JPEG compression and other modalities at 2:1 lossless compression. These juke boxes can archive all the images generated by the hospital over a period of approximately 15 years (which, incidentally, is more than twice the time period recommended for archival of adult images by the Royal College of Radiologists in Great Britain).

The image information and patient demographic data are stored separately from the images using a general purpose database (Sybase). This use of a commercial database management system increases data storage and retrieval efficiency. The general purpose database handles image retrieval queries (via default and site configurable worklists and folders) and allows control of workstations, user privileges, and exam characteristics. The separate image and database networks allow the fast specific transfer of image data on optical fibers, while retaining database access speed. The preparations for an image transfer are accomplished over the control network between the workstation and the VAX database host, whereas the image itself is transferred from the ISU to the workstation over the dedicated image network, a proprietary protocol using optical fibers.

There are a total of approximately 168 image display workstations in the hospital; ten of these are diagnostic workstations located in the imaging department. The graphical user interface of the workstations is currently based on the user-friendly Macintosh operating system, with pull-down menus, a mouse, and keyboard shortcut key commands. The diagnostic workstations have either four or two display monitors, in portrait mode (better suited to the review of chest images). Their resolution is 2K (2048 × 1536 pixels) or 1K (1280 × 1024 pixels). The clinical review workstations situated in the clinics, seminar rooms, and on the wards have one and, in some cases, two monitors of 1K resolution (870 × 1152 pixels) in landscape mode. Exactly the same software and image manipulation soft copy tools are available on all the workstations throughout the hospital.

PACS Software

A complete PACS must be able to replace the traditional roles of conventional film-based radiology (namely, image acquisition, transmission, storage, and display) with an entirely filmless electronic network in which the resultant digital images are viewed on workstation monitors. The Hammersmith PACS demonstrates that hardware technology is now sufficiently advanced to implement a hospital-wide PACS that:

- Can satisfactorily acquire images using computed radiography equipment (as well as the specialist digital modalities).
- Has rapid enough (<2 seconds) image data transmission, sufficiently large short- and long-term and archival storage for the hospital throughput, and adequate monitor luminance (228 cdm^{-2}) for image display.

If merely replacing the roles of conventional film were the only purpose of a PACS, then the considerable expense and complexity of such a system would not be justified. However, a PACS offers a number of important advantages over film, the most valuable of these being to provide an efficient image data management system, including benefits such as the elimination of lost images and the almost immediate concurrent access to images by multiple users. Other advantages of PACS include the benefits of photostimulable phosphor plate (PSP) technology and CR, such as the reduced patient radiation exposure, as well as the potential for teleradiology (Leckie, Walgren, and Vincent et al., 1994).

In order for a PACS to maximize its benefits as an efficient image data management system, it is clear that:

- The entire hospital must operate without film.
- Soft copy images must be displayed with their associated reports and with relevant historical images.
- Computed radiography (the bulk of any hospital's imaging workload) must form an integral part of the PACS.

Thus any partial or "mini" PACS falls short of this goal. Given that the concept of a hospital-wide PACS has been implemented, incorporating all modalities and examination reports, the major challenge facing all PAC systems now is the design of sufficiently sophisticated software to manage the vast amount of data acquired onto the PACS. The aim should be that soft copy reporting and viewing of images by radiologists and other clinicians should not only emulate previous normal working practices using hard copy film, but also improve upon them wherever possible.

The Hammersmith PACS software features have been designed jointly by hospital radiologists liaising with vendor engineers specifically to address these clinical requirements. The four key software features are prefetching, worklists and folders, and default display protocols (DDPs), and dictation macros.

Prefetching

Efficient automated prefetch software is essential for any large-scale PACS to be clinically operable. It ensures that any image likely to be required by the user has already been retrieved from the central long-term archive (or from the appropriate storage server in a distributed PACS architecture) to reside in the short-term server (ISU), so that it appears almost immediately on the workstation when requested. Sophisticated prefetch algorithms can virtually eliminate the need for any images, other than ad hoc requests, to be fetched manually from the long-term archive, and thereby avoid the delay that this would entail were the fetch to occur at the time when the images are desired for viewing. Rapid radiological reporting of high quality cannot be performed without simultaneous comparison of the current examination with quickly available earlier studies, where these exist.

Prefetching can only work if there is seamless integration between the hospital information system (HIS) and PACS, and between the radiological information system (RIS) and PACS (Reynolds, Mosley, Fitzpatrick et al., 1993). Although this need only be unidirectional integration, from HIS/RIS to PACS, for prefetching to be satisfactorily achieved, bidirectional integration among all three systems would be ideal for greater flexibility and to allow ready propagation of any changes made on one system to the others.

Prefetch can trigger on a number of events scheduled on HIS or RIS. The previous images on any patient scheduled for elective admission are prefetched from the long-term archive between midnight and 9 AM the night before his/her admission or review appointment, when traffic over the network is light. If the patient is due for a radiological examination, then the prefetch is triggered by the RIS. If the patient is scheduled for an elective admission or outpatient clinic appointment, the prefetch is triggered by the HIS. Patients to be reviewed in clinicoradiological conferences are listed on the HIS, and their previous images are thus prefetched even though these patients themselves are not actually attending the hospital. Thus only patients who arrive unexpectedly at the hospital (e.g., as emergency admissions) have not had their previous images fetched (if any exist). These patients do not pose a problem because when a new examination is scheduled, a prefetch request is automatically triggered, so any old images will have arrived on the ISU short term storage by the time the patient has been examined by the doctor.

Intelligent prefetch involves more sophisticated configurable prefetching rules limiting the number and type of previous images prefetched for patients (Wilson, Smith, and Rice, 1994). Prefetch criteria can be configured only to retrieve images of a specific body part, modality, number of years, number of studies, or certain combinations thereof. Hammersmith is currently limiting the intelligent prefetch for radiological reporting to retrieve just the three most recent examinations of the same body part. Intelligent prefetch is of practical value in retrieving only previous studies likely to be of value for comparison with the current study, thus saving space on the short-term storage unit.

Worklists and Folders

Worklists and folders organize the huge amount of image data acquired onto PACS into clinically useful and manageable subdivisions (Allison, Martin, Reynolds et al., 1994). From the engineer's viewpoint, worklists and folders are almost identical entities; for the medical user, however, they are rather different concepts. Worklists represent work to be done (i.e., unreported examinations), subdivided into categories such as modality or work type (e.g., unreported CT or barium meals). Folders represent work that has already been performed, now visible through one or several different folders selected for relevance in various different clinical settings. No images physically move anywhere in the database nor are they duplicated. This increases performance and saves disk space. Folders merely represent different views of the same data. Images are included automatically within some folders (e.g., the modality and body part folders) but must be manually transferred to others, such as the academic or demonstration folders. Folders are generally sets of images, but they also group exams, patients, locations, and so on.

Worklists solve a number of problems. They subdivide the workload into manageable portions that can be usefully accessed by radiologists. Without such subdivisions, it would be very difficult for a radiology department to function efficiently. A radiologist wishing, for example, to review all the barium studies he/she performed that afternoon needs to be able to call up quickly a list of all those studies grouped together, rather than having to search for them randomly distributed among the mass of computed radiography examinations also acquired that day.

Worklists cater to the specialist radiologist, such as the pediatric or chest radiologist, wishing to report only specific types of examinations that can be automatically grouped together into a specialized worklist using, for example, procedure code or referring specialty as an identifying tag. One advantage of storing the database separately from image files in a PACS is that the database can be easily used to create new customized worklists deemed clinically helpful. A list of patients by location might be used to access, for example, a worklist of all the patients in the neonatal unit.

Worklists facilitate running a department in which there are radiologists in training. The subdivision of work means that radiologists can be assigned a category of reporting work that matches their level of competence. When used in conjunction with the macro software, trainees can systematically either display and remove examinations from the worklists (after reporting them), or can just display them (allowing further review with a senior colleague later). Worklists also allow prioritization of examinations to be reported. Intensive care or accident and emergency images might be considered more urgent than outpatient clinic examinations, and the former worklist can therefore be reported first.

Folders also solve a number of problems by organizing reported images into different groupings appropriate to various clinical settings. The clinical folder is an example of a single patient folder that is particularly useful in the outpatient department. It provides a thumbnail sketch of the patient's relevant imaging history to date. It is the equivalent of the clinical summary in the case notes. The clinical folder automatically contains a configurable number of the most recent computed radiographic images, as well as any relevant images from specialist investigations (such as a CT scan) illustrating relevant pathology that may be manually added to or removed from the folder. Thus the clinician is provided, at a glance, with a complete radiological summary on the patient for quick and easy reference.

Folders also solve the problem of specialist clinicians desiring ready access to a particular type of image. For example, the orthopedic surgeon in a busy fracture clinic or on a ward round, who wants to review the progress of a healing ankle fracture in a chronic asthmatic, is not interested in seeing the numerous chest images the patient has had performed in the past, because they are not relevant to the current clinical problem. The "extremities" body part folder may be accessed under these circumstances to display the ankle images without the chest images.

Folders cater to the needs of teaching, research, and clinical demonstration. Images desired for teaching or research purposes can be transferred to academic folders issued to individual clinicians/radiologists. Such folders are visible only when logging onto PACS with that individual's user password. Every patient is provided with a demonstration and conference folder. The demonstration folder can be assembled by a nonradiological clinician or radiologist before a ward round or hospital case presentation and is a simple means of demonstrating representative images pertinent to the case under discussion. This allows the nonradiological users to save image attributes, such as text annotation, for later reference without affecting the source examination, which is configured only to allow changes to be saved by radiologists. The purpose of a patient's conference folder is to provide a repository of images deemed relevant by the radiologist which can be quickly reviewed at clinicoradiological conferences when the patient's management is being discussed. The conference folder is most useful in patients with complicated, often chronic, diseases who return regularly for follow-up and are under the multidisciplinary care of several different clinical teams. The presence of a well-prepared conference folder saves the radiologist from having to reselect the most relevant images from numerous studies each time the patient is reviewed.

One very important aspect of good radiological practice, which must not be overlooked when changing to a soft copy imaging environment, is quality control. The quality assurance folder is a means of accessing all images that are rejected on PACS. These may then be analyzed by the departmental physicist/radiation protection adviser, or reviewed by tutors teaching trainee technologists about technique. To guarantee a quality assurance program, no image can be rejected on the Hammersmith PACS without a reason for rejection being annotated on the image, and all rejected images pass into the quality assurance folder by default. Hammersmith Hospital's reject rate with PACS is now approximately 3 percent compared with 7.5 percent previously when using film.

Default Display Protocols (DDPS)

This software concept refers to the arrangement of images on monitors so that they will appear, by default, distributed across the workstation monitors in a way optimal for viewing and reporting, thereby obviating any further image rearrangement by the viewer (Beard, 1990; Strickland, and Allison, 1995). Even after the initial learning curve, there is a risk that soft copy reporting may take longer than hard copy reporting because so much more information is extractable from every image using soft copy tools to manipulate the images. It is thus vital that radiologists spend as little time as possible dragging images from one monitor to another and rearranging them in an appropriate viewing order.

It is important to remember that PAC systems are designed by computer engineers and physicists who have no knowledge of radiologists' normal working practices. Thus it is crucial that there is close liaison between clinical radiologists and software engineers in the initial design of DDPs.

Such DDPs need to be carefully designed to fit best the number and type of images being displayed, the imaging modality used, the body part imaged, and, possibly, the clinical setting in which the images are to be viewed.

Two DDPs have been designed and implemented on the Hammersmith PACS: the general chest DDP and the intensive therapy unit (ITU) "trend" DDP. They both display images across monitors so that the current image appears on the righthand monitor and sequentially older images appear on successive monitors to the left; the number of images simultaneously visible varies depending on the number of monitors on the workstation. Other previous exams, if they exist, can be brought to the foreground on the smaller workstations, if desired.

There are several differences between the general chest and the ITU DDP (Strickland, Allison, Reynolds et al., 1995). For example, the general chest DDP displays all images full screen (one on one) by default, with one examination painted per monitor. In the ITU DDP, the viewer is usually trying to assess a subtle incremental change occurring daily, or faster; therefore, it is useful to have a greater number of images simultaneously displayed. Thus, in this ITU DDP, the left-hand monitor becomes a superfolder, automatically defaulting to a higher image up-count (4:1 for a four monitor workstation, 6:1 for a two monitor workstation). Subtle changes in a radiological image are best appreciated by comparison with a gold standard. In the ITU DDP, the image at or up to 48 hours preceding the patient's current admission appears by default as the first image in the series to act as a gold standard. There has to be a balance so that the number of past images displayed is not so great that it imposes an unacceptable time delay on the painting of the entire DDP. The ITU DDP is likely to prove useful in any clinical setting in which a subtle trend in a disease state is being sought, and is already also being used to display fracture clinic images. A variety of tags may be used to elicit this trend DDP, such as the patient's location (e.g., the intensive therapy unit, the neonatal unit) or referring specialty (e.g., the renal transplant team).

A DDP for comparative viewing of cross-sectional imaging (CT and MR) is currently under development for a future software release. Each examination is divided into subsections (DICOM series) comprising pre- and postcontrast enhancement, or different MR imaging sequences. These can then be manually matched for corresponding anatomical level, temporarily locked together and scrolled in synchrony.

Dictation (Reporting) Macros

This is a software concept which allows radiologists to work rapidly and efficiently through any selected list of unreported exams. A single keystroke displays the current exam with its clinical history on the PACS workstation, with a configurable number of relevant past exams (of the same body part and modality) according to the DDP. After dictation, the same single keystroke closes all displayed exams, saving any changes, marks the current exam dictated, thereby removing it from the worklist, and automatically displays the next unreported exam from the same list in the same fashion.

Acceptance of PACS by Users

Nonradiologist Clinicians

The Hammersmith PACS has been very enthusiastically accepted by non-radiological clinical users who greatly appreciate the huge time saving that results from the ready accessibility of any image at any workstation throughout the hospital, day and night, regardless of how many other users may be looking at the same image simultaneously elsewhere in the hospital. The quality of these doctors' lives (especially true for the more junior doctors) has been markedly improved by never having to face the crisis situation of a patient's key images being missing when they are urgently needed for a ward round, clinic visit, or operating list. This factor has a number of sequelae. No time need now be wasted in arranging for repeat imaging examinations to be performed merely because the relevant study is lost or misfiled. Clinical decisions and management can proceed more rapidly because the images are available to the requesting clinician as soon as they are verified onto PACS, without the clinician having to seek them in the radiology department, or the patient having to wait to collect the films before returning to clinic.

Four large overhead projectors (Barco) have been a useful recent addition to the PACS equipment. These projectors slave directly off one of the monitors (either landscape or portrait) on a 1K workstation and project that monitor display onto a large overhead screen for audience viewing. This apparatus has significantly enhanced the public image of PACS among hospital clinicians, because it is very important that all members of the audience should be able to see the images being discussed, not merely those (usually more senior) doctors sitting in the front row nearest the PACS workstation. An added benefit of the large-screen projector is that the images are projected higher than the physical level of the workstation, and thus are not partially obscured by the radiologist operating the workstation. Two of these projectors are situated in the radiology department and used for clinicoradiological conferences and departmental meetings; the other two are in the largest of the hospital lecture theaters, and are used for staff rounds and other more formal presentations to large audiences.

PACS training has been a difficult area. Although a comprehensive PACS training program has been implemented in the hospital, it has proved an uphill struggle trying to get clinicians to attend the training sessions for which they have been scheduled. Some computer-literate doctors feel they do not need training, but the majority of doctors fail to attend their training sessions because other commitments are given priority and they feel they can pick up the basics of PACS training by asking colleagues informally. The attitude of most nonradiologists is that, provided they know how to call up, display, and perform basic manipulations upon the images they require, there is no need for them to learn a more refined technique of using PACS. The result is that some aspects of the very sophisticated PACS installed at Hammersmith are underused by clinicians. Consequently, these doctors may not be accessing and displaying images in the most efficient way, yet have achieved a level of competence in operating PACS which allows them to function satisfactorily in the clinical setting.

Technologists

The technique of computed radiography (CR) has proved quite challenging for technologists, especially those in training or on temporary attachments in the department. They must become familiar with a considerable amount of new machinery and learn some new techniques. It has become clear that technologists must receive instruction and gain a reasonable level of understanding of the physics of CR if they are to be able to analyze the reason for obtaining an image of poor quality and make the appropriate correction in technique. Features specific to CR must be understood, such as choosing the correct body part algorithm, not coning the field of view excessively, covering more than one third of the imaging plate with nonoverlapping exposures, and so on. The quality assurance folder that retains rejected images, allowing later analysis with a physicist, has helped promote a better understanding of the technical reasons explaining the generation of a poor-quality CR image and enables these to be corrected.

The wide latitude of the photostimulable phosphor imaging plates compared with conventional film screen makes CR a forgiving technique in difficult radiographic areas, such as mobile films on the ITU. Thus, it is important to check that the wide latitude is not masking too high an exposure, and regular checks must be made on the S (sensitivity numbers) being used to reflect dose. This should be instituted as part of the department's quality assurance program. Entry of the exposure mAs and kV have been made compulsory.

PACS has introduced some changes into the technologists' role. They have now become responsible for typing in the patients' clinical histories directly onto PACS so that these details appear in conjunction with the images when viewed by the reporting radiologist, making the radiology department paperless. Technologists must be disciplined in verifying rapidly the images they have acquired, as this step is essential before an examination can appear on PACS worklists.

Radiologists

Radiologists are the most demanding and least forgiving users of the PACS, because they have to work with the system all day every day. Thus, they set higher standards than the average clinician for image quality and presentation.

PACS results in a complete change in the work habits of radiologists. Training in use of the system is essential. At Hammersmith, the greatest resistance to the use of PACS was encountered at the introduction of soft copy reporting, when the learning curve was steepest. This learning phase only lasted a short while (a few weeks) and was obviously shortest for those radiologists who performed the most soft copy reporting and rapidly became familiar with the system.

PACS has been well accepted by the radiologists only since achieving a paperless environment in conjunction with the introduction of the dictation/review macros for CR soft copy reporting. This means that the radiologist no longer has to key in the patients' names or read request forms, because sequential examinations to be reported are automatically displayed from the worklists (with related previous images), simultaneously accompanied on screen by the typed clinical history for the exam to be reported. This software and mode of working with PACS has enabled soft copy reporting to be as fast as, and often faster than, conventional hard copy film reporting.

Radiologists, who are familiar with all the sophistications and complexities of the system, are the users who exploit PACS to its full capacity. Because PACS increases efficiency in their daily work, they have become adept users of advanced features, such as using keyboard command keys rather than the slower mouse controlled pull-down menus, using DDP to compare old images, thereby avoiding having to display them separately, and so forth. It is vital to radiologists that display times are sufficiently rapid (below 3 seconds) to make electronic reporting feasible. Software concepts such as prefetching are essential to achieve this.

Conclusion

The Hammersmith Hospital is now almost completely filmless. It has proved that current PACS hardware is sufficiently fast and reliable to run a hospital-wide PACS. At Hammersmith, the architecture and organization of the PACS rely on centralized long- and short-term storage, with separate storage of image files and text data. The sophisticated software implemented on the

Hammersmith PACS includes the concepts of intelligent prefetching, worklists and folders, and default display protocols. These have been essential to the successful acceptance of PACS by radiologists and general clinicians. It is already clear, although difficult to prove with statistical significance, that the hospital-wide PACS at Hammersmith is improving clinical efficiency; this, in combination with the benefits of computed radiography, is contributing to better patient care.

Acknowledgment. The author is grateful to Marc J. Deshaies for reading the manuscript.

References

Allison DJ, Martin NJ, Reynolds RA, Strickland NH. Clinical aspects of PACS. Proc 18th International Congress of Radiology 1994, 813–819.

Beard D. Designing a radiology workstation: a focus on navigation during the interpretation task. J Digit Imaging 1990, 3, 152–163.

Glass HI, Reynolds RA, Allison DJ. Planning for PACS at Hammersmith hospital. In Proceedings of the Nordic Symposium on PACS, Digital Radiology and Telemedicine. Stockholm, SPRI, 1993, pp. 37–50.

Glicksman R, Wilson D, Perry J, Prior F. Architecture of a high performance PACS based on a shared file system. Proc SPIE Med Imaging 1992, 1654, 158–168.

Leckie RG, Walgren HN, Vincent S et al. Clinical experience with teleradiology in the US military. Proc SPIE Med. Imaging 1994, 2165, 301–311.

Strickland NH, Allison DJ. Default display arrangements of images on PACS monitors. Brit J Radiol 1995, 68, 252–260.

Strickland NH, Allison DJ, Reynolds RA, Crowell J, Schuurmans M, Keller S. Organization of intensive therapy unit images on PACS monitors. Proc SPIE Med Imaging 1995, 2435, 278–285.

Wilson D, Smith DV, Rice BV. Intelligent prefetch strategies for historical images in a large PACS. Proc SPIE Med Imaging 1994, 2165, 112–123.

21

PACS in Academic Medical Centers

H.K. HUANG

Academic medical centers (AMCs) contributed substantially to early PACS research and development (R&D) by utilizing existing medical imaging, computers, networking, software, and database technologies in PACS applications. They also drove the imaging manufacturers to change from a philosophy of a single modality to one of total system integration.

In this chapter, AMCs are defined as having multiple functions including pre- and postgraduate education, research, patient care, and community service. Medical centers that provide residency training but do not have a medical school are not classified as AMCs. It is fair to say that most early PACS research and development efforts originated in AMCs; and it is also fair to say that AMCs were not the first to make successful daily use of large scale PACS for primary interpretation. Despite this deficiency, AMCs have played an important role in PACS research and development (R&D) for the last 15 years and will continue to do so.

Early PACS R&D in AMCs

The term digital radiology was introduced by the University of Arizona in the early 1970s (Capp et al., 1981). However, the concept was conceived before its time; technological development was not ready to support such a revolutionary change. The first major contribution from AMCs in PACS was the organization of the first International Conference and Workshop on PACS in Newport Beach, California, in January 1982 sponsored by the International Society for Optical Engineering (SPIE). This conference stimulated the continuous R&D efforts of PACS.

AMCs involved in early PACS R&D include those at the University of Kansas, University of Arizona, University of Pennsylvania, Georgetown University, University of Washington, Leiden University, Utrecht University, University of Pittsburgh, University of California Los Angeles (UCLA), and University of Ottawa. Most of these AMCs worked on various components of PACS: the laser film digitizer, laser film printer, computed radiography (CR), computed tomography/magnetic resonance/ultrasound (CT/MR/US) interface to PACS, high-resolution display monitor, workstation design, graphic user interface, large storage device, parallel transfer disk technology, communication networks, teleradiology, and PACS evaluation (Huang, 1996). Most of these R&D efforts contributed to later PACS implementation. In the early days, system integration and clinical implementation were not R&D topics; each AMC concentrated on its own component expertise. The importance of these two components was not apparent until the deployment of large-scale PAC systems.

The first large-scale PACS implementation was the Hokkaido University Medical Information System project in Japan (Irie, 1991). With the help of Fuji Medical Systems and Nippon Electronic Corporation (NEC), the university hospital installed a large scale PACS based on CR technology in 1989. Next, in 1991, UCLA developed the first large scale PACS in house for clinical use (Huang, Taira, Lou et al., 1993). The implementation of these two systems in two AMCs using two different approaches formulated the three implementation strategies of PACS in later years (Huang, 1992).

The first implementation method is based on a multidisciplinary team with technical know-how within the institution. The team becomes a system integrator; it writes specifications, designs the system, and selects components from various manufacturers. It also develops the system software, interfaces the system to imaging modalities and databases, implements the system in the clinics, trains the user, and performs service and maintenance. In the second method, the institution assembles a group of experts to write specifications and contracts a manufacturer to install and to maintain the system. Later, manufacturers gained enough experience from AMCs in PACS to develop a turnkey solution for hospitals which is considered the third method. These three methods gradually cross boundaries, and the separation between them has become less clear in recent years.

PACS Implementation in Academic Medical Centers

According to Bauman, Gell, and Dwyer (1996a, 1996b),

"A large scale PACS has to satisfy four criteria:

1. Daily clinical operation;
2. Three or four modalities on the PACS;
3. Workstations inside and outside of Radiology department; and
4. The PACS must handle a minimum of 20,000 exams annually."

Applying these criteria to survey data obtained in 1995, Bauman, Gell, and Dwyer (1996a, 1996b) identified 23 large-scale PAC systems in the world. Twelve of them were in AMCs. (Since the survey was performed, many more large-scale PACS have come online.) These AMCs can be divided into two categories: PACS managed internally and those managed by a single manufacturer. Let us examine some commonalties between these types of AMCs.

First, consider the PACS implementation method. The first group, PACS managed internally, includes the Universities of Brussels, Geneva, Pennsylvania, Pittsburgh, and California at San Francisco. Each institution in this group has a large R&D team and functions as the system integrator, thereby collaborating with multiple vendors. The PACS implementation method adopted was the first kind. The second group includes Brigham and Women's Hospital and the universities of Florida, Graz, Hokkaido, Osaka, and Virginia. Each of these also has an R&D team, but on a smaller scale. They chose the second PACS implementation method and depended on one single manufacturer—Kodak (two), Siemens (one), NEC (two), and E-Med (one), respectively—to manage the system.

Second, consider the question, Do these AMCs use PACS for primary interpretation? If we divide the frequency of use for primary interpretation into four categories (i.e., all, much, some, and none), then all AMCs' PACS belong to the "some" category, whereas other medical centers belong to the "all" and "much" categories. An explanation of this phenomenon is that academic freedom prevails in all these AMCs, even in terms of patient care, thereby making it difficult to mandate the use of PACS for everyday clinical use. In nonacademic medical centers, on the other hand, a direct order from the executive or management level can sometimes expedite the process. This result may seem to tarnish AMCs' contribution to PACS. However, the role AMCs play should be in their innovation and R&D, which helps demonstrate the feasibility of PACS and, in turn, stimulates its implementation in other medical centers by manufacturers.

A Case Study: PACS Implementation at UCLA and UCSF

This section reviews the research, development, and implementation of PACS as experienced at UCLA (Huang, Taira, Lou et al., 1993) and UCSF as of 1996 (Huang, Andriole, Bazzill et al., 1996; Huang, Wong, Lou et al., 1996). Six subsections provide information on assembling the R&D team and budgeting, infrastructure design, clinical consensus, implementation, clinical experience, and lessons learned.

Assembling the R&D Team and Budgeting

In the early 1980s, PACS was only a concept; R&D efforts were limited and small in scale. Most research focused on modeling, designing a specific module, or on certain key technologies in a complete PACS. UCLA took a pragmatic approach and assembled a large team with the goal of implementing a large-scale PACS inhouse for daily clinical use. The following major components were identified as keys to a successful implementation of a large scale PACS:

- Conversion of conventional radiographs to digital format.
- Data integrity.
- Digital interface to computed tomography (CT), magnetic resonance (MR), and ultrasound (US) scanners.
- Fast networks.
- High-resolution workstation design.
- Image compression.
- Infrastructure design.
- Clinical requirements.

In the early 1990s, when UCSF implemented PACS, most of the aforementioned components were understood and some solutions were available. Clinical experience gained at UCLA and data from other systems (Osteaux, 1992) prompted the realization that PACS should be integrated in the total healthcare enterprise instead of being treated as a radiology system. For this reason, UCSF added several key components to its hospital-integrated PACS. These components are mostly related to system performance:

- Open architecture and connectivity.
- Standardization.
- Interface to hospital information systems (HIS) and radiology information systems (RIS).
- Reliability and fault tolerance.
- Training, service, maintenance, and upgrades.

The methods used to assemble the teams at UCLA and UCSF were quite different. The former was dictated by environment, the latter by choice. At UCLA, the team was assembled internally from faculty, postdoctoral fellows, and graduate students of the Medical Imaging Division in the Department of Radiological Sciences. PACS was frontier research then, and it was not difficult to recruit talent to work on PACS. In the later stages of the project, when the large-scale PACS was implemented in the clinics, it was obvious that professional engineers, programmers/analysts, and technologists were needed for system stability and quality assurance. Additional personnel qualified in these areas were recruited to the team. At the peak, more than 25 individuals were involved in the project.

A core team of seven people from the UCLA PACS project relocated to UCSF by choice in October 1992. This team included experts in system integration, CT/MR/CR interface, networking, display workstation, and database architecture. People with backgrounds in computer science and system programming were recruited later to fulfill the system integration requirement. The maximum number of persons involved in the system implementation was 12.

There was no budget allocated to PACS by the institution when the project started at UCLA in 1982. Small-scale projects related to PACS components were supported primarily by private industry and the National Institutes of Health (NIH). Three early sources of support merit mentioning: an NIH research grant for digital viewing stations in radiology; Konica for the laser scanner and printer; and Philips Medical Systems for computed radiography (CR). Their support provided the seed money that enabled the UCLA team to apply successfully for an NIH program project grant on PACS in radiology and for matching funds from the Department of Radiological Sciences. The total spent on the UCLA PACS project was approximately $5 million; of this, the majority went to R&D and approximately one quarter to implementation. Approximately $1.5 million of the total came from the department. The total did not include some faculty salaries that came directly from the university.

The total spent implementing the UCSF hospital-integrated PACS from October 1992 to March 1996 was approximately $2.3 million. Of this, approximately $1.5 million came from the university and the balance from extramural grants and contracts. The money was used to purchase two CRs, one digitizer, one US PACS module, one optical disk library, one optical fiber asynchronous transfer mode (ATM) network, a mirrored database, and four 2K and three 1K workstations.

Infrastructure Design

The design and implementation of PACS infrastructure at UCLA took three years, from 1988 to 1991. The infrastructure included a fiber optic system connecting three buildings located at various parts of the campus; a three-tiered communication system with Ethernet, fiber distributed data interface (FDDI), and a proprietary 1 gigabit/second network; and a dual PACS controller located in two different buildings. It also included a mirrored database, minimum fault tolerance, and system integration software. Unfortunately, the concepts of standardization and connectivity were not realized then. As a result, the PACS remained a closed system in 1992.

The design and implementation of the PACS infrastructure at UCSF took 18 months, from 1992 to 1994. There are several basic differences between these two infrastructures. First, the UCSF infrastructure, shown in Figure 21.1, retains many of the features of the UCLA infrastructure, including a communication network (in this instance, two-tiered, using ATM and Ethernet), PACS controller, mirrored database, and fault tolerance. Second, it incorporates standardization, open architecture, and connectivity concepts so that the infrastructure will not become obsolete and can support future growth. Third, it provides an interface for the hospital information system (HIS) and radiology information system (RIS). Fourth, the system integration software has an intelligent archive server, with image routing, stacking, prefetching, studies grouping, and optical disk management functions. Fifth, the infrastructure has a server to support desktop PC users, so they can access PACS images and data (Ramaswamy, Wong, Lee et al., 1994). Figure 21.2 shows the concept of a server for distributing PACS and related data to desktop computer users. Perhaps the most unusual feature of the infrastructure is the interface engine, designed to

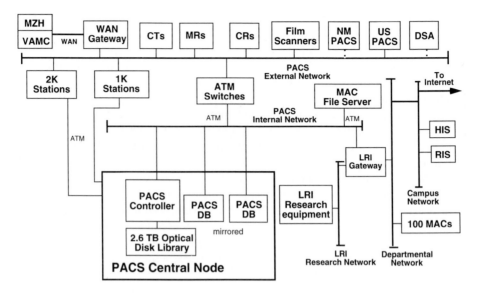

FIGURE 21.1. The UCSF PACS infrastructure. The HIS/RIS are connected to the infrastructure through the campus and departmental networks. The WAN gateway connects the infrastructure to Mt. Zion Hospital (MZH) and VA Medical Center (VAMC) through an ATM OC-3 ring. The PACS external network is standard Ethernet. PACS internal network is ATM with Ethernet as a back up. The Laboratory for Radiological Informatics (LRI) can access PACS data for large-scale clinical studies described in the Medical Image Informatics Infrastructure Design section. Mac users can access PACS data through the Mac file server. (Legend: - - - - - - not yet connected) (from Huang et al. 1996).

allow integration with PACS modules or components from other manufacturers in the future.

Clinical Consensus

Both UCLA and UCSF considered clinical consensus a very important step in PACS implementation. Before the UCLA infrastructure was implemented, two PACS modules were installed, one in the pediatric radiology section and the other in the coronary care unit, as a means of obtaining clinical consensus. These two modules were continuously modified and refined, based on clinical feedback. Workstation installations at various diagnostic sections and wards were implemented one section at a time. A prototype version was first installed at the research laboratory with clinical input. Each type of workstation normally went through three revisions before it was placed in the clinic. A similar approach was used at UCSF, with one notable difference. The cycle between prototype and clinical version was shortened because of the experience the core team brought with them from UCLA.

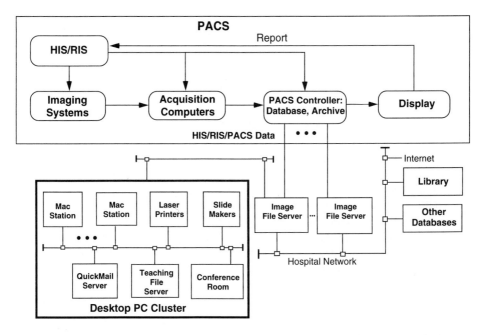

FIGURE 21.2. Concept of a PC server for distributing PACS and related data to desktop PC users. Each file server can access images and related data from PACS and other databases. The desktop PC cluster is an example of a specific image file server serving desktop PC users.

Implementation

The implementation strategy has changed over time, from "Do it all by ourselves" to "Collaborate with as many vendors as possible while remaining as the system integrator." Both UCLA and UCSF chose not to use one single manufacturer's technology. Both worked selectively with multiple vendors based on their strengths. Both designed and implemented their own infrastructures prior to installing workstations in clinical sections. At UCLA, workstations were installed in the following order: pediatric radiology inpatient, coronary care unit (CCU), genitourinary radiology, neuroradiology, pediatric radiology outpatient, and pediatric intensive care unit (ICU). At UCSF, the order was as follows: neuroradiology inpatient, pediatric radiology, neuroradiology outpatient, medical surgery ICU, pediatric ICU, cardiac ICU. Macintosh computers wereconnected to the departmental network. We also connected a commercial Ultrasound PACS module to the infrastructure.

The partnership of UCSF with ISG Technologies (Toronto, Canada) to develop and install the ICU workstation illustrates the collaborative model both AMCs use in working with manufacturers. UCSF selected ISG for the following reasons:

- Their workstation user interface demonstrated at the 1994 RSNA annual meeting.
- Their similar hardware platform.

Under the partnership, ISG contributed the graphical user interface software and UCSF provided the basic workstation architecture. They worked together on image communication between the UCSF PACS controller and ISG workstation software using DICOM. The software went through three revisions, with ICU physician input. By the end of the project, UCSF possessed five copies of the software: three for intensive care units (ICUs) with a minimum charge, one for quality assurance, and one for future research. The agreement gave ISG the right to market the software. Under this model, UCSF received functional ICU workstations at minimal cost, while ISG got a marketable product. We learned the technology together.

The implementation strategy at UCSF and UCLA differs from that used elsewhere. Its advantage is that the two AMCs are in control of their individual destiny; the disadvantage is that they must do almost everything themselves, including system maintenance.

Clinical Consensus

The clinical experiences in implementing largescale PACS at UCLA and UCSF have been mentioned elsewhere (Huang, Andriole, Bazzill et al., 1996; Huang, Taira, Lou et al., 1993; Huang, Won, Lou et al., 1996). However, one major success factor, best described as user's willingness to try, has not been discussed before. Examples exist at both AMCs.

At UCLA, the section chiefs in both GU and pediatric radiology wanted PACS workstations installed in their sections. They were willing to try and had the patience to go through several workstation revisions without complaints. The clinical staff worked with the technical staff as a team. As a result, both sections used the workstations as the primary reading tool in 1992.

At UCSF, the US section wanted to read from the workstation from the very first day the core team relocated to San Francisco. The team worked with them side by side, raising the money needed to purchase an US PACS module from a vendor and collaborating with the vendor to interface the module to the PACS infrastructure. One week after the module was online, the US section went digital and used the workstations for all primary diagnosis. Currently this section archives all digital images, printing only six images on a sheet of 8- × 10-inch film for a patient's file.

When the core team arrived at UCSF, ICU physicians knew that their colleagues at UCLA were using PACS workstations and expressed their desire to have them also. At that time, UCSF had no computed radiography (CR) and no high-speed network. During the two years it took to install two CRs, set up the ATM network, and develop a second generation workstation for ICU use, the ICU physicians were most patient and contributed their ideas on how the workstation should be. Immediately after the installation, the workstation was in use. Regrettably, because the project was not funded by the institution, only three workstations could be installed.

The situation in neuroradiology was somewhat different. A very large section, its physicians cover four hospitals in the San Francisco Bay area, including UCSF's second campus at Mt. Zion Hospital (MZH). When they expressed the need for teleradiology service between UCSF nor MZH, the team worked with them to apply for extramural support, obtained the money needed for the ATM wide area network connection, and implemented two workstations, one each in the inpatient and outpatient reading areas.

The users in these five clinical sections all made important contributions to the success of PACS. Unlike other medical center, neither UCLA or UCSF had large sums of money allocated for PACS installation. Both AMCs implemented the infrastructure and workstations by raising money as needed.

Lessons Learned

The core team working to implement PACS at UCLA and UCSF learned three valuable lessons:

- Secure sufficient funds before starting each of the implementation phases. Most large-scale PACS in other medical centers have been installed with sufficient initial funds and a continuous annual budget for maintenance and upgrade from the medical center. UCLA and UCSF raised funds as the projects moved along. This strategy created anxiety at several critical moments.
- Assemble two teams if possible. In most imaging companies, all products go through two distinct phases, engineering and production. As an AMC, UCSF assembled an R&D team that was always in the engineering phase to fine tune the system. This team was reluctant to perform maintenance and service when the system became operational in 1995. Yet because there was no second team, the R&D team had to stretch to meet the responsibilities for continuous engineering work and for daily operations.[1]
- Realize that it may not be possible to satisfy everyone. In an AMC, colleagues tend to treat a PACS implementation as an R&D project and request workstation connections to the PACS for their specialty. At UCSF, the team could not fulfill most of the requests due to budget and manpower constraints. Some clinicians understood the team's difficulty, but some did not. This created some embarrassing moments.

---

[1] Since April 1996, the USCF PACS research and development team has split into two units: a clinical team takes care of the daily PACS operation and continuous clinical growth; and a research team continues R&D effort on PACS and related topics.

Future PACS Research

After 15 years of R&D efforts, the imaging community understands and has resolved most PACS-related issues in engineering, system integration, operation, and cost analysis. Two areas for future PACS development remain: the role of AMCs in both digital mammography and medical image informatics infrastructure design.

Digital Mammography

One last missing link in a filmless radiology department is the conversion from film-based mammography. Digital mammography requires a very high spatial resolution digital image of up to $4K \times 5K \times 12$-bits. This level of resolution necessitates a new image acquisition device for direct digital output, a high-resolution workstation for display, a large disk space for storage, and a high-speed communication network for image transmission. Existing mammography technology cannot satisfy some of these requirements. Early applications acquired data by digitizing conventional mammography films. This approach severely limits the potential of digital mammography because the resultant images can contain no more radiographic information than the standard films from which they are produced. Indeed, most current digitized images are slightly inferior in quality to their corresponding parent films, accounting in no small part for the general lack of clinical acceptance of digital mammography applications.

Direct digital mammography can overcome most of these problems and at the same time provide features not available with standard mammographic imaging (Sickles, 1993). During the past several years, the concentrated efforts from the National Cancer Institute and the United States Army Medical Research and Development Command, have resulted in the development of some prototype direct digital mammography systems. This is a joint effort between academic institutions and the private industry. Some of these systems are ready for clinical evaluation (Nelson, 1995).

Image acquisition and display are major components in a digital mammography system. The basic requirement for general use is the ability to portray the entire breast with such fine detail that tiny structures, such as malignant microcalcifications, are readily retained by the acquisition and made visible by the display. Furthermore, because routine mammographic interpretation involves four images of a current examination compared with four images from a prior examination, digital workstations either must include at least eight monitors or utilize monitors providing sufficiently fine detail that two or more whole-breast mammograms are displayed per monitor (Lou, Huang, and Breant, 1992). As including full-field direct digital mammography in PACS is a very expensive R&D effort involving contributions from manufacturers, government funding agencies, and clinical sites, we anticipate AMCs will play a major role in this development.

Our involvement in this R&D effort is to explore teleradiology mammography or telemammography applications (Lou, Sickles, and Huang, 1997). Radiologists who work in several different offices or hospitals will be able to monitor and interpret examinations that are carried out in a nearby or even at a distant location or locations. This will permit radiologists with the greatest interpretive expertise to manage and read in real time all mammography examinations, an operational procedure far superior to the alternative of choosing between deferred interpretation by expert readers or real-time interpretation by general radiologists (Sickles, 1992; Sickles, Ominsky, Sollitto et al., 1990). Real time is defined in this context as a very rapid turnaround time between examination and interpretation. In addition, mammography screening in mobile units will be made more efficient, not only by overcoming the need to transport films from the site of examination to the site of interpretation, but also by permitting image interpretation while patients are still available for repeat or additional exposures. Furthermore, telemammography can be used to facilitate second-opinion interpretation, in effect making world-class mammography expertise immediately accessible to community-practice radiologists.

Medical Image Informatics Infrastructure Design

The second area through which AMCs can contribute to the continuous growth of PACS is the medical image informatics infrastructure design (MIII) (Huang, Wong, Pietka, 1997). A PACS involves system integration of multimodality images and health information systems originally designed for improving radiology operations. As it evolves, PACS becomes a hospital image management system with a voluminous image and related data file depository. A properly designed MIII can take full advantage of the enormous volume of data from PACS and other related medical databases to achieve new levels of clinical, research, and educational applications that could not be performed before because of insufficient data. The infrastructure design can only be originated from AMCs because it requires the involvement of a multidisciplinary team to initiate the process. Other medical centers may not have sufficient manpower and resources to launch the concept.

Our effort in this area of research is to design and implement a MIII within the current existing PACS framework shown in Figure 21.3 (Wong and Huang, 1996). Our current MIII is comprised of the following components: medical images and associated data (including a PACS database), image postprocessing, data/knowledge base management, visualization, graphical (or multimedia) user interface, communication, and application oriented software. Databases of PACS and other related health information systems, comprised of patient demographic data, medical images, and diagnostic reports, constitute the data source in the MIII. This data is organized and archived with standard data formats and protocols, such as DICOM for image and HL7 for text. This input data component

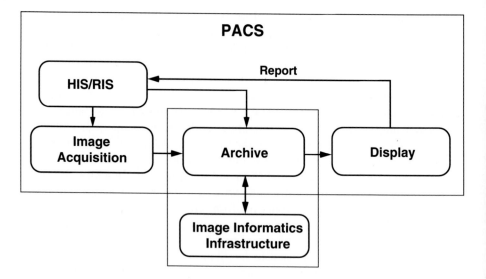

FIGURE 21.3. Medical Imaging Informatics Infrastructure (MIII) design based on an existing PACS framework.

can be designed as an input server, which extracts relevant data from the PACS database either automatically or manually. The server can have a generic architecture with specific types of data extraction software for a given application. Within this MIII, we have been able to launch several large-scale longitudinal and horizontal clinical projects with data derived from PACS and other related databases. Some of these projects are:

- Bone age assessment with a digital hand atlas (Pietka and Huang, 1996; Pietka, Kaabi, Kuo et al., 1993;)
- Effectiveness of therapy treatment planning using spiral CT images (Zhu, Lee, Levin et al., 1996)
- Noninvasive surgical planning using multimodal neuroimages (Wong, Soo Hoo et al., 1996)
- Collaborative consultation with high-resolution images from PACS database (Wong and Huang, 1996). Figure 21.4 shows steps involved and Figure 21.5 illustrates a teleconference session with PACS data

This MIII can also support the current concept of using the Web server to distribute PACS data through Internet and Intranet.

Summary

During the early years of PACS research and development and more recently as well, AMCs have contributed many technological advances for PACS

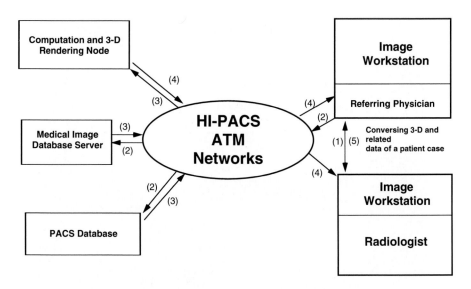

FIGURE 21.4. Collaborative consultation with high resolution images from PACS database. Video conference uses "Store and Forward," whereas collaborative consultation allows query to large databases, perform high speed computation, and return results with high resolution images almost in real time. Steps are as follow: (1) Referring physician (RP) requests for a consultation session with the radiologist. (2) RP sends request to HI-PACS networks searching images from PACS database and related medical image database server. (3). Data return from the server and the PACS database and are sent to the computation and 3-D rendering node. (4) Computational results return to both the RP and radiologist workstation almost in real time. (5) Collaborative consultation in process (from Huang, 1996).

implementations, including the use of optical disks for long-term archive, high-speed networking, interfacing to imaging acquisition devices, display workstation design, and system integration. The experiences of two AMCs, namely UCLA and UCSF, in implementing large-scale PACS offer valuable lessons. Moreover, AMCs are playing and will continue to play an important role in the development of digital mammography.

AMCs have also contributed to the research frontier through the design of medical image informatics infrastructure (MIII) based on the existing PACS framework. Implementation of the medical image informatics infrastructure is the next logical step after the PACS is in place. With the MIII, we can advance our biomedical knowledge to new levels of application in longitudinal and large-scale horizontal clinical studies, and to initiate novel research and educational programs. All of these would result in a better health care delivery system. We can consider MIII as life after PACS.

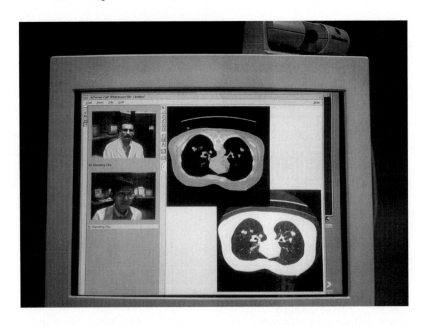

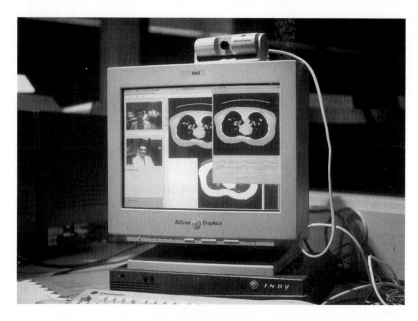

FIGURE 21.5. Collaborative teleconferencing. (Top) Referring physician at upper left window; Radiologist at lower left window. (Bottom) Referring physician at lower left window; Radiologist at upper left window. High-resolution CT images from PACS database are retrieved for consultation.

Acknowledgments. The author would like to thank all individuals who have contributed to the UCLA and UCSF PACS implementations. The PACS development at UCSF has been partially supported by the following: NLM contract N01-LM-4-3508; NLM contract N01-LM-6-3547; NCHS BPA 50257C-95, National Center for Health Statistics;US Army Medical R&D DAMD 17-94-J-4338; US Army Medical R&D DAMD 17-96-C-6111; US Army Medical R&D DAMD 17-94-J-4196; US DHHS 282-97-0057; Lumisys (equipment); Fuji Medical Systems USA, Inc. (equipment); Abe Sekkei, Japan (equipment); Philips Medical Systems DPA 109; and California Breast Research Program 1RD-0148.

References

Bauman RA, Gell G, Dwyer SJ. Large scale picture archiving and communication systems of the world. Part 1. J Digital Imag, 1996a, 9(3), 99–103.

Bauman RA, Gell G, Dwyer SJ. 1996b. Large scale picture archiving and communication systems of the world - part 2. J Digital Imag, 9(4), 172–177.

Capp MP et al. Photoelectronic radiology department. Digital Radiography, Proceedings of the Society of Photo-Optical Instrumentation Engineers, 1981, 3A, 2–8.

Huang HK. Three methods of PACS research, development, and implementation. RadioGraphics, 1992, 12, 131–139.

Huang HK. PACS: Picture Archiving and Communication Systems in Biomedical Imaging. New York, VCH/Wiley & Sons, 1996.

Huang HK, Andriole K, Bazzill T et al. Design and implementation of PACS: the second time. J Digital Imag, 1996, 9(2), 47–59.

Huang HK, Taira RK, Lou SL et al. Implementation of a large scale picture archiving and communication system. J Comp Med Imaging and Graphics, 1993, 17(1), 1–11.

Huang HK, Wong AWK, Lou SL et al. Clinical experience with a second generation PACS. J Digital Imag, 1996, 9(4), 151–166.

Huang HK, Wong STC STC, Pietka E. Medical Image Informatics Infrastructure Design and Applications. Medical Informatics 1997, 22(4), 279–289.

Irie G. Clinical experience: 16 months of hi-PACS in picture archiving and communication systems. In: Huang HK et al. (eds). Picture archiving and communication systems, NATO ASI series F, volume 74. Berlin, Springer-Verlag, 1991, pp. 183–188.

Lou SL, Huang HK, Breant CM. A 2K Radiological Image Display Station. Radiology 1992, 185(P), 146.

Lou SL, Sickles EA, Huang HK et al. Full-field Direct Digital Telemammography: Technical Components, Study Protocols, and Preliminary Results. IEEE Trans. on Inform Tech Biom 1997, 1(4), 270–278.

Nelson MT. A clinician's view of digital mammography. Proceedings of the 4th International Conference on Imaging Management and Communications. IMAC, 1995.

Osteaux M. A second generation PACS concept. Berlin, Springer-Verlag, 1992.

Pietka E, Huang HK. Epiphyseal fusion assessment based on wavelets decomposition analysis. J Comp Med Imaging Graphics 1996, 19(6), 465–472.

Pietka E, Kaabi L, Kuo ML, Huang HK. Feature extraction in carpal bone analysis. IEEE Trans. Medical Imaging, 1993, 12, 44–49.

Ramaswamy MR, Wong AWK, Lee JK et al. Accessing a PACS text and image information through personal computers. Am J Roentgenology, 1994, 163, 1239–1243.

Sickles EA. Quality assurance: How to audit your own mammography practice. Radiol Clin North Am 1992, 30, 265–275.

Sickles EA. Current status of digital mammography. Proceedings of the 7th International Congress on Senology (Excerpta Medica International Congress Series). Amsterdam, Elsevier, 1993.

Sickles EA, Ominsky SH, Sollitto RA et al. Medical audit of a rapid-throughput mammography screening practice: methodology and results of 27,114 examinations. Radiology 1990, 175, 323–327.

Wong STC, Huang HK. A hospital integrated framework for multimodality image base management, IEEE Trans. System, Man, and Cybernetics 1996, 26(4), 455–469.

Wong STC, Soo Hoo K, Knowlton RC. Use of image coregistration and visualization techniques to study relationships between MEG neurophysiology and FDG-PET metabolism in epilepsy imaging. Proc Medical Imaging, SPIE 1996, 2709, 280–289.

Zhu XM, Lee KN, Levin DL et al. Temporal image database design for outcome analysis. J Comp Med Imaging Graphics 1996, 347–356.

Glossary

DAVID S. CHANNIN AND PAUL J. CHANG

A

ACR-NEMA A joint committee of the American College of Radiology and the National Electrical Manufacturers' Association that has developed the DICOM standard for medical image communication. The DICOM standard documents are distributed by NEMA, 1300 N 17th St, Ste 1847, Rosslyn, VA 22209; (703) 841-3200 or *www.nema.org*.

ANSI American National Standards Institute. A private-sector, nonprofit, membership organization that facilitates the development of standards and is the sole U.S. representative to the ISO. The ANSI is also the party responsible (in the United States) for assigning universal identifiers for use in DICOM communications. Although these identifiers can be provided by the system vendors, institutions may want to obtain their own. The ANSI is at 11 W 42nd St, New York, NY 10036; (212) 642-4900 or *www.ansi.org*.

ATM Asynchronous transfer mode. A relatively high-speed, low-level networking protocol usually but not exclusively based on fiber-optic wiring. Typical network speeds are 100 Mbits/sec to 2 Gbits/sec. Information (data and voice) is broken into small pieces called cells, which are routed over the ATM network. Advantages of this technology, in addition to its high speed, are its combined use in voice, data, and multimedia communications and its ability to provide (different) guarantees of quality of service. Although ATM is not yet completely accepted as a standard, interoperability between differing vendors is very high.

Authentication The process whereby the identity of a computer user is verified electronically. A user typically enters a user name into a computer system and is prompted for a password. The password authenticates the user to the system. There are many mechanisms for authentication, many of which provide more security than just a password.

B

Backbone A larger network that connects smaller networks. For example, the Internet is usually considered to consist of a high-speed backbone

---

[1] Originally published by David S. Channin and Paul J. Chang, "Part Five: Glossary," in RadioGraphics, September-October 1997, Volume 17, Number 5, pages 1310–1315. Reprinted with Permission from the Radiological Society of North America

operated by the major telecommunication and Internet service providers; this backbone connects slower, smaller segments of the Internet. An analogy can be made to a corporate intranet, which might have a high-speed central network with slower, smaller subsidiary networks to individual work groups.

Bandwidth   A measure of the amount of information that can be transferred across a communication channel. Bandwidth is usually measured in bits or bytes per second with the appropriate prefix (kilo-, mega-, or giga-) added as necessary. Because networks operate at multiple layers, the different layers may "perceive" differing amounts of bandwidth over the same channels. Usually, the lower levels have more bandwidth available to them than the application level due to overhead introduced by the intervening layers. Of importance to the user is the available bandwidth at the application program level rather than the theoretical bandwidth available from the channel. This net bandwidth effect must be taken into account when the planning networks.

Baud   The signaling rate of a communication channel in symbols per second. This unit roughly coincides with bits per second. Originally a measure of telegraph signaling speed (equivalent to one morse code dot per second), the baud was proposed at the 1927 International Telegraph Conference. The baud is named after French engineer J. M. E. Baudot (1845-1903), who constructed the first successful teleprinter.

Big endian   One way data are stored and transmitted within the context of the DICOM standard. In a big endian format, the most significant bit is sent first; in a little endian format, the least significant bit is sent first. The distinction arose (and is maintained) because of the way different hardware platforms (ie, the processing chips themselves) deal with the digital data. The nature of the transmission in DICOM (ie, little endian vs big endian) is negotiated between the client and the server at the start of the communication session.

Bit   A binary digit (0 or 1) (cf **byte**).

Bridge   A network connectivity device used to interconnect two or more segments of a network. More advanced than a repeater, a bridge looks at each packet individually and decides if the packet should be allowed across the bridge. Technically, a bridge is a network layer 2 (data link layer) device, as opposed to a repeater, which is a layer 1 (physical layer) device, or a router, which is a layer 3 (network layer) device.

Byte   Eight bits, enough to store one character. A kilobyte is 1,024 bytes ($2^{10} = 1,024$). Two kilobytes is approximately one typed page of text; 10 kbytes is equivalent to a finely typed page of text (eg, in a dictionary); 100 kbytes is the size of an uncompressed (cf **compression**), low-resolution (640×480 pixels) color image on the Web. A megabyte is technically 1,048,576 bytes ($1,024 \times 1,024$ or 2^{20}), roughly the amount of information that can be stored on the original 3.5-inch floppy disk. (Later 3.5-inch floppy disks can hold almost 2 Mbytes.) Five megabytes is roughly the size of the complete works of Shakespeare; 10 Mbytes is the size of a single diagnostic-quality digital radiograph of the chest (uncompressed); 40 Mbytes is roughly the size of a single digital mammogram (uncompressed). A CD-ROM can store approximately 680 Mbytes. A gigabyte is 1 billion bytes ($1,024 \times 1,024 \times 1,024$ or 2^{30}), which is the same as 1,000 Mbytes or 1 million kbytes. One gigabyte is equivalent to 2 minutes of full-motion video (uncompressed) or 50 posteroanterior and lateral radiographs of the chest. A terabyte is 1 trillion bytes ($1,024 \times 1,024 \times 1,024 \times 1,024$ or 2^{40}) or 1,000 Gbytes. Two terabytes is roughly the amount of image data generated in 1 year by a small teaching hospital. A petabyte is 1,000 Tbytes.

C

CCITT   Consultative Committee for International Telephony and Telegraphy. A working group of the International Telecommunications Union that develops standards for international voice, data, and radio communications.

CD-ROM   Compact disk, read-only memory. An optical disk used to store approximately 680 Mbytes of digital information. There are several data format standards for writing information to CD-ROMs. These include standards for audio, video, and data. The most common standard for data storage is the ISO 9660 format, which is readable by many platforms. The term *High Sierra* used in the context of CD-ROMs refers to the location of a workshop, the purpose of which was to modify the standard slightly.

Certificate   A digital document usually provided by a recognized, trusted third party that contains information identifying the user to a computer system.

Client   A computer program that communicates (usually via a network) with a remote system and requests information from this remote system (the server) or the computer system on which this program executes. For example, a client workstation such as a personal computer might run a client program such as a Web browser. A thick client is a client workstation (eg, a personal computer or advanced workstation) that has significant local processing, memory, and storage capacity. A thin client is a client workstation that has minimal local processing or storage and merely acts as a sophisticated interface to network resources (servers).

Compression   Mathematical reduction of the size of a piece of data to reduce the amount of time needed to transmit the data or the amount of space needed to store it. There are two broad categories of compression algorithms: loss-less and lossy. Loss-less compression techniques mathematically reduce the size of a piece of data so that the process can be mathematically reversed perfectly. There is no loss of information. In lossy compression, some degradation of the data occurs that cannot be reversed. Loss-less compression techniques can reduce the size of an image and then restore the image perfectly. However, with lossy compression, there will be loss of image information that can never be completely reversed. Lossy algorithms are still attractive because in general they produce much higher levels of compression (10-30:1 compression vs 2-5:1 compression).

Concentrator   A networking device that multiplexes connections so that increased bandwidth can be created or shared. For example, a concentrator might merge four separate 2,400-baud modems into one 9,600-baud channel. Occasionally, this term is casually used to refer to a network repeater.

CORBA   Common object request broker architecture. CORBA is a definition of a standard way for client-server systems from different vendors to communicate information in the form of objects. CORBA is being developed by the Object Management Group (OMG). A subcommittee of the OMG (CORBAmed) is defining how medical information objects, including those defined in HL7 and DICOM, can be communicated successfully in a heterogeneous, networked client-server environment. The OMG is at 492 Old Connecticut Path, Framingham, MA 01701; *http://www.omg.org*.

D

DICOM   Digital Imaging and Communications in Medicine. An industry standard for the transmission of medical images and related information. ACR-NEMA is responsible for the ongoing development of the standard. The standard is both object oriented and client-server. Services are defined in terms of SOPs (service-object pairs). The SOPs define not only the service to be provided but the data on which a particular service will operate (cf **SCP** and **SCU**).

Digital signature   An electronic signature to a message so that the originator of the message can be at least as well identified as if he or she had physically signed the message. In particular, a digital signature is a peculiarity of certain mathematical methods of encryption. In public key cryptography (a popular and robust method used for the majority of high-level digital security needs, including the Internet), the user has a private code number and a related (in some complex mathematical sense) public code number. If someone wants to send the user an encrypted message, the sender uses the public code to encrypt (render illegible) the message; only the legitimate recipient has the private code to decrypt (render legible) the message. Due to symmetry of the mathematical algorithms used, the message can be signed by first passing it through a private code and then through someone else's public code. The recipient uses his or her private code to decrypt the message, then uses the sender's public code to decrypt the message again. Because only the sender could have used the sender's private code to perform the first encryption, the recipient can be certain that the message is from the sender. Much of the complexity of this transaction is hidden from the user, and the code numbers required for the transaction (often large) are usually stored in certificates.

DNS   Domain name service. An application program just like any other except that it is usually run by other programs to look up addresses on the Internet (although it can be run manually). When a user of a program (eg, a Web browser) types in the fully qualified domain name of a site to visit (eg, *www.rsna.org*), it is unlikely that the user's computer will know the Internet address of the requested site. Instead, the Web browser program requests the address from the Internet service provider's machine. If that machine does not know the address, a hierarchical search is conducted in real time until a machine is identified that believes it knows the address of the machine in question; this information is returned to the user's computer. This looking up of the Internet address of a machine explains the momentary pause that typically occurs before information is transferred from a Web site being visited for the first time.

Domain   The domain is a portion of the name of a machine on the Internet (or an intranet). It identifies, in some not always direct way, the owner of the machine or at least the party responsible for the machine. To locate a computer on the Internet, the machine must have a fully qualified name. The fully qualified name can then be translated into the IP address of the machine by the DNS. This process is analogous to looking up someone's telephone number in the telephone book but is much more automated. The first part of the fully qualified name of a machine is the specific machine's local name. The second part of the machine's name is the domain name, and the third part is the top-level domain name. For example, there are many computers named "bob" on the Internet. Within any given domain, however, there can be only one computer named "bob." Thus, "bob.toyota" would be unique within the "toyota" domain. The last part of a fully qualified domain name is the top-level domain. Until recently, there were only a handful of top-level domains ("edu" for educational sites, "org" for nonprofit organizations, "gov" for the U.S. government, and "com" for commercial organizations). There are now proposals to create many more top-level domains, and this will likely occur in the coming years. Thus, "bob.toyota.com" would be a fully qualified domain name, indicating a computer named "bob" within the "toyota" domain, which itself is in the "com" top-level domain.

DVD   Digital versatile (video) disk. A new, industry-standard, 5-inch-diameter optical disk that can store approximately 5 Gbytes (almost 10 times as much as a CD-ROM). The DVD has already been adopted for use in the music and motion picture industries and will likely become a standard for information storage.

E

Ethernet   Originally developed by Digital Equipment, Xerox, and Intel, the Ethernet is a low-level networking standard, adopted by the IEEE as standard number 802.3. This standard, in common use in local area networks, defines certain kinds of wiring and the electric signals that must be sent over them. Many high-level protocols, including TCP and IP, can run over this low-level protocol.

F

Firewall   A computer system that connects two or more networks with the intent of securing or isolating one network from another. The "filtering" performed by the firewall can occur at one or more levels or the network protocols.

FTP   File transfer protocol. One of the original, high-level protocols designed for reliable transfer of files from one computer to another via the Internet. The protocol requires the permission of the sender and the recipient. Anonymous FTP is a variant of FTP in which the permission of the recipient (get) or the sender (put) is implicitly given by logging into the remote system under the user name "anonymous." A tremendous amount of information, programs, graphics, and so on can be accessed by using anonymous FTP from a myriad of machines. A database of the anonymous FTP sites and their contents (called "Archie") is now available via the Web.

G

Gateway   An imprecise term referring to devices (hardware or software) that interconnect protocols or networks. For example, an Internet gateway might be nothing more than a router or a firewall. On the other hand, a mail gateway might be a high-level application that connects two mail systems.

H

HIS   Hospital information system. One or more computer systems in a hospital that handle the information necessary to operate a health care facility. Such information systems usually include admission, discharge, and transfer (ADT) information; billing systems; pharmacy systems; scheduling; and materials management.

HL-7   Health Level 7. A nonprofit organization founded in 1987. Its aim is to develop standards for the electronic interchange of clinical, financial, and administrative information among independent health care-oriented computer systems (eg, HISs, clinical laboratory systems, enterprise systems, pharmacy systems). This organization is working on version 3 of the HL-7 standard. HL-7 is at 3300 Washtenaw Ave, Ste 227, Ann Arbor, MI 48104; (313) 677-7777 or *http://www.mcis.duke.edu/standards/HL7/hl7.htm.*

HTTP   Hypertext transfer protocol. The high-level Internet protocol that defines the World Wide Web. Web browsers speak to Web servers via this protocol. The format of the information exchanged via this protocol is hypertext markup language (HTML), which includes the information in the message and instructions on how to display the message. Thus, Web pages can be written in HTML, then transferred from server to browser via the HTTP protocol. One need not understand the intricacies of the HTTP protocol to develop Web pages in HTML.

Hub A device that connects segments of networks (analogous to the hub of a wheel). The term is imprecise and could refer to devices of different network layers, such as repeaters, bridges, or routers.

I

IEEE Institute of Electrical and Electronics Engineers, the largest technical professional society in the world.

Internet The set of computers in the world that are connected by many different wiring schemes and fall under many different jurisdictions yet all use agreed-on high-level protocols to communicate information over TCP/IP lower layers.

Intranet A private Internet. If segments of the intranet are connected by public networks (ie, two corporate intranets connected by a commercial provider), the term extranet or virtual private network (VPN) may be applied.

IP Internet protocol. A low-level protocol for assigning addresses to packets of information. There are many protocols for doing so, but IP has become the de facto standard due to its worldwide prevalence on the Internet and in intranets. The addresses consist of four numbers each between 0 and 255 separated by dots (eg, 192.191.23.2). Fortunately, names can usually be used to identify machines on the Internet and the conversion to their IP addresses is performed automatically (ie, by the DNS).

ISDN Integrated Services Digital Network. A set of communications standards intended to eventually replace the telephone system. The ISDN allows a single wire or optical fiber to carry voice information, digital network services, and video.

ISO International Organization for Standardization. A worldwide federation of national standards bodies from some 100 countries. Established in 1947, the ISO is a nongovernmental organization. Its mission is to promote the development of standardization and related activities in the world with a view to facilitating the international exchange of goods and services and to developing cooperation in the spheres of intellectual, scientific, technologic, and economic activity. The ISO produces international agreements that are published as International Standards (3). The ISO developed the seven-layer model of computer networking known as the open systems interconnection (OSI) model, on which much of modern computer networking is based.

J

Java   An object-oriented programming language designed specifically to take advantage of network computing and to be platform independent. Java is used to develop an application (called an applet) that can then execute (within security constraints) on any computer on a network by using data located anywhere on the network.

L

LAN   Local area network. You own the wires connecting the computers. With a wide area network (WAN), somebody else owns the wires.

Little endian   See **big endian**.

N

Nonrepudiation   A security function whereby it is impossible for the sender of a message to deny that the message was sent (similar to a digital signature).

O

Object   Information objects. The term *object oriented* refers to a new way of thinking about information and new methods of manipulating information objects. In traditional information processing, computer programs are implementations of algorithms that operate on data. In an object-oriented paradigm, pieces of information that in some way represent a collection are grouped with program pieces that execute on the information within the object. Thus, the object contains not only a piece of information but the necessary methods of manipulating that information. For example, the elements of patient name, address, and telephone number can be grouped into an object called "patient demographics." A new instance of the object can be created and told to store the name "john smith." Later, that same object can be told to change the name. In this way, logically grouped pieces of information can behave in similar ways and the relationship between objects can be implied in how the objects are defined. A patient object might contain a demographics object, a laboratory object, an image object, and so on. There are many advantages to the object-oriented model, including the ability to communicate the objects conveniently in a networked environment and elimination of the dependence for processing from a specific platform.

OC-3 through OC-12   The *OC* refers to "optical carrier," a unit of measurement of the bandwidth of fiberoptic networks based on SONET (synchronous optical network). SONET is a broadband networking standard based on point-to-point optical fiber networks that provides a high-bandwidth "pipe" for supporting ATM-based services. The number after *OC* refers to the multiplier used to determine the bandwidth of the particular network. For example, OC-3 refers to 3 × 51.84 or 156 Mbits/sec.

P

Packet   A small piece of information. In most computer networks, the messages to be transmitted are broken into packets. The packets are then routed over the network to the destination, where they are reassembled. The exact size and format of the packet depend on the protocols involved.

PACS   Picture archiving and communication system. A broad term that encompasses a number of computing systems and their components used to capture, transfer, store, and display digital information in a medical imaging environment.

PPP   Point-to-point protocol. One of two low-level protocols that simulate an IP network over a modem. The other protocol is serial line IP (SLIP). Modems were originally developed for point-to-point communications (ie, between a terminal and a mainframe computer). To emulate a computer network, a piece of software running on the sender's and the receiver's computer system must make the point-to-point modem connection appear as if it were a piece of network cabling.

Q

Query/Retrieve   In the generic sense, query/retrieve is a pair of database transactions that occur frequently in database applications. A query is made of a database to find a certain piece of information, then a retrieve operation is performed to obtain it. In the context of medical imaging, query/retrieve is one of the services defined by the DICOM standard. Devices that allow query/retrieve to be performed are servers (cf **SCP**), whereas those that make such requests are clients (cf **SCU**).

R

RAID   Redundant array of inexpensive disks. A method of arranging multiple, cheap disk archives so that the amount of storage, the speed of access, and the redundancy of the information can be markedly increased. The disk storage mechanism becomes much more reliable than that of a traditional single (large)-disk system. There are five levels of RAID storage, which have trade-offs in terms of size, speed, and redundancy.

Repeater   A device that propagates electric signals from one cable to another. A low-level device, a repeater interconnects devices on a network in a simple manner, much as a "power strip" connects multiple electric devices. A repeater operates at the physical layer (electric signals) of network models.

RIS   Radiology information system. One or more computer systems in a radiology department that handle the information necessary to operate the radiology facility. Typically, an RIS manages patient, physician, and resource scheduling for radiologic procedures; film file room operations such as film tracking; and radiologic reporting functions (including electronic signature reports). The RIS, HIS, and PACS must be able to exchange information because the information content of these systems may not overlap significantly (ie, one system may contain information of importance to another that the other system cannot obtain elsewhere).

Router   A computer system that connects one or more networks and direct packets of information from one network to another. This is a middle-layer function. In fact, routers communicate with each other to select the best path for packets to take and thus allow the Internet (and intranets) to adapt dynamically to changing environments on the network. For example, if a portion of the Internet ceases to function, the routers on the remaining portions of the network will agree to route traffic around the damaged area.

S

SCP   Service class provider. The DICOM term for a server program.

SCU   Service class user. The DICOM term for a client program. DICOM defines a set of services that can be provided. Clients that request these services are called service class users.

Server   A computer system that delivers information on request from a client.

SLIP   See **PPP**.

SMTP   Simple mail transport protocol. One of many high-level protocols for exchanging mail messages on the Internet. SMTP, the de facto standard, was recently enhanced by multimedia Internet mail extensions (MIME) that allow mail to include graphics, audio, video, and so on. Another extension, the post office protocol (POP), was developed to serve mail to computers that may not be permanently available on the Internet (ie, that are turned off or disconnected from the Internet for long periods).

T

TCP   Transmission control protocol. A protocol for breaking information into smaller pieces known as packets. The de facto standard for packet formation and assembly on the Internet.

U

UTP   Unshielded twisted pair. This term refers to a specific type of copper wiring commonly used in local area networking.

W

WWW   World Wide Web. The set of Internet computers that agree to exchange information via the HTTP protocol.

References

1. The free on-line dictionary of computing. http://wombat.doc.ic.ac.uk/foldoc/index.html.
2. http://www.mcis.duke.edu/standards/HL7/hl7.htm
3. http://www.iso.ch/infoe/intro.html

Index

Health Informatics Series
(formerly Computers in Health Care)